Modern Medicine

Modern Medicine: Biomedical Devices, Medical Gases, Radiopharmaceuticals, New Drug Discovery, Volume 2 discusses the procedures of drug approval and regulatory requirements that must be met according to the United States Food and Drug Administration (FDA), the European Medical Agency (EMA), and the Central Drug Standard Control Organization (CDSCO). In the rapidly evolving landscape of modern medicine, groundbreaking innovations have emerged that are reshaping the way we approach healthcare. *Modern Medicine* delves into the cutting-edge realms of medical devices, medical gases, radiopharmaceuticals, and new drug discovery, offering a comprehensive exploration of these transformative fields that are revolutionizing patient care and medical practices.

- Discover the future of healthcare technology, and uncover the intricate world of biomedical engineering, where state-of-the-art devices seamlessly merge with the human body to monitor, diagnose, and treat ailments.
- Dive deep into the utilization of medical gases for respiratory conditions, pain management, and even novel applications in regenerative medicine.
- Unravel the mysteries of radiopharmaceuticals, a fusion of molecular imaging and therapy that offers unprecedented insights into the inner workings of the human body.
- Embark on a journey through the intricate process of drug discovery, where groundbreaking research and cutting-edge technologies are yielding therapies that were once deemed impossible.

Modern Medicine is a must-read for medical professionals, researchers, students, and anyone intrigued by the remarkable intersection of science, technology, and patient well-being. Join us on a journey to the forefront of medical innovation, where the unimaginable becomes reality, and the future of healthcare takes shape before our eyes. The chapter on regulatory implications for the approval process in this book will be the most useful resource for researchers and students, particularly those with backgrounds in pharma, forensic medicine, regulatory affairs, or those who aspire to succeed in drug research. Additionally, the information contained in this volume of the book could be of great interest to researchers working in the pharmaceutical and health industries.

I0031589

Modern Medicine: Biomedical Devices, Medical Gases, Radiopharmaceuticals, New Drug Discovery, Volume 2 is a companion volume to *Life Sciences Research to Product Development: Regulatory Requirement Transforming, Volume 1* (2024), by the same authors.

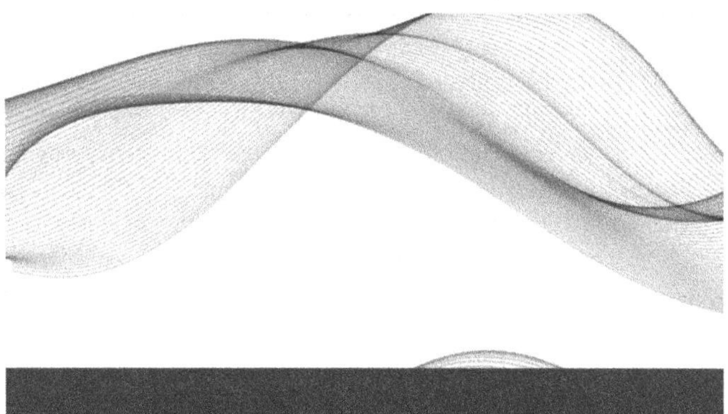

LIFE SCIENCES RESEARCH TO PRODUCT DEVELOPMENT

REGULATORY REQUIREMENT TRANSFORMING, VOLUME 1

Pronobesh Chattopadhyay and Danswrang Goyary

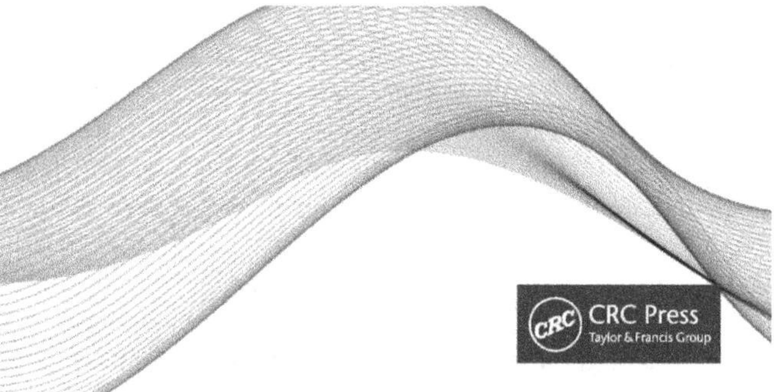

Modern Medicine

Biomedical Devices, Medical Gases, Radiopharmaceuticals, New Drug Discovery, Volume 2

Pronobesh Chattopadhyay and
Danswrang Goyary

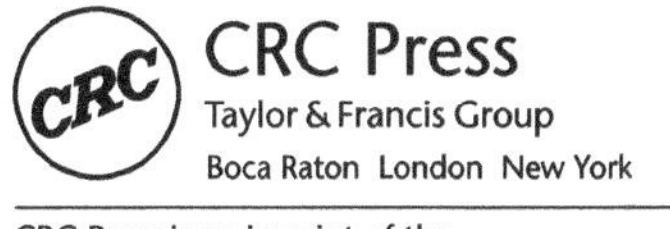

CRC Press is an imprint of the
Taylor & Francis Group, an **informa** business

First edition published 2024
by CRC Press
2385 NW Executive Center Drive, Suite 320, Boca Raton FL 33431

and by CRC Press
4 Park Square, Milton Park, Abingdon, Oxon, OX14 4RN

CRC Press is an imprint of Taylor & Francis Group, LLC

ISBN: 9781032503004 (hbk)
ISBN: 9781032503042 (pbk)
ISBN: 9781003397854 (ebk)

DOI: 10.1201/9781003397854

Typeset in Times
by Deanta Global Publishing Services, Chennai, India

Contents

Acknowledgement

The authors express their happiness to bring out successfully this Volume 2 and give thanks to almighty God for the enlightenment, strength, and knowledge to write this book. They also express their heartfelt gratitude to their loved ones, especially their parents, spouses, and children, who provided unwavering encouragement and support throughout the writing of this book. They also extend their thanks to many people who have directly or indirectly contributed to making the writing of this book possible.

The authors are also grateful to Dr. Y.D. Bhutia, Scientist-E, Dr. Sanjeev Karmakar, Technical Officer-B, Mr. Sumit Kishore, Technical Officer-A, and Mr. S. Rahaman, STA –B of the Division of Pharmaceutical Technology, DRL, for their ever-ready help and support in acquisition of practical and technical know-how of regulatory processes through working together and long association since the inception of the Division of Pharmaceutical Technology in Defence Research Laboratory, Tezpur (Assam), as well as all the staff who contributed to the successful completion of writing this book. The authors are also indebted to their friends and colleagues who have been instrumental in building their career in the field of life sciences regulatory aspects and making this book a reality and for their unwavering encouragement and warm companionship.

The authors would also like to express their deep gratitude to all students for their help, especially Mr. Mohit Kumar, JRF for his consistent assistance in manuscript formatting.

The authors are indebted to their research collaborators for their unflinching trust, infinite affection, and uncompromising honesty, which were major driving forces behind the writing of these volumes. They are deeply grateful for the constructive suggestions received during various project meetings and reviews which inspired them to create these volumes with a sense of purpose, duty towards society at large, and hope for the future.

The authors are also thankful to the Director, DRL, Tezpur, Assam for providing space and opportunity to write this book and acknowledge all senior officials of DRDO for their relentless support to write this book on life sciences product development and managing its regulatory processes.

The authors gratefully acknowledge Dr. Renu Upadhyay, Ms. Jyotsna Jangra, CRC Press and Ms. Jayanthi Chander, Deanta Global Publishing Services, for their patience, guidance, advice, editing and ever-ready help in making the successful preparation of this book possible.

In conclusion, the authors express their heartfelt gratitude to their most treasured readers. They take great satisfaction in telling the narrative and are hopeful that it has been well received by their dear readers.

P. Chattophadhyaya, Ph.D., FNASc, FICS
D. Goyary, Ph.D.

Preface

The authors take great pleasure in releasing their current efforts, an in-depth guide on the regulatory ramifications of the pharmaceutical research approval process. This book serves as a highly beneficial resource for persons who possess expertise in pharmaceuticals, forensic medicine, regulatory affairs, or those who aspire to excel in the field of drug development. The chapters encompassed within this work present a methodical and concentrated approach to comprehending the progression of new drugs. The procedure commences with the utilization of computer-aided tools for the virtual design of molecules, followed by laboratory synthesis to ensure both efficacy and safety. The information provided herein adheres to authentic scientific methods, specifically tailored to meet the requirements of researchers and students who are seeking a deeper understanding of the drug research domain.

Furthermore, the process of approving biomedical equipment is a multifaceted undertaking that exhibits variation among various countries and areas. In this book, we provide a comprehensive outline of the standard procedure and essential prerequisites for obtaining approval in significant regulatory countries, including the United States and the European Union. Although not exhaustive, this information will serve as an excellent initial resource for researchers and students investigating the regulatory aspects of medical devices.

The emerging field of telemedicine, characterized by the distant provision of healthcare services, introduces distinct factors to be taken into account regarding data privacy and ethical principles in the medical domain. This book offers a detailed examination of the fundamental elements pertaining to data confidentiality and medical ethics in the practice of telemedicine, taking into account the variations in rules across different countries and jurisdictions.

In addition, given the essential function that compressed medical gases fulfil in the provision of healthcare services, it is imperative to comply with regulatory guidelines and implement rigorous quality control protocols to safeguard their safety, quality, and appropriate utilization. Though there may be variations in specific legislation across different countries or regions, this book provides a thorough overview of the fundamental elements pertaining to the regulations and quality control measures for compressed medical gases.

This book examines the regulatory framework governing radiopharmaceuticals in India, as outlined in the Drug and Cosmetics Act of 1940. The legislation, in conjunction with the Drug and Cosmetics Rules of 1945, regulates the production, importation, distribution, and commercialization of pharmaceuticals, including radiopharmaceuticals, inside the nation. This book provides a comprehensive and instructive review, making it a helpful resource for gaining a thorough understanding of the regulatory environment pertaining to radiopharmaceuticals in India.

The Abbreviated New Drug Application (ANDA) and the Biological Licence Application (BLA) processes are of great significance in the United States for generic pharmaceuticals and biological goods, respectively. The present publication elucidates the regulatory paths pertaining to Abbreviated New Drug Applications (ANDA) and Biologics Licence Applications (BLA), thus furnishing readers with a full comprehension of the approval procedures associated with these essential pharmaceutical classifications.

Not only that, but the book also goes into great detail about the rules that govern biosimilars, which include nucleic acid-based recombinant medicines, recombinant therapeutic enzymes, and proteins. This publication aims to elucidate the regulatory approval process for biosimilars by highlighting their ability to exhibit similarities to a reference biological product while simultaneously maintaining safety, efficacy, and quality. This study acknowledges the existence of variations between countries and areas as it examines the legislation pertaining to biopharmaceuticals, genetically modified foods, vaccine development, and environmental protection laws. Furthermore, the book explores the significance of the Institutional Biosafety Committee (IBSC) in guaranteeing safe handling and utilization of genetically modified organisms (GMOs) and other potentially perilous biological substances.

Finally, it is important to note that the regulatory approval process for orphan drugs, which are specifically developed to treat rare diseases or ailments that impact a limited number of patients, is comprehensively addressed. This book aims to provide researchers and students with a full grasp of the regulatory framework pertaining to orphan pharmaceuticals, acknowledging the significance of promoting the advancement and accessibility of treatments for these infrequent medical conditions.

In summary, this book functions as an essential resource for researchers and students, offering comprehensive insights into the regulatory ramifications within the domain of drug development. Due to its emphasis on rigorous scientific methods and strict adherence to regulatory frameworks, this resource is considered indispensable for professionals working in the fields of pharmaceuticals, forensic medicine, regulatory affairs, and the herbal medication sector.

Pronobesh Chattopadhyay, Ph.D, FNASc, FICS
Danswrang Goyary, Ph.D

Author Biographies

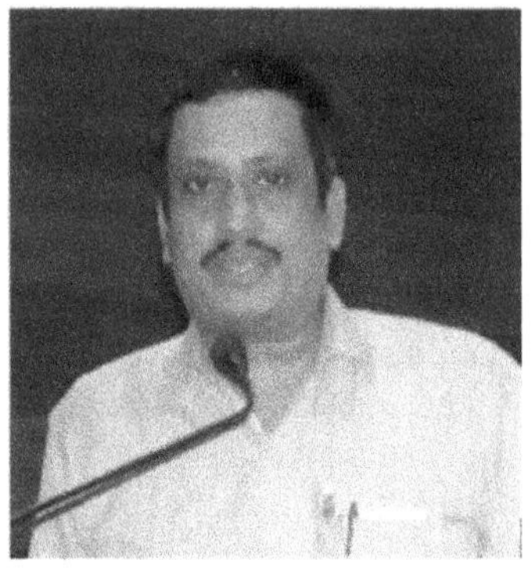

Dr. Pronobesh Chattopadhyay, Ph.D., FNASc, FICS is a pharmaceutical scientist in the Defence Research Laboratory (DRDO), Tezpur. His working areas are chemical pharmacology, toxicological interaction on expression, chemical target to TRPV, AdipoR1, AdipoR2, c-Jun kinase pathway in lungs and eyes, and these resulted in exploration to development of many defense products. He was instrumental in developing many defense products which are successfully used by India's armed forces. A notable technology like the "chili grenade" developed from Bhot Jolakia (one of the hottest chilies in the world) has been transferred (transfer of technology) to three industries and is presently used successfully by many law enforcing agencies in India. He also developed protective gear for ultra-violet protection which is stable at –50 C for armed forces deployed in Siachen Glacier; and he has contributed to the development of many products for protecting the armed forces deployed in jungle warfare. He is a Fellow of the National Academy of Sciences India (NASI) and Fellow of Indian Chemical Society (FICS). He has published more than 170 research papers and five book chapters, and filed 15 patents, three of which have been granted. He has received many awards, including the Gandhi Young Technology Innovation Awards under Biotechnology Industry Research Assistance Council (BIRAC), Laboratory Scientist Awards, Technology Awards from DRDO etc. He is a regular reviewer of ethnopharmacology, toxicology, and biochemical pharmacology, and Elsevier publishing house recognized him as a potential reviewer. Twelve Ph.D. degrees and three postdoctoral degrees have been awarded under his supervision, and 25 postgraduate students completed their dissertations.

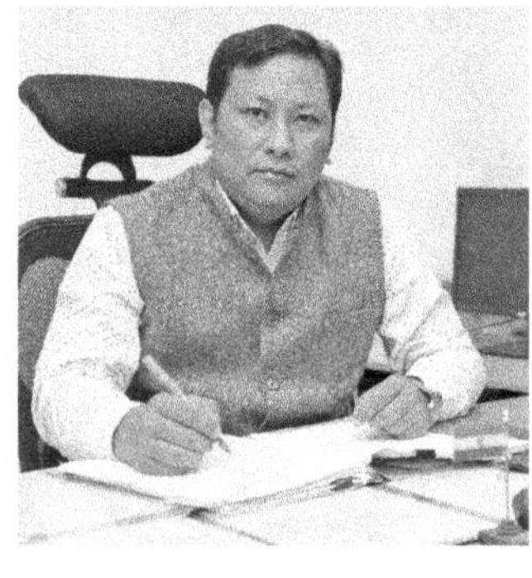

Dr. Danswrang Goyary, Ph.D., graduated in Biotechnology, Completed M.Sc. and Ph.D. in Biochemistry from North Eastern Hill University (NEHU), Shillong, India. He qualified NET-JRF (UG-CSIR) in 2002 and received a fellowship for his doctoral degree. He started his professional career at Defence Institute of Bio-Energy Research (then Defence Agricultural Research Laboratory), Haldwani (Uttarakhand) as a scientist in the year 2005 and extensively contributed in the fields of life sciences and bio-pharmaceuticals of defence importance as a biochemist.

Dr. Goyary is presently working in Defence Research Laboratory (DRDO), Tezpur. He is actively involved in studying the mechanism of different kinds of wound healing, haemostasis, and is associated with the development of defence products such as chili grenades, snake repellent, high SPF sunscreen, impregnated fabrics for disease vector and insect control etc. He has contributed more than 50 publications in peer-reviewed journals, secured two patents, supervised three Ph.D. students, and guided more than 15 postgraduate students. He has received laboratory awards such as Technology Group awards, Science Day oration award, Technology Day oration award etc. He is a member of many committees such as institutional animal ethical committees (IAEC) and institutional biosafety committees (IBSC).

Disclaimer

The contents of this book are for informational purposes only and are not intended to be legal advice. This book is not intended as a substitute for consultation. The publisher and the authors strongly recommend that you consult with your legal firm, advocate, or regulatory authority before beginning any exercise for approval. The authors are not legal advocates or regulators, and they represent that they have no expertise to exercise for regulatory clearance. Thus, the information and/or documents contained in this book do not constitute legal advice and should never be used without first consulting with a professional to determine what may be best for your individual needs. Further, this book does not constitute legal advice, and no attorney–client relationship is formed, and the publisher and the authors assume no responsibility for errors, inaccuracies, omissions, or any other inconsistency herein and hereby disclaim any liability to any party for any loss, damage, or disruption caused by errors or omissions, whether such errors or omissions result from negligence or any other cause. The opinions and assertions presented in this book are exclusively those of the authors and may not necessarily reflect the views of their respective connected or affiliated institutions or the publishers, editors, and reviewers involved. The book is exclusively intended for educational purposes, to the best of the author's knowledge and belief, and does not guarantee or endorse any assertion or information provided here.

Pronobesh Chattopadhyay, Ph.D., FNASc, FICS
Danswrang Goyary, Ph.D.

17 New Drug or Investigational New Drug Applications' (INDA) Approval Process with the Drugs and Cosmetics Act

17.1 INTRODUCTION

The beginning of drug discovery journey may be traced back to the laboratory, when researchers first began to understand the cellular and molecular underpinnings of disease. These days, modern medications are becoming increasingly sophisticated and are only developed after the disease processes and diseases pathways have been well understood. As a result, modern drug research focuses on genes or proteins that could interfere with disease prevention in the same way as hybridoma technology does, either by acting as an agonist or an antagonist of a critical receptor. Understanding drug research required deep understanding to begin with the knowledge of nature, such as herbal medicine, and is now moving towards computer-based methods with, which may result in the production of 10,000 lead molecules, of which only 10–15 molecules have the potential to be therapeutic. Recently, several new promising molecules have won the race to identify new drugs. These include Ocrevus, developed by Roche for the treatment of multiple sclerosis, and sarilumab, developed by Regeneron and Sanofi for the treatment of rheumatoid arthritis. The search for novel drugs can be a difficult episode, especially when it comes to obtaining regulatory permission and a financial return on investment.

17.2 DIFFERENT TYPES OF INVESTIGATION NEW DRUG APPROVAL

1. Investigational New Drug (IND)
   Prior to the approval of the drug, the drug may be manufactured or delivered for the clinical study, and the IND application is essentially granting authority for such purposes. The three different types of IND are considered here.

DOI: 10.1201/9781003397854-1

2. An Investigator IND
   A trained medical practitioner may submit a research IND application of either an unapproved drug or an approved drug for the treatment of a new indication or in a new patient group. The physician is in authority of the submission of the application and the investigation, as well as the distribution and administration of the experimental drug.
3. Utilisation in Case of Emergency IND
   Under the direction of the drug regulatory authority, even without the submission of an IND application, an experimental drug may be used if there is no other option available and the situation is considered an emergency.
4. Treatment IND
   Although conclusive clinical tests have not yet been conducted by the regulatory body, an investigational medicine may show promise in the treatment of life-threatening illnesses. This is despite the fact that the IND therapy has not yet been established. In most cases, investigational new drug (IND) applications are research (non-commercial) types, and the regulatory body is given adequate time to understand the drug's safety when it is used in crisis situations. The application for IND requires a significant amount of data. According to the US Food and Drug Administration (FDA) and in accordance with Section 312 of Title 21 of the Code of Federal Regulations (CFR), the sponsors are required to submit a large number of documentation in order to receive clearance for their clinical trial. Documents such as an investigator's brochure, an exploratory trial plan, and an introduction statement regarding the compounds are required in order for the FDA to grant approval. The investigator's brochure is a vital document that should include information on protocols, chemistry, the manufacturing process, pharmacology, preclinical safety, and any other relevant information.
5. New Drug Application (NDA)
   The NDA is the predecessor or successor of the Investigational New Drug Application (INDA), and it is used when the drug in question has the credentials necessary to demonstrate that it is safe and effective in accordance with the regulatory standards for marketing approval. The NDA is intended for solely commercial purposes, and, as a result, many other types of data must be provided, such as review data, chemistry, pharmacology, medical, biopharmaceutics, safety and statistics.
6. Over-the-Counter (OTC) Drugs
   This class of medications is a significant one, and its potential market share is rapidly expanding. There are many therapeutic categories of pharmaceuticals that are considered over-the-counter and sold without a prescription. These drugs range from headache treatment to food and drugs that manage weight control.
7. Biologic Licence Application (BLA)
   Vaccines, toxoids, or any products developed from the microorganism by recombinant technology are regarded to be the biological products that are

used in the Public Health Service (PHS) Act in US or Drug Cosmetic Act in India.

8. Abbreviated New Drug Application (ANDA)
   This category of pharmaceuticals is also known as generic drugs, and the term "abbreviated" refers to the fact that the drugs in this category do not need to include preclinical or clinical evidence to prove that they are safe and effective. This category of medication has already been made available on the market, and the original patent has expired. Comparable to an innovative drug in terms of its efficacy, quality, and safety, this medication has the same potency, strength, and dosage as the original medication. All medications, both brand-name and generic, can be found in the "Orange Book," published by the FDA, which is also referred to as "Approved Drug Products with Therapeutic Equivalence Evaluations."

17.3 RULE OF THE DRUG APPROVAL PROCESS IN INDIA

The major law that controls the regulation of drug-related activities in India, including the manufacture, storage, import, sale, and distribution of medications and cosmetics, is called the Drug and Cosmetic Act of 1940 and Rules of 1945. These two pieces of legislation were passed in 1940 and 1945, respectively. The controlling power is known as the Central Drugs Standard Control Organization (CDSCO), and the Drugs Controller General (India) is the primary authority responsible for the regulation of drugs across the entire country of India. Schedule Y gives explicit directions regarding the required data and clinical trials, and Schedule Y was inducted in 1988 and revised as required from then on. Because of stringent regulatory requirements, such as Good Clinical Practices (GCP) and Good Laboratory Practices (GLP), and government controls through the regulatory authority to achieve the best health care in terms of safe and high-quality drugs at affordable prices to the public, the Indian pharmaceutical industry is considered to be the third largest industry in the world. The quality of the product is a direct result of these requirements. The Drugs and Cosmetics Act of 1940 and Rules of 1945 regulated the distribution and retail sale of pharmaceuticals and cosmetics. The regulations are put into effect by the CDSCO, which operates under the Drugs Controller General of India (DCGI), which is part of the Ministry of Health and Family Welfare. In India, as said the CDSCO to regulate pharmaceuticals, cosmetics, and medical devices. In addition, the CDSCO possesses the authority to regulate and grant approval for the marketing of medications, as well as the monitoring and approval of clinical trials, new drug applications, and drug manufacture and importation.

The registration process is addressed in a number of important provisions in the Drugs and Cosmetics Act of 1940 and the Rules of 1945 which are as follows:

1. Rule 122A: In this section, the licensing authority is the deciding authority for the import of drugs in the public interest from other countries on the basis of the clinical efficacy already demonstrated by trials in other nations.

In addition, this rule adopted the provision of waiver of clinical studies for new drugs that are already being used in other countries.

2. Rule 122B: Provisions are made in this section for application for the approval to manufacture new drugs other than the drugs designated under Schedule C and C (1).
3. Rule 122D: Provisions are made in this section for the import or manufacture of fixed-dose combinations of two or more drugs, as defined in rule 122E. The necessary fees in addition to the data needed are described in Appendix VI of Schedule Y.
4. Rule 122DA: Provisions have been made in this section for the application for the grant of authority to conduct clinical trials for a new drug or an investigational ("experimental") new drug.
5. Rule 122 of the DAB: Provisions are made in this section for the payment of compensation in the event that clinical trial participants become physical injured, sustain injuries.
6. Rule 122E: Within this part, the term "Novel Drugs" refers to any new substance with therapeutic values or new claims, as well as any new route of administration for an approved drug. This is applicable is the fixed-dose combination in this section.
7. Rule 122DB: This is the rule that mandates that regulatory authorities be informed in advance if the person who is importing the good or making the medical product or drugs does not comply with any of the requirements that are attached to the licence or approval. It is an opportunity to import drugs in order to meet the shortfall requirements before the order is cancelled or suspended.
8. Rule 122DC: It is the appeal against the cancel order that was passed by the licensing agency, and it has the provisions for appealing within sixty days from the date that such an order has been passed.

   Section 2.4 (a) of Schedule Y: In accordance with the provisions of the Drugs and Cosmetics Act of 1940 and the Rules of 1945, clinical tests must be conducted on any molecule that was discovered in India.

   Section 2.4 (b) of Schedule Y: In accordance with the provisions of the Drugs and Cosmetics Act of 1940 and the Rules of 1945, clinical tests must be conducted on any molecule that was discovered in India.

   Section 2.8 of Schedule Y: According to the Drugs and Cosmetic Act of 1940 and the Rules of 1945, pharmacokinetic studies may be required (Bioequivalence studies).
9. Registration Certificate: The certificate is issued in accordance with Rule 27A, listing the substances that were defined as drugs in Section 3b of the Drugs and Cosmetic Act, 1940 and Rules 1945 in the format that was prescribed by Form 41. The registration, which includes any locations where drug are imported or manufactured, is required. The submission of an application for approval of a new drug in accordance with Rule 24A, following confirmation that all conditions of the registration certificate have been met, will result in the granting of the licence.

17.4 SOME IMPORTANT APPLICATION FORMS FOR REGISTRATION

1. Form 10
   This is the form that is used for the grant of an import licence for a drug, while Form 10A is the form that is used for drugs that are on Schedule X. Form 8 of the application is to be filled out by the importer, and Form 9 is to be filled out by the authorised Indian distributor. After the imported medical device has been registered in India by a foreign vendor, the distributor is required to register to himself by obtaining an import licence using Form 8. In order to comply with the customs clearance provisions that were enacted in accordance with Rule 24, registration is required to be made mandatory.
2. Form 11
   This licence allows for the importation of small amounts of drugs and medical equipment for inspection, testing, or analysis. The licence is called a "Test Licence for Import." This does not involve any kind of business activity and the provisions that have been enacted are in accordance with Rule 33.
3. Form 17
   This form is used for importation of any medical equipment and small amounts of drugs including biotech drugs, vaccines, new drugs, and diagnostic kits, for the sole purpose of examination, testing, or analysis. Such imported items could not be used for any kind of commercial purpose.
4. Form 19
   This is an application to grant a licence to stock, exhibit, distribute, or sell drugs other than drugs specified in Schedule X.
5. Form 19A
   This is an application for renewal of a restricted licence to stock, exhibit, distribute, or sell drugs at retail through a dealer without engaging the services of a qualified person.
6. Form 19B
   The purpose of this application is to request the granting of a licence to stock, exhibit, distribute, or sell homeopathic medicines.
7. Form 19C
   The purpose of this application is to request the granting of a licence to stock, exhibit, distribute, or sell those drugs specified in Schedule X.
8. Form 20
   The purpose of this application is to request a licence to stock or exhibit or for the sale or distribution of a drug in retail, excluding those drugs specified in Schedules X, C, or C (1).
9. Form 21
   License for stocking, exhibiting, selling, or distributing a drug in retail, excluding the drugs specified in Schedules C or C (1).
10. Form 21B (For Sutures, Ligatures, and *In-vitro* Diagnostic Devices)
    The licence may be issued initially or renewed for dealers in drugs who do not employ the services of a qualified person in order for them to stock, exhibit, offer for sale, or distribute drugs by retail.

11. Form 24
    The purpose of this application is to request a licence for manufacture for stock, exhibit, distribution or sale of drugs other than those specified in Schedule X or C C (1).
12. Form 24A
    The purpose of this application is to request the granting of a loan licence for manufacture for stock, exhibition, distribution, or sale of drugs other than those specified in Schedule X, C, or C (1).
13. Form 24B
    This is an application to grant a licence for repacking for stock, exhibiting, or distributing, or selling of a drug that is not specified in Schedule X, C, or C (1).
14. Form 24C
    This is an application to grant a renewal licence for repacking homeopathic medicines for stock, exhibiting, or distributing homeopathic medicines, or selling homeopathic medicines.
15. Form 24F
    This is an application for the grant or renewal of a licence to repack for stock, exhibiting, distributing, or selling drugs listed in Schedule X.
16. Form 25
    This is for approval or renewal of a licence for approved premises to manufacture drugs for sale or distribution in accordance with Schedule M. This form is not to be used for drugs listed in Schedules C, C (1), or X of the Drugs and Cosmetics Rules, 1945. The application must be submitted using Form 24, through the owner/responsible person.
17. Form CT26
    This is an application form for the manufacture of an unapproved new drug. This form is for the manufacture of an unapproved new drug for the treatment of life-threatening conditions in seriously ill patients when no other options have been explored. In addition, the consent to use the drug must be obtained in writing from the patient or the patient's legal heirs in the location where the drug is going to be used. Within ninety calendar days of the date of application, the form will be reviewed by the Institutional Ethics Committee (IEC) at the Government Hospital, after which it will be forwarded by the IEC to the Central Licensing Authority (CLA) for manufacturing such a type of drug, via Form CT 27.
18. Form 27A
    The purpose of this application is to request the granting or renewal of a license loan licence to repack for stock, exhibition, distribution, or sale of drugs listed in schedules C and C (1) with the exception of drugs listed in Schedule X.
19. Form 27B
    The purpose of this application is to request the granting or renewal of a license to repack drugs for stock, or to exhibit, distribute, or sell drugs that are listed in Schedules C, C (1), or X.

20. Form 27C
    The purpose of this application is to request the granting or renewal of a licence to operate a blood bank, which may include the processing of whole blood and/or the preparation of blood components.
21. Form 27D
    The purpose of this application is to request the granting or renewal of a licence for manufacturing for sale or distribution of large volumes of parenteral, sera, and vaccines, excluding the drugs specified in Schedule X.
22. Form 27DA
    The purpose of this application is to request the granting or renewal of a licence for manufacturing for sale or distribution of large volumes of parenteral, sera, recombinant DNA (rDNA) -based drug, and vaccines, excluding the drugs specified in Part XB and Schedule X.
23. Form 27E
    The purpose of this application is to request the granting or renewal of a licence to manufacture, sell, or distribute blood products, which includes the processing of whole blood and/or the preparation of blood components.
24. Form 28
    The approval of an authorised premises to produce, for sale or distribution, a drug and, if appropriate, a drug that is mentioned in Schedules C, C (1), or X of the Drugs and Cosmetics Rules.
25. Form 29
    This form is also called the "Test Licence for Manufacturing." According to the assertion, the testing licence necessary to manufacture pharmaceuticals for the purposes of analysis has been granted. After the test, a licence application could not be manufactured any drug for use and GMP (Good Manufacturing Practices) provisions had to be implemented in accordance with Rule 33. The test licence did not require any GMP conditions.
26. Form 30
    This is for an application to be used solely for the purpose of testing, analysing, or examining a pre-grant proposal.
27. Form 31
    This application is for the grant or renewal of a licence to manufacture, sell, or distribute cosmetics.
28. Form 31A
    This is for an application for the granting or renewal of a loan licence to manufacture, sell, or distribute cosmetics.
29. Form 36
    This is for an application for grant or renewal of approval for carrying out tests on behalf of licensees for the manufacture of drugs or cosmetics for sale, or raw materials used in the manufacture thereof.
30. Form 44
    This is for the grant of permission for a clinical trial of any new drug, fixed dose mixture, or already-approved drug that can be imported or made according to rules 122A, 122B, 122D, and 122 DA. The completion of a

Form 44 is necessary for the development of new drugs, and for obtaining permission to carry out research calls for a substantial amount of information.

31. Form 45

    In pursuance of the provisions of rules 122 A, 122 D, and 122 DA, a licence for the importation of a drug, including any necessary raw materials, may only be issued if the licensing authority has established that the molecule in question is safe and not flawed. This determination must be made before a licence may be granted for the importation of a drug.

32. Form 46

    Rules 122B, 122D, and 122DA state that a licence for making a new drug, including the raw material, can only be given if the licensing authority is sure that the molecule is safe and not flawed. Form 46A is used for making new bulk drug substances.

17.5 APPROVAL PROCESS AND REQUIRED DATA OF NEW DRUG

The regulation and approval process is made easier because it can now be completed online using the "Sugam" Gateway, and a time schedule for the method of evaluation has been well defined. In addition, the necessary components of the document have been thoroughly outlined. Rule 21 of the Drug and Cosmetics Act of 1945 states that any chemicals, pharmaceuticals, or bulk drugs that have not been used considerably and have never been recognised by the licensing authority as being effective and safe may only be used with the approval of the licensing authority if they have stated claims or are using a restricted amount of a molecule. Also, according to Rule 21, any drug can be approved by the CLA under certain claims. However, any drug where any changes have been made since the drug has been approved, such as a new claim, a modified dosage form, an extended claim, a delayed or sustained release, or a new route of administration, is considered to be a new drug. In addition, two or more individual drugs that have been approved in India but that have been changed to a fixed-dose combination or any change in any approved ratio with a modification claim or an improved claim, as well as a modified dosage form, extended claim, delayed or sustained release or route of administration, are considered to be new drugs. The biological molecules, such as vaccines, sera, or toxoids, stem cell therapies, and medications generated from rDNA, must be classified as new drugs, unless they fall into one of the other categories. After a period of four years following the initial approval, the compounds are eligible for consideration as new therapeutic candidates. The following category has been established as an investigational novel drug according to the definition.

1. A new chemical entity or molecular entity (NCE/NME) that was developed in India.
2. New salts or new formulations that have already been approved or commercialised in other countries but have not been approved in India.
3. A new claim or indication, a change in dosage form, or method of administration for a drug that has already been approved, or a change of status of

a drug from one that is prescribed to one that may be purchased over the counter.

4. Combinations of two or more drugs that are either new or have a fixed dosage.
5. Granted permission to sell in India within a period of four years.
6. The import and registration process: During the first stages of the drug approval process, the following three types of quality information or dossiers are necessary for approval which are included in the regulatory dossier, data relating to pharmaceuticals, and animal studies or pre-clinical studies.
7. Clinical Trial Document (CTD): Any changes made to a drug product after it has been approved must first undergo clinical testing to determine whether or not it is safe and effective. The International Council for Harmonisation of Technical Requirement of Pharmaceuticals for Human Use (ICH), in which Japan, the European Union, and the United States took part, developed a standard dossier for the required documents for the approval procedure. This document is known as the Common Technical Document (CTD). In 2009, the CDSCO in India mandated that the CTD be regarded as one of the mandatory technical conditions for the licensing of biological goods.
   - 7.1. Information Regarding Drugs: The information required is pertaining to the drug, including its dosage form, composition of the formulation (if it is a fixed-dose combination), active and inert ingredients, pharmacological classification of the drug, suggested application of the drug, and patent status of the drug.
   - 7.2. Requirement for the Submission of Data—Authorisation to Market a New Drug: The information and subsequent data are necessary on the chemical entity and information, pharmacology, preclinical toxicology, data from stability and dissolution experiments or kinetics, clinical pharmacology (Phase I), related published or review articles, exploratory clinical trials (Phase II), and confirmatory clinical trials (Phase III). In addition, data such as the regulatory status in other countries, product monographs, drafts of labels, and marketing information regarding cartons are necessary. Other pieces of information, such as the risk-to-benefit ratio in accordance with ISO 14971, the accessible therapeutic action, and the medical need of the country, are also required to be submitted.
   - 7.3. Approval to Produce a New Drug Formulation that has Already been Approved: It is necessary to have the information and subsequent data regarding the bioavailability or bioequivalence, as well as the identity of the investigator or facility, the raw material suppliers, and the results from the stability research.
   - 7.4. Obtaining Authorisation to Manufacture Bulk Drug Substances: The information and following data are necessary regarding the manufacturing methods, quality control, analytical data, stability, and animal

toxicity data. Additionally, the information must be including about the stability.

7.5. A Licence to Produce Fixed-Dose Combinations: The information and following data are necessary regarding the manufacturing methods, quality control, analytical data, stability, and animal toxicity data. Additionally, the information must be including about the stability.

7.6. Subsequent Permission for Manufacturing for New Indication or New Dosage: It is necessary to have information regarding the granting of approval for drugs that have already been approved, as well as therapeutic justification for a new dosage form, as well as quality parameters for safety, efficacy, and effectiveness.

17.6 PERMISSION TO IMPORT A NEW DRUG ACCORDING TO PROVISION 122A

Permission is granted by the licensing authority in accordance with clause (b) of rule 21. The application made in Form 44, with prescribed fee, and later applications can be made for any modified dosage form or with new claims along with a further additional fee and the appropriate data. The importer has to ensure that the clinical trial data are generated as per Schedule Y (Appendix II) along with requisite data as per annexure –I of Schedule Y.

The central licensing relaxes the safety data like animal toxicology, reproduction studies, perinatal studies, teratogenic studies, mutagenicity, and carcinogenicity, etc., if the drug is available or approved in another country and in the public interest the drug can be inducted. The authorisation to import the medicine is granted by Form 45 and/or Form 46.

1. Type of New Drug Approval

   In India, a new drug approval is considered as follows

   1.1. Clinical Trial Permission

   This is for an application requesting permission to conduct Phase I, Phase II clinical studies for exploratory purposes after Phase I clinical trials are completed, and followed by Phase III confirmatory clinical trials, which come after Phases II and I are completed. To complete the entire process, Form 44 is applicable under Rule 122DA of the Drug and Cosmetics Act.

   1.2. Approval for a Licence

   Rules 122A, 122D, and 122DA are applicable for the manufacture of a finished formulation, and the applicable form is Form 45. Usually, the product has successfully completed the clinical trials in India and generated post-marketing clinical data.

   1.3. Licence for Import of Raw Material

   Form 45 A is an authorisation for a licence to import raw material or bulk substance that is considered to be a new bulk drug substance, and this constitutes conformity with rules 122A and 122DA.

1.4. Authorisation for Formulation of a New Drug
Form 46 is utilised for the purpose of granting permission or approval for the manufacture of a new drug formulation, and this action ensures compliance with Rules 122B, 122D, and 122DA.
1.5. Authorisation for Manufacturing of Raw Material or New Bulk Drug Substance
In this case, the requisite data are filled as per Form 46A for approval for the manufacturing of raw material or new bulk drug substance, and it ensures conformity with Rules 122B and 122DA.
1.6. Registration Certificate for a Medical Device
In this case, the requisite data are filled as per Form 41 and used to obtain authorisation or approval for a registration certificate for a medical device. Obtaining this clearance is a necessary step in the process of gaining approval to sell products on the Indian market. The product falls under the "notified device" category; hence, it is required to be registered with the CDSCO, using Form 40. The registration certificate is valid for three years pursuant to Rule 24A.

17.7 AUTHORISATION TO CARRY OUT CLINICAL TRIALS FOR A NEWLY DEVELOPED MEDICINE (SECTION 122D)

In accordance with the provisions of Clause (b) of the Rule, clinical trials of new pharmaceuticals cannot begin unless the relevant licensing authority, the CDSCO, has given their approval. The required application Form 44, along with the prescribed fees and the necessary data as described in Schedule Y, must be submitted to the licensing authority as part of the application for authorisation to conduct a phase I clinical trial. In addition, the relevant data must be submitted in accordance with the requirements of Schedule Y.

Phase II clinical trial, also known as exploratory clinical tests, are allowed for a new drug trial by the licensing authority after they are satisfied by the data from Phase I trials. After the phase II clinical trial is complete, and on the basis of the data emerging from Phase II as well as the data emerging from Phase I, permission is granted to conduct either Phase III confirmatory clinical trials or Phase III trials of a new drug. This trial is also known as multi-centric study. After the clinical trial is over and there are no reports of problems, it will be possible to obtain or make a new drug on the premises without paying a separate fee. After the end of the clinical trial without any adverse reports, it will no longer be necessary to pay a separate fee in addition to the application for permission to import or manufacture a new drug on the premises. In addition, at the time of approval, payments payable to the Central Government or State Government institutes involved in clinical research have those fees waived earlier in the trial Phases I to III in order to facilitate the running of studies for academic or scientific reasons.

The licensing authority shall issue approval in Form 45 or Form 45A or Form 46 or Form 46A, with the criteria that are mentioned therein, after analyzing the data that has been supplied by the host institute.

17.8 PERMISSION TO PRODUCE A NEW DRUG IN SCHEDULES OTHER THAN C OR C (1) (122B)

It is impossible to manufacture any drug without first receiving permission from the CLA specified in Clause (b) of Rule 21. The same rules also stated that application authorisation of the manufacture of the new drug and its formulations should be submitted to the licensing authority using Form 44, along with the prescribed payments. The clause for a new drug also extended to the modified dosage form or with new claims of dosage forms and the application Form 44, separate fees are required.

According to the first paragraph of Sub-rule 21 of Rule 21, in order to get clearance from the licensing authority CLA, it is required to submit the data as per the Schedule Y. This includes the findings of any clinical trials that were conducted in the country as per the schedule described in defined in Schedule Y. Additionally; it is required to submit the clinical trials in the format that is given in Appendix II.

After the fulfilment of the requirements, the licensing authority granted the permission in the format of Form 46 and/or Form 46A, subject to the conditions. The state licensing authority permitted manufacture of a new drug under Sub-rule (1) when application has already been approved by the central licensing authority. Rule 21 includes a clause that states the drug may be used if it is deemed to be in the public interest. In this scenario, the clinical trial requirements may be waived so long as they are consistent with the published literature from another country in which the drug was approved. Tier III toxicology data, such as animal toxicology, teratogenic studies, perinatal studies, reproduction studies, mutagenicity and carcinogenicity studies, and others, may be modified or relaxed if the drug has been used for an extended period of time in other countries.

In addition to Form 44 and in accordance with the requirements of Schedule Y, the following information must also be submitted with page numbers.

1. New Drug Approval
2. Part I: New Drug Particulars
    - The Name of the Drug
    - The Content of the Formulation Expressed as a Percentage
    - Dosage Form—Liquid, Solid, Semi-solid, etc.
    - Specification for Analytical Procedures and Quality:
    - Active Ingredients and Other Ingredients.
    - Categorisation of the Drug in Accordance with its Pharmacological Action
    - Potential Clinical Applications of the Drug
    - Specifications for the Raw Materials or Bulk Drug Substances, as Well as Their Sources
    - Patent Status
3. Part II: Information Regarding Research and Development
    - Specifics regarding the chemical and pharmaceutical industries.
    - The pharmacology involved or the mechanism of action.
    - The study of toxicology in animals and in pre-clinical settings (Phase O)

- Human Trial/Safety Data (Phase I).
- Initial Investigational Clinical Trials (Phase II).
- Confirmatory Clinical Trials, which should include the Phase III trials proven with the published/review paper.
- Dissolution data.
- A study on the bioavailability as well as the stability of the data.
- The regulatory environment in other countries.
- Information regarding marketing.
- A Monograph on the Product
- Primary Drafts of Labels and Leaflets
- Approval for Test Licence where analytical data tax generated

17.9 APPLICATION FOR PERMISSION TO IMPORT A NEW DRUG

According to Regulation 122-A, the import of drugs and medical devices is permissible, and registration is essential. However, importation of drugs or medical devices is prohibited unless it is done with the authorisation of the licensing authority and in accordance with the terms of that licence. The application must be submitted to the licensing authority, using Form 44, and it must be accompanied by the necessary fees. According to the regulation, the necessary are required fees for a subsequent application from the same application, such as one with a modified dosage form or with new claims, or for the import or sale of the pharmaceuticals within one year of the first application, are reduced. The necessary data or information is required according to Schedule Y of Appendix 1 or Appendix 1A. A clinical trial must first be conducted in the country before a new import drug may be authorised, and the results of the clinical trial must be reported to the Schedule's Appendix-II. On the basis of the established literature on the new drug, the licensing authority may, in the case of a national emergency or in the interest of the public, waive the requirement for a local clinical trial. If the drug has been used for long periods of time in the other country, the licensing authority may decide to waive certain aspects of animal toxicity, including studies on teratogenicity, reproduction, mutagenicity, perinatal studies, and carcinogenicity, if the reason is sufficiently compelling. The licensing authority grants permission to import new drugs using Form 46 or 46A, while permission to import large quantities of drugs is granted using Form 45 or 45 A, each with its own set of particular additional restrictions.

17.10 DOCUMENTS FOR REQUIREMENT FOR THE APPROVAL OF IMPORTING DRUGS

This is a certificate for the registration of an Indian agent for importing or manufacturing a drug acquired from a foreign vendor. In addition, the power of attorney must be apostilled, and the foreign manufacturer and the Indian agent must jointly verify the drug's legal implications with the Indian embassy in the country of origin. In most cases, the application might be submitted to DCGI using the format of Form 40.

1. Schedule DI Certificate: A Schedule DI Certificate, signed and stamped by the manufacturer, must be deposited with the Licensing authority. Schedule DI typically refers to certain provisions in the Drugs and Cosmetics Act, and the certificate may contain specific details about the drug.

Signed and stamped by the manufacturer, it must be deposited with the Licensing authority.

The schedule DI has following components.

1.1. Specific information regarding the manufacturer and the manufacturing facility
1.2. Specifications of the manufactured pharmaceuticals that are required to be registered
1.3. An undertaking or declaration that includes the following affirmation, which must be stated
1.4. Affirmation of the Rules 74 and 78, as well as the Provisions made in Part IX of the Drugs and Cosmetics Rules, 1945
1.5. Meets the requirements for potency, quality, and purity outlined in Chapter III and Part IV of the Drugs and Cosmetics Rules, 1945, as well as any subsequent revisions to those regulations
1.6. Report of any alternation form of registration certificate, encompassing the drug's production process, packaging, labels, testing, and certification. This report must include all of the aforementioned details
1.7. The immediate action clause must be put into effect without delay in the event of any adverse reaction, such as a regulatory limitation, the removal of the product from the market, or the revocation of authorisation, and/or a report that is not of standard quality

2. Requisite documents for the approval conditions of DI are listed in Table 17.1.

TABLE 17.1
The Documents Required for Approval of D-I

1	Application letter	
2	Information related to administration including the owner, key personal	
3	Table of contents (Modules 1 to 5)	
4	Form 40 and TR 6 Challan with prescribed fees	
5	Application related to the responsible personnel	
6	Name, address, telephone, fax, e-mail address of the following responsible persons/officer	
	6.1	Active drug substance or API and finished formulations manufacturer
	6.2	Official responsible for the overall operation
	6.3	Indian authorised agents for importing from foreign country
	6.4	Official accountable for the distribution of batches of drug products

- 6.5 Authorisation certificate of the market for imported pharmaceuticals
- 6.6 Pharmaceutical company that manufactures the medicine
- 6.7 Additional manufacturer(s) involved in the manufacturing process

7 Information about product

- 7.1 The whole name of the drug, including any commercial, proprietary, or trade names
- 7.2 Common name or non-proprietary name of the drug product
- 7.3 Composition (according claim in label)
- 7.4 Dosage and strength per dosage unit
- 7.5 Dispensing requirements
- 7.6 The route by which the medication is administered
- 7.7 Conditions pertaining to storage

8 Summary of Product Characteristics (SPC)

9 Labelling of products according to the guidelines established in the Drugs and Cosmetics Rules of 1945. The labelling of the product must adhere to the regulations outlined in the primary package, the secondary package, and the package leaflet.

10 A quick summary of the manufacturer's research profile

- 10.1 The name of the drug products or pharmaceutical medicine that was manufactured by the manufacturer
- 10.2 The commercial activities of the manufacturer in the market
- 10.3 The acknowledgment of the power of attorney
- 10.4 Affirmation that the authorised signatory is present and accounted
- 10.5 A plant registration or approval or establishment license that has been notarised and was issued by the Ministry of Health or National regulatory authority of the country
- 10.6 Approval copy of permission for the drug to be manufactured and/or marketed in the country of origin
- 10.7 A notarised Certificate of Pharmaceutical Product (CPP) as per WHO GMP certification scheme or Certificate of Good Manufacturing Practices (cGMP) combined with the Free Sale Certificate (FSC) from the nation of origin for imported Drug Products
- 10.8 A copy of permission to produce the bulk drug in the country of origin or to import the drug into India for marketing purposes.
- 10.9 The price at the domestic in India, as well as the price in the country of origin.
- 10.10 Market authorisation of the countries where import permission has been granted and status of withdrawal, if any
- 10.11 Copies of patented inventions marketed in other countries
- 10.12 A plant master file that has been properly notarised
- 10.13 Experts list
- 10.14 Evaluation and verification of the product's quality
- 10.15 Non-clinical and clinical data
- 10.16 Environmental risk assessment
- 10.17 Information pertaining to pharmacovigilance
- 10.18 Information concerning clinical trials
- 10.19 Samples from three different batches that have been produced consecutively, in a quantity sufficient for triple testing
- 10.20 Manufacturer undertaking as earlier described

3. Schedule DII Certificate

In accordance with the Drugs and Cosmetics Rules, 1945, the new drugs are referred to in Rule 122-E, and the licencing power grant is specified in Rule 122-A. In accordance with the D II, a new drug is required to have a concise overview as well as clinical documentation, in addition to complying with the rules of 122-A. The following documents (Table 17.2) must be submitted in order to obtain a Schedule D III certificate:

TABLE 17.2
The Following Documents Must Be Submitted in Order to Obtain a Schedule D III Certificate

1	The complete name of the drug, the drug class, and a brief description of the medicine's therapeutic use	
2	A certificate permitting the sale of the drug and an additional document confirming that it obtained regulatory approval in either the country of origin or the country of sale. In addition to the CEP (EDQM certificate), the issuing country's National Regulatory Authority (NRA) must also provide a declaration and certification attesting to the origin country's drug products' compliance with WHO GMP regulations	
3	List of countries and dates for which marketing or import approval has been received	
4	A list, including the relevant date, of the nation's whose marketing approval or import permit has been revoked or cancelled	
5	A list, including the relevant dates, of the countries in which marketing authorisation or import approval has not yet been granted	
6	The price of the drug when it is sold on the local market is stated in the currency that is most commonly used in the country of origin	
7	List of patents by country	
8	Information on the chemical and pharmacological ingredients of the drug	
	8.1	The chemical or pharmaceutical name of the active ingredient, CAS number, non-trade secret name, and molecular structure and physical properties
	8.2	Dosage form, quality, quantity, and composition—both active ingredients and excipients—are required for a pharmaceutical formulation
	8.3	Dosage form and composition, including the active medication or substances and the excipient (s)
	8.4	The name of the company that supplies the active ingredient(s) as well as their address should be included
	8.5	Tests of impurity profiles using reference materials and standards
	8.6	Experiments to evaluate the impurity profile utilising standards and references
	8.7	Describe a detailed description of the production procedure, including a flow chart.
	8.8	A complete testing technique that must be approved by the registration authorities in the country of origin and must include either references to pharmacopeial standards or in-house specifications for the testing facility
9	Data on stability, including accelerated and real-time stability as well as other forms of stability.	
10	Dimensions of the package as well as any inserts that it may contain	
11	The presence of a number expression as well as a bar code on the packaging, both the labels and the cartons	
12	Precautions to be taken to ensure the safety of containers and closures	

13 The terms and conditions that apply to storage

14 Samples must be sent in triplicate, be packed at the outlet, and come with a batch Licence. It is also important to provide additional samples and reference substances with batch certifications that specify the shelf life and storage conditions of the reference substance at the time when registration is required

15 It is required to supply batch-specific test reports and certificates, in addition to five consecutive production batches that must be supplied in order

16 Labelling as required by Rule 96 of the 1945 Federal Food, Drug, and Cosmetic Act

17 Package leaflet

18 The process that should be followed in order to securely handle the drugs

19 Specifics of the report on the PMS study

20 Details regarding the biological and pharmacological effects of the medication are included below

  20.1 Biological examination of the raw materials

  20.2 There are two products that are considered intermediates: biological control testing

  20.3 Three biological quality control checks for final pharmaceutical items

  20.4 The consistency, satiability, and effectiveness of the final pharmaceutical items

  20.5 Tests to establish sterility and quality standards 17.10.3.20.6 tests to check for pyrogen, in addition to the requirements

  20.6 Tests to check for pyrogen, in addition to the requirements

  20.7 Tests to determine the acute and subacute toxicity of the substance

  20.8 Bioavailability and bio-equivalence data

  20.9 An analysis of the potential threat that rDNA products represent to the environment

21 Additional data

  21.1 Pharmacology and pre-clinical toxicity

  21.2 An overview of the pharmacological actions, including pharmacokinetic data to determine absorption, metabolism, distribution, and excretion.

  Report on sub-acute and long-term toxicology studies, as well as possible impacts on reproduction, the environment, and cancer.

  21.3 Data from clinical trials

22 Information on drug labelling and packaging

23 Labels should be in accordance with the drugs and cosmetics rules, 1945

24 Documents relating to clinical efficacy and trial

25 The therapeutic indications must be listed in each of the official languages in the product's booklet. The accompanying brochure included information on the active component, any additional pharmaceutical excipients, and any possible incompatibilities. The leaflet also contains information on drug interactions, the product's shelf life after opening the container, the product's shelf life after packaging, the product's shelf life after diluting or reconstituting, and the product's shelf life after it has been opened for the first time.

26 Specific information:

Any changes to the manufacturing procedure, testing procedure, designing, packaging, labeling, sale pack, or any other documentation must be reported to the licensing authority within thirty days and must be approved by the licensing authority.

17.11 PLANT MASTER FILE

The free sale Certificate, Pharmaceutical Products (CPP), as per the WHO GMP Certification Scheme, must be included in the plant master file. This certificate must be given by the National Regulatory Authority (NRA) of the country of origin, and it must also include the CEP (EDQM certificate).

Site Master File is a document that is kept at the licensed premises and contains factual and precise information regarding excellent manufacturing procedures.

1. Information of the Firm
2. Licence for Pharmaceutical Manufacturing
3. Other Simultaneous Manufacturing
4. The Quantity of Products That are Allowed to be Manufactured Using the Same Ingredients
5. Process Flow and Procedure.
6. Total Number of Employees Involved in Production, Storage, Quality Control, and Distribution
7. Outsourcing for the Scientific, Analytical or Other Technical Assistance for Manufacture and Analysis
8. Provide an In-depth Description of the Quality Management System
9. Specifications of the Product have been Submitted for Registration with Foreign Nations

17.12 PERSONNEL

Submit the following papers as part of the application: The designated duty and organisational chart, containing the qualifications, experience, and responsibilities for engagement in the plant operation, including production, quality assurance, and distribution, are to be recorded. Keep a record of things like upkeep and distribution, as well as human resources and training. Also, the documents pertaining to individual health, as well as personal hygiene and clothing, etc., are also to be recorded.

17.13 PREMISES

The following documents are required to be submitted because Schedule M of the Drug and Cosmetics Act of 1940 applies, and it is applicable. Briefly, the following documents are required.

1. The design plan of the production regions with the scale of production.
2. Specifications on the structure and the materials used, including the fittings and fixtures.
3. A description of the ventilation system, along with a diagrammatic representation of the important regions that may be in danger of airborne pollution.
4. Classification of the room, filtration unit, and other components necessary for sterile production.

5. A special location has been set aside for the treatment of highly toxic, dangerous, and sensitising materials for before disposal.
6. A description of the water system along with schematic drawings of the sewage disposal system.
7. Specifics of the preventative maintenance performed on the operation and the recording system.

17.14 EQUIPMENT

1. A condensed description of the primary apparatus utilised in production and quality control laboratories (a list of apparatus that is necessary).
2. Provide a description of the scheduled preventative maintenance programme for the recording system as well as the equipment.
3. Calibration and credentials, comprising the setup and recording systems for the validation of computerised systems.

17.15 SANITATION

The cleaning and sanitising of the instruments must be done on a regular basis.

17.16 DOCUMENTATION

The production, in-process quality control, final quality control, and instrument validation aspects of the documentation and organisation of the operating procedure must be submitted. In addition, documents such as distribution systems, such as the process of distribution chain and product retrieval of withdraws system, need to be deposited.

17.17 PRODUCTION AND INVENTORY

A synopsis of the steps involved in the manufacturing process, complete with flowcharts and diagrams that highlight the most crucial variables also required to be included, are the procedures for the processing of the raw material. Furthermore, this study examines the quality control protocols pertaining to the initial supplies and bulk products, as well as the logistical processes involved in handling starting materials, packaging materials, bulk products, and finished goods. These procedures encompass several aspects such as sampling, quarantine, release, and storage. Also worthy of notice is the administration of materials that were deemed unacceptable. In addition, the validation of the policy process and the methodology should be mentioned.

17.18 QUALITY CONTROL

An abstract of the quality control procedures that have been established and the activities that make up the quality control are to be provided. The release of finished products is another aspect of process quality control that needs to be discussed.

17.19 LOAN LICENCES FOR MANUFACTURING

It is necessary to evaluate the GMP maintenance procedure in depth, as well as the licensee loan application process.

17.20 DISTRIBUTION METHOD, CUSTOMER COMPLAINTS, AND PRODUCT WITHDRAWAL

Information about the storage information, distribution, and procedure of retrieval, as well as the process of managing or retrieval of the complaints.

17.21 SELF-INSPECTION

Details about an experienced and unbiased outside inspector as well as a description of the manufacturer's self-inspection system are required in order to evaluate the manufacturer's compliance with GMP.

17.22 EXPORT OF DRUGS

Specifics about all exported products, including any complaints, product withdrawals, or recalls. The supporting documentation for the particulars is to be enclosed.

1. Site plan including the equipment layout, men and material flow, and pressure differential lay-out.
2. Details of Heating, Ventilation, and Air Conditioning (HVAC) with covered areas, including the filtration level and classification as per small membrane filtration (SMF) standard.
3. Details about the water system, such as how the incoming water is cleaned, how the quality is controlled, and how the outgoing water or sewage is treated.
4. Make a list of all the employees, including their titles, qualifications, and years of experience.
5. Standards and cultures for reference are available.
6. Give information about the production, testing, and utility equipment.

17.23 RULES FOR IMPORTING

After getting a registration certificate or approval from CDSCO through Form 41, an Indian agent can apply for an import licence through Form 10 and get a shipment from a foreign seller sent to India. The following documents are needed in addition.

1. Form 8: Fully filled and submitted by the Indian Agent along with the required fees for a licence to import drugs (not eligible for Schedule X) under the Drugs and Cosmetic Rules, 1945.

2. Form 9: The Indian agent can apply for an import licence by filling out a form that is signed by an authorised agent and confirmed by the Indian embassy in the country of origin. The copy must be notarised, and the wholesale licence copy of the Indian dealer must also be notarised.

17.24 DRUG APPROVAL IN USA

Drug clearance to the US is similar to India. Any New Drug Application (NDA) must pass both the preclinical safety test and all clinical trials to show that it is safe and works. For the FDA to give their final approval of the licence, they need the standard technical document.

17.25 FDA CLEARANCE NEEDS TO BE BASED ON A STUDY

Technical section: Technical section is a record of how drugs are tested for quality and how things change as they are made. It is comprised of the following components:

1. Pre-clinical pharmacology and toxicology section
2. Clinical pharmacokinetics and bioavailability section
3. Microbiology section
4. Clinical data part
5. The part on statistics
6. Use on children, section
7. Use of the drug in paediatric patients
8. Samples and labelling
9. Part of the case report

Archival Copy: This is the source that FDA reviewers use as a reference. It has the tabulations and case report forms for clinical studies. It has the following things in it:

1. Fill out form FDA 356
2. Put the page number in the index
3. A brief overview of the clinical study
4. Copy for review: This is called the changes made to the processes during the review process. It has the following things in it:
5. Index
6. Fill out Form 356h from the FDA
7. Cover letter copy
8. Letters of permission
9. Copy of the description of the application

The FDA maintained communication with the sponsor and held at least two meetings with the sponsor during the review process. In most cases, the meeting takes place after the completion of the Phase II clinical trial, and then again prior to the submission of an NDA, in which case it will be referred to as a pre-NDA meeting. The review team is going to look at the results, examine them, and decide whether the application should be approved or not.

17.26 COMMON TECHNICAL DOCUMENT (CTD) FOR APPROVAL OF NEW DRUGS

The standard technical document (CTD) was made to meet the needs of internationally accepted guidelines, and India, the US, the EU, and other important regulatory agencies all accept it. CTD has five Modules.

1. Module I: Administrative/Legal Information
2. Module II: Summaries
3. Module III: Quality Information (Chemical, Pharmaceutical and Biological)
4. Module IV : Non-Clinical Information
5. Module V : Clinical Information

17.26.1 Module I: Administrative/Legal Information

It is a regional requirement, and, according to the various regulations, this module might be established by the regulatory authorities in the relevant regions. In most cases, Module I (Table 17.3) is sectioned down into the following categories:

TABLE 17.3
Module I Is Sectioned Down into the Following Categories

1	Specifics regarding the governance of the organisation
2	Form 44, along with the required payment, must be filled out and submitted.
3	Documents of a legal and statutory nature
3.1	Required documentation licence and necessary approvals
3.1.1	Form 11 applicable if an imported drug product
3.1.2	Form 29 applicable if an indigenous drug
3.1.3	No objection letters/approval for clinical trial
3.1.4	Clearance from the Genetic Engineering Appraisal Committee (GEAC) for any biotechnology or genetic drugs
4	To be notarised legal papers relevant to the application include the following:
4.1	A copy of the plant registration or approval certificate that was issued by the Ministry of Health or the National Regulatory authority of the nation in which the plant originated
4.2	A copy of any approval that demonstrates that the drug can be manufactured and/or sold in the country of origin, if there is such permission
4.3	An original or a copy of the Pharmaceutical Product Certificate, often known as the PPC, in accordance with the WHO GMP certification programme for imported drug products
4.4	A copy of the Free Sale Certificate (FSC), which must come from the nation of origin for any imported pharmaceutical products
4.5	Certificates of Compliance with Good Manufacturing Practices (CGMP) from all other manufacturers engaged in the production of the vaccine
4.6	The NRA will provide a batch release certificate for products that are imported

4.7 Undertaking to declare (as per Annex A)

4.8 A copy of site master file

4.9 Certificate of analysis from Central Drug Laboratory (India) of three consecutive batches.

4.10 Product Permission Document (PPD)

5 Coordinates related to the application

5.1 Specific information regarding the name and address of the drug product's manufacturer, along with their contact information including their phone number, fax number, and email address

5.2 Specifics regarding the name, address, and means of communication of the accountable authority, including their phone number, fax number, and email address

5.3 Specifics on the authorised agent's name and address in India, including any applicable contact information such as a phone number, fax number, or email address (for pharmaceutical products that have been imported)

5.4 Information regarding the producer or official responsible for releasing batches of drug product, including their full names and addresses, along with their contact information (telephone numbers, fax numbers, and email addresses), if available

5.5 Specific information regarding the maker or official of the drug product, such as their name and address, as well as their contact information, including their telephone number, fax number, and email address (for imported drug products)

5.6 Specific information regarding the name and address of the drug substance's manufacturer, along with their contact information including their phone number, fax number, and email address

5.7 Specific information regarding the other manufacturer(s) that are a part of the production process, including their names, addresses, and contact information (i.e., phone numbers, fax numbers, and email addresses)

6 General information on drug product

6.1 Name of drug product, including any proprietary, commercial, or trade names for the product

6.2 Common name, non-proprietary name, or product name of the drugs

6.3 Contents that make up the drug (according to the information provided on the label)

6.4 The amount of strength or concentration present in each dose unit

6.5 If there is a requirement that the product be dispensed before usage

6.6 Method of administration (Route of administration)

6.7 Commercial presentation

6.8 Storage condition

6.9 A detailed account of the product's characteristics

7 Labelling of products in accordance with the Drugs and Cosmetics Rules of 1945

7.1 Initial labelling on the primary package

7.2 Labelling of secondary package

7.3 The insertion label of the packaging, written in English

7.4 Information for prescriptions or a literature insert for medical practitioners

7.5 Packaging for transporting shipments to India, providing details on box sizes and packing volumes

7.6 An overview of production as well as process variable control

7.7 In the event that the drug is granted a patent, the patent status can be extended to other nations

7.8	Conditions that must be met in order for new drugs to be approved for use in other countries
7.9	In the event of imports, a list of Nations with pending imports is provided
7.10	The price in INR for the domestic market, or an equivalent amount in other currencies if the drug is also sold in other countries
7.11	A synopsis of the research and development efforts undertaken by the manufacturer
7.12	A summary of the manufacturer's commercial endeavours in both the domestic and international markets
7.13	Details concerning the involvement of any and all experts
7.14	Evaluation and classification of potential environmental hazards
7.15	Drug product samples: The reference samples consist of approximately 50 clinical doses, or double the quantity, and are stored in an airtight container

17.26.2 Module II: Summaries

It is essential to have adequate knowledge of Module II in order to comprehend the drug profiles' summaries, as these modules contain the abstracts of the pharmacologic classes, modes of action, and clinical applications. In addition to that, these modules provide information regarding the mode of drug administration, as well as safety, dosage strengths, and recommended indications.

In Module II, the most essential facts are written down on just one page, together with a brief introduction, pharmacology, pharmacokinetics, and toxicity. The following Table 17.4 constitutes a synopsis of the material covered in Module II:

TABLE 17.4
The Following Constitutes a Synopsis of the Material Covered in Module II

1 Module II Introduction: As previously stated, the summary or abstract of the safety, dose, method of administration, pharmacology, safety, pharmacokinetics, and related toxicological is provided.

- 1.1 Summary of quality
  - 1.1.1 A quick overview of the active pharmaceutical ingredient
  - 1.1.2 A quick summary of the pharmaceutical product
  - 1.1.3 Application of details in appendices
- 1.2 A brief overview of the non-clinical investigations
  - 1.2.1 Statement of compliance with GLP requirements
  - 1.2.2 A brief overview of the non-clinical tests
  - 1.2.3 Pharmacology of the drugs, including hypotheses regarding the mechanisms of action of drugs
  - 1.2.4 The pharmacokinetics of different drugs
  - 1.2.5 The pharmacology and toxicology of drugs
  - 1.2.6 Conclusions for drugs
  - 1.2.7 Bibliography for different drugs
- 1.3 Summary of non-clinical studies
  - 1.3.1 The protocol is followed while introducing non-clinical investigations
  - 1.3.2 A brief look at the pharmacology

- 1.3.3 A synopsis of the data provided in tabular form addressing the pharmacology
- 1.3.4 A synopsis of the pharmacokinetic data presented in tabular form (if relevant)
- 1.3.5 An abbreviated version of the pharmacokinetics summary (if it applies)
- 1.3.6 Toxicology
- 1.3.7 In tabular forms of toxicology, the range of dose, LD50, and other information should be mentioned

1.4 Brief of clinical studies

- 1.4.1 Introduction to clinical research
- 1.4.2 Discussion and development of the product
- 1.4.3 A synopsis of the immunogenicity
- 1.4.4 Efficacy in a nutshell
- 1.4.5 An overview of the safety
- 1.4.6 Risk-benefit analysis
- 1.4.7 A list of the published works

1.5 Summary of clinical studies

- 1.5.1 Introduction as well as a brief summary of the findings
- 1.5.2 Contents
- 1.5.3 A summary of the clinical research conducted on immunogenicity
- 1.5.4 A summary of the efficacy trials conducted in clinical settings
- 1.5.5 A summary of the safety studies conducted in clinical trials

17.26.3 Module III: Quality Information Including the Chemical, Pharmaceutical, and Biological

The tabulated brief description that is required for the registration procedure is included in Module III, which has been written in accordance with the M4Q guideline. The document is written to comply with the minimum standards for the quality of the chemistry, manufacturing, and controls of both the drug substance and the drug product (Table 17.5).

TABLE 17.5
Description that is Required for the Registration Procedure Is Included in Module III

1 The active ingredients contained

2 In the event that several drugs are combined, or a combination dosage form is used, information regarding the individual drug component must be provided as well as information regarding the drug substance itself.

3 It is necessary to provide information regarding the starting materials and the raw materials used in the dosage development process.

- 3.1 The specific name of the drugs product, which may include one or more trade names or names that are not proprietary
- 3.2 The molecular formula, the structural formula, and the relative molecular weight are all things that need to be addressed
- 3.3 It is necessary to discuss the characterisation and description of the drug substance

- 3.4 It is necessary to provide a general description of the drugs as well as the history of the starting material
- 3.5 It is necessary to describe the biological products as well as the production of antibiotics and microbial stains
- 3.6 System of seed/master/working banks
- 3.7 Embryonated eggs as well as various types of cell substrates
- 3.8 An overview of the various types of raw materials
- 3.9 Certificates of analysis bearing the signatures of both the manufacturer and the applicant for registration

4 Manufacturing process for drug substance
- 4.1 Manufacturer(s)
- 4.2 Detailed of the production procedure
- 4.3 Diagrammatic representation of the production process
- 4.4 Identifying the most important stages of the process and the controls
- 4.5 The manufacturing process is subjected to validation.
- 4.6 The development of the manufacturing process.
- 4.7 Detailed explanation of the deactivation or purification procedure
- 4.8 Detailed explanation of the purifying procedure
- 4.9 Detailed explanation of the conjugation procedure
- 4.10 Enhancement of the active ingredient's stability
- 4.11 Reprocessing
- 4.12 Procedure for filling the active ingredient, controls during the manufacturing process
- 4.13 The selection of key steps to be taken and their justification
- 4.14 Detailed explanation of the batch identification system

5 Identifying characteristics of the drug substance
- 5.1 The physicochemical characterisation of the substance
- 5.2 Biological characterisation
- 5.3 Impurities, if there are any

6 Quality control of drug substance
- 6.1 Details regarding the constituents of drugs
- .6.2 Controlling quality through techniques for analysis
- 6.3 Procedures for analysis, as well as validation
- 6.4 The analysis of batches, as well as the uniformity of analyses

7 Container closure system
- 7.1 Both primary and secondary packaging in accordance with the IS standard
- 7.2 Packaging evaluation and quality assurance

8 Stability of drug substance
- 8.1 The study's methods, its findings, and its conclusions. Usually, follow the ICH recommendation or the Schedule Y of the Drug and Cosmetics Act
- 8.2 Post-approval stability program
- 8.3 Conditions for storing and moving drug substances

9 Drug product
- 9.1 Formulation of the pharmaceutical product
- 9.2 Detailed explanation of the manufacturing process for drugs
- 9.2.1 Active drug substance(s)
- 9.2.2 Complete drug product

9.2.3 Final formula and composition qualitatively/quantitatively
9.2.4 The procedure or operation of making
9.2.5 Container, closing method, and compatibility with the drugs all need to be considered.

10 Manufacture of drug product
10.1 Address and contact information of the manufacturer(s)
10.2 Formulation for batches, including the quantitative formula
10.3 Detailed explanation of the production procedure together with an associated flowchart
10.4 Process variable control. Specific information regarding the essential and intermediate stages of the manufacturing process.
10.5 The procedure for the evaluation and certification of the manufacturing
10.6 Identification of the batches, as well as a description of the system

11 The formulation's excipients, such as adjuvants, preservatives, stabilisers, and others, described in detail
11.1 Specifications
11.2 Analytical methods and processes
11.3 Methods of analysis are subjected to validation.
11.4 Justification of the requirements and specifications
11.5 Use of novel adjuvant, preservatives, stabilisers, and excipients

12 Control of finished drug product
12.1 Particulars of the manufactured version of the drug product
12.2 Procedures for the analysis of the completed pharmaceutical product
12.3 Report of analysis validated by the producer and the applicant

13 Finished pharmaceutical product
13.1 The validation of the already used analytical techniques.
13.2 A comprehensive analytical analysis regarding the uniformity across all batches
13.3 Analysis of the impurities, including their characteristics and concentrations
13.4 Justification of the requirements and specifications

14 Stability of drug product
14.1 The protocol, the guidelines, the findings, and the conclusions of the stability research.
14.2 Thermostability testing, diluents and reconstitution details, and stability testing of freeze-dried items, where applicable
14.3 Stability after the post-approval phase
14.4 Preservation of the cold chain and contingency plans
14.5 Specifications for the production of a drug product, including the master formula, batch record, and documentation for set release, as well as the equipment and facilities used to produce the drug
14.6 Assessment of danger and potentially hazardous substances

---

17.26.4 Module IV: Non-clinical information

It provides the safety evaluation together with the final non-clinical study results and describes them based on the ICH guideline. The facts on a drug's safety during its duration of use are provided by non-clinical research and critical analysis (Table 17.6).

TABLE 17.6
Description that is Required for the Registration Procedure Is Included in Module IV

1 The findings of studies: in a nutshell
2 A discussion on the pharmacology of the finished product or drugs
3 Investigations into the pharmacodynamics and immunogenicity of the product
4 Pharmacokinetics of the products including the bioavailability of the drugs
5 Additional pharmacokinetic studies, as well as investigations into the impact of potential novel adjuvants and administration methods.
6 Toxicology
    6.1 Specifics regarding the animals: Research into and justification of the use of animals as a model, including specifics on the age of the species, the size of the group's dose, the method of administration, and the control groups. Monitored parameters, local tolerance
    6.2 If necessary, additional types of toxicology testing can be performed, such as immunological tests, tests for genotoxicity and carcinogenicity
7 Additional toxicity studies of the new formulation are necessary if new adjuvants, stabilisers, additives, etc. are utilised
8 Special considerations of the toxicity studies
    8.1 Examination of the "shedding" (excretion) of microorganisms in the context of attenuated vaccinations
    8.2 New adjuvants, stabilisers, additives, more methods of delivery, and new combined vaccinations all require toxicological testing
    8.3 References

17.26.5 Module V: Clinical information

The clinical information is necessary in Module V for evaluating the pharmaceutical formulation, pharmacokinetics and pharmacodynamics, clinical pharmacology studies, clinical safety, clinical efficacy, synopses of the individual investigations, and final copies of complete clinical study reports. The studies for the clinical trial are carried out in accordance with the ICH guidelines. The following items (Table 17.7) should be supplied for Module V of the clinical summary:

TABLE 17.7
The Following Items Should Be Supplied for Module V of the Clinical Summary

1 Contents and reports of clinical studies
    1.1 An overview of the Phase I study
    1.2 An overview of the Phase II trial
    1.3 An overview of the Phase III trial
    1.4 A bridging and conclusive from the studies
2 Considerations about the clinical facts
3 Additional information about the adjuvants and the human trials
4 Studies in Phase IV and either a pharmacovigilance plan or an adverse event reporting system
5 Studies demonstrating the lack of sufficiency to validate the bioavailability in conjunction with other combination vaccines
6 Studying the effects of co-administration with other vaccinations with regard to their safety
7 Listings of each patient individually as well as case report forms
8 The bibliographical references for the information

17.27 RAW MATERIAL OR BULK DRUG SUBSTANCES ALREADY APPROVED IN THE COUNTRY

Manufacturing procedures, quality assurance, analytical specifications, stability reports, and data on the medication's toxicity in animals are only a few of the many documents needed for approval when producing raw material or bulk drug compounds through bulk synthesis.

The following documentation (Table 17.8) is needed to move forward with the approval procedure.

TABLE 17.8
The Following Documentation Is Needed to Move Forward with the Approval Procedure

1	Information about the company and the drug application
2	Drug name
3	Classification (Therapeutic) Class of the drug
4	Initial approval date and details approval number
5	The application must be made on Form 2626 by the authorised authority
6	Fees that are required by regulation
7	Included are forms 25 and 26 for a manufacturing licence for raw materials, as well as forms 29 for bulk drugs
8	Included for importation is a copy of the drug sale licence in Form 20B and Form 21B
9	Information about pharmaceuticals and chemicals, like the IPUAC or CAS number
10	Flowcharts as well as specific information regarding the manufacturing process
11	Check the procedure and the in-process control, as well as the report control
12	Record of production batches
13	The procedure for the report of validation
14	Specifications of the drug supply in bulk, as well as techniques of analysis and a validation report
15	Specifics regarding the naming and amounts of any impurities that may be present
16	Purity of the enantiomers, as well as the structural isomer
17	The presence of residual solvents as well as other volatile impurities (OVI) and the methods for their quantification
17	The structural elucidation methods and the data can be presented
19	Conformity of the certificate of analysis with a minimum of three batch requirements
20	Data on the long-term stability of three separate lots, as required by Schedule Y of the Food and Drug Administration. Details concerning the batch number, the batch size, the date the product was manufactured, the date the process was started, as well as the packaging details, are included in the rules
21	Material safety data sheet
22	The characterisation of the reference product
23	Draft label specimen
24	The subacute toxicity of the drug in two different animals
25	CD of TL/IPC test report

17.28 FIXED-DOSE COMBINATION (SECTION 122-D) OF A NEW DRUG (FORMULATION) ALREADY APPROVED IN THE COUNTRY

Fixed-dose combination of two or more pharmaceuticals that have already been approved, as defined in Clause (c) of Rule 122 E as a new drug and separate applications are required using Form 44 for approvals by the licensing authority, as described in Clause (b) of Rule 21 as is required in Appendix VI of Schedule Y. In a manner analogous to that of the approval of a new drug, the authorisation to manufacture or import the drug is granted by submitting either Form 45A or Form 46 when all of the required data have been provided. The justification of a fixed dose combination with a therapeutic advantage should be included in an application, and this reason should be supported with authentic literature from peer-reviewed journals or textbooks. In addition, the data on the pharmacokinetics and pharmacodynamics of the fixed dosage forms, as well as the data on the safety and effectiveness of the combination of dosage forms, must be included in the combination dosage form data.

The consideration of the approval is conditional upon the submission of the following information (Table 17.9):

TABLE 17.9
The Consideration of the Approval Is Conditional upon the Submission of the Following Information

1	Clear indication of the application's purpose, whether it be for manufacturing or importing, is required
2	Applicant's full name and mailing address
3	Name of the drugs, as well as the constituent parts of the brand-new drugs
4	The new drugs or combination formulation's dosage form and indication
5	The rationale for the recommended dose form from a therapeutic perspective
6	Specifics regarding the country's authorisation of each newly developed drug
7	Approved dosage form of the new drug in the country
8	Composition of each individual new drug that has been approved for use in the country as well as indications for use that have been authorised
9	Application on Form-44 by an appropriate authorised authority
10	Fees that are prescribed and come in the form of challans from the Treasury
11	Forms 25/28/26 for a valid manufacturing licence have been enclosed
12	Form 29 for a valid test licence has also been enclosed
13	Enclosed the Form 46A/45A and source of bulk drugs along with current regulatory status
14	Included in this package are Forms 46A and 45A, as well as the source of bulk drugs and the current regulatory status
15	Specifics regarding the active components, including the amounts that are now present as a percentage
16	Brief the chemical and pharmacological information
17	Specification of the active pharmaceutical ingredient, including the impurity profile

18	Analysis and verification procedures for the report
	Detailed of overdose, pharmacodynamics and pharmacokinetic characteristics, duration of shelf life, incompatibilities, packaging details, storage conditions, and instructions for handling
19	Conformity of the certificate analysis for each of the previous three batches in consecutive order
20	Formulation-related data
21	Forms of the manufacturing recipe that are considered master forms
22	The procedure for manufacturing/the manufacturing of the master record
	Report on product development, including an analysis of excipient compatibility and a study of force degradation. Specification of the finished product, including a profile of any impurities
23	Method of investigation for the finished product
24	Method of analysis and validation report for the completed products
25	Conformity of the analysis reports for three batches and three validation batches in conjunction with a finished product certificate
26	Checking both the process itself and the specifications as part of quality control.
27	Data regarding the stability of three distinct lots, as required by Schedule Y of the Drugs and Cosmetics Rules, along with information regarding the batch number, batch size, date of manufacturing, date of initiation, and packaging particulars
28	The dissolution and release characteristics of the oral dose form
29	Release and dissolution profile comparison with the marketed oral dosage form
30	Comparative analysis and pharmaceutical equivalency with international brand(s) or Indian brands that have been approved, if relevant
31	The insert of the packaging must include all of the generic names of the active ingredients, as well as the dosage form(s), dose, applications, and route of administration of a certain medication. Furthermore, it is imperative to include information regarding contraindications, cautions, safety measures, interactions between drugs, adverse consequences, use in special populations, an accidental
32	Draft of the label and the container as a specimen
33	Regulatory standing in various other nations
34	The current status of authorisation for the proposed dosage form or alternative method of administration in other countries, as well as copies of approval in key countries, are both required
35	In the event that a drug or similar combinations of drugs are removed from the market for any reason
36	While importing pharmaceutical products, are required to have a free sale certificate (FSC) or a certificate of pharmaceutical product (COPP)
37	Procedure for testing bioequivalence or bioavailability
38	An overview of the study
39	Biographical information and research activities as per Schedule Y Appendix VII
40	Volunteers should be given an informed consent form in accordance with Schedule Y in the event of a clinical experiment. This document should include the subjects' addresses, qualifications, occupations, and annual incomes, as well as the provision of audio-visual recordings
41	A declaration of conformity or undertaking by the sponsor in accordance with the remuneration requirement of Rule 122 DAB
42	Copies of letters of permission from the "Ethics Committee" together with registration information for the Ethics Committee
43	Bioequivalence research exemption, if needed (justification required)
44	In the event of parenteral administration, sub-acute toxicity information is necessary

17.29 ALREADY-APPROVED DRUG (RULE 21) TO BE USED AND PROPOSED TO BE MARKETED AS A "NEW ROUTE OF ADMINISTRATION"

According to Clause (c) of Rule 122 E, an approved drug that will be used in the treatment of a condition by alternating the route of administration is also known as a new drug. A separate application is necessary in accordance with Clause (b) of Rule 21, which states that new drugs must meet certain criteria. The completed Form 44, as indicated in Appendix VI of Schedule Y, must be submitted to CDSCO for approval. The application also needs to include the approval number along with the date and a reason for the use of new dosage forms that have a therapeutic advantage. This justification needs to be supported by legitimate literature that has been published in journals or textbooks that have been pre-reviewed. In addition to that, data on the new route of administration's safety and efficacy, as well as the quality control criteria, are required. The following information (Table 17.10) is required for determining approval:

TABLE 17.10
The Following Information Is Required for Determining Approval

1	The application's purpose, such as producing or importing, must be explicitly stated
2	Name and address of the applicant
3	The new drug's name and each of its constituents
4	The new drugs or combination formulation's dosage form and indication
5	The therapeutic recommended dosage forms and rationale
6	Details of the individual new drug approval in the country approved dosage form
7	Approved dosage form of the individual new drug in the country
8	Individual new drug composition approved in the country and approved indication
9	The competent authority submits an application on Form 44
10	Treasury challans are used to collect prescribed fees
11	Include the Form 25/28/26 for a valid manufacturing licence
12	Include the Form 29 for a valid test licence
13	Include the Form 46A/45A for supply of pharmaceuticals in bulk and the regulatory status
14	Copy of manufacturing licence form from bulk medication supplier and consent letter for supply
15	Specifics about the active components, including the percentage basis present
16	Brief data on chemicals and pharmaceuticals
17	API specification, including impurity profile
18	Analytical procedure and report validation
19	Analysis of certificate conformity for three consecutive batches
20	Formulation information
21	Master versions of the manufacturing ingredients
22	The creation of a master manufacturing record (MMR) for a pharmaceutical product involves documenting the procedures and specifications for manufacturing. The MMR serves as a comprehensive guide for the production process. Here are the general procedures for creating an MMR, focusing on the growth of a product, ingredient interactions, and finished product specifications

23 Analysis of the finished product
24 Analysis method and validation report of finished goods
25 Conformity of the analysis reports for three batches or three test batches with a finished product certificate
26 In-process quality control checks and standards
27 Stability data for three different lots according to Schedule Y of the Drugs and Cosmetics Rules, including the batch number, batch size, date of manufacture, date of initiation, and information about the packaging
28 Dissolution release curve for the oral dose form
29 Comparison of the oral dosage form's approved formulation's breakdown and release profile
30 Pharmaceutical equivalence with foreign brand(s) or approved Indian brand(s) and comparative evaluation, if necessary
31 On the insert of the package, all of the generic names of the active components, the composition, the dosage form or forms, the dose, the indications, and the method of administration must be mentioned. Also included should be the contraindications, warnings, precautions, drug interactions, unwanted effects, use in special populations, overdose, pharmacodynamics and pharmacokinetics, expiration dates, incompatibilities, details about the package, storage requirements, and handling guidelines
32 Sample drafts of the label and container
33 Regulation in other countries
34 The current status of authorisation for the proposed dosage form or new mode of administration in other countries, as well as copies of approval in key countries, are required
35 In the event that drug products or similar combinations of drugs are removed from the market for whatever reason
36 When importing pharmaceutical products, it is necessary to have a free sale certificate (FSC) or a certificate of pharmaceutical product (COPP)
37 Bioequivalence or bioavailability study protocol
38 Synopsis of the study
39 In addition to the biodata, a synopsis of the study that the investigators are now conducting in accordance with Appendix VII of Schedule Y
40 In the event of a clinical trial, the volunteer must be provided with an informed consent form in accordance with Schedule Y. This document must include the subjects' addresses, qualifications, occupations, and annual incomes, as well as audio-visual recordings
41 Provision requiring conformity or undertaking by the sponsor in regard to remuneration in accordance with Rule 122 DAB
42 Copies of letters of permission from the "Ethics Committee" together with registration information for the Ethics Committee
43 Exemption from the bioequivalence studies, if necessary, and supported by justification
44 Information on the drug's sub-acute toxicity is necessary in the event that it is administered parenterally
45 Included are 11 sets of technical literature (where relevant), namely ten soft copies and one hard copy for the experts' review. Each attachment must have a size that is less than or equal to 20 megabytes (MB) and must be correctly indexed

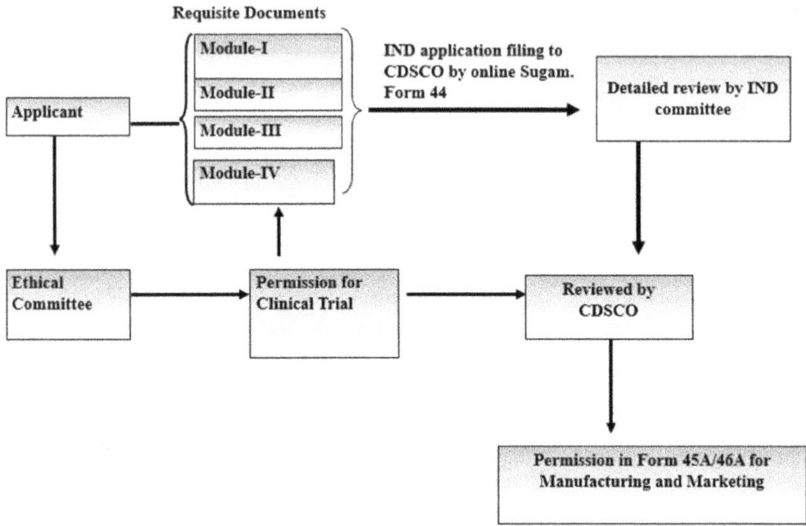

FIGURE 17.1 Approval process for NDA or INDA in India.

17.30 APPROVAL PROCESS AS A DEFINITION OF "NEW MEDICATION" FOR USE IN NEW INDICATION AND THE INDIVIDUAL COMPONENT PREVIOUSLY APPROVED UNDER RULE 21 OF DRUGS AND COSMETICS RULES, ALSO KNOWN AS REPURPOSING DRUGS

According to Clause (c) of Rule 122 E, a new drug is an approved drug that will be used in a new indication or treatment of a different disease. As was mentioned earlier, a separate application is required for approvals from the licensing authority, as per Clause (b) of Rule 21, described in Form 26, which is required in Appendix VI of Schedule Y. A manufacture or import license can be obtained through Form 26 or Form 25, which is analogous to the licensing process for new drugs. The following information (Table 17.11) is necessary in order to take the approval into consideration:

TABLE 17.11
The Following Information Is Necessary in Order to Take the Approval into Consideration

1	It is essential that the application's goals, whether they be manufacturing or importing, be stated fairly explicitly
2	Provided name and address of the applicant
3	The dosage form and indication that were used for the newly developed drugs or combination formulation
4	Therapeutic justification for the currently proposed dosage form
5	Specifics regarding the approval of the individual new drug in the country
6	Specifics about each new medicine being approved in the country

7 The approved dosage form of the individual new drug in the country
8 The approved composition of the individual new drug in the country as well as the approved indication for use in the country
9 Submission of an application to CDSCO on Form 26 by the Competent Authority
10 Fees that are required to be paid and are presented in the form of challans from the Treasury
11 Form 25/28/26 for valid manufacturing license must be enclosed
12 Included is a completed Form 29 for a current test license
13 Enclosed the Form 26A/25A and source of bulk drugs along with current regulatory status
14 A copy of the manufacturing license form submitted by the bulk drugs supplier along with a consent letter for supply
15 Specifications of the active components, including the percentage of every component present
16 Summary of chemical and pharmaceutical information
17 The specification of the API (Active Pharmaceutical Ingredients), including the impurity profile
17 The approach taken for the analytical and validation analysis of the report
19 Conformity of the certificate analysis for three batches that have been produced in succession
20 Information pertaining to the formulation
21 The manufacturing recipe in its master forms
22 Procedure for manufacturing/master manufacturing Record Report on product development, including an analysis of excipient compatibility and a study of force degradation. Specification of the finished product, including a profile of any impurities
23 Procedure for the analysis of finished products
24 Report on the analytical method and validation of the completed products
25 Conformity of the analysis reports for three batches and three validation batches together with a finished product certificate
26 Quality control check while the product is being manufactured and the specifications
27 The stability data of three distinct lots in accordance with Schedule Y of the rules governing drugs and cosmetics, including information on the batch number, facts about the packaging, the date of commencement, the manufacture date, and the batch size
28 Profile of dissolution and release for the oral dose form
29 Comparative dissolution release profile with the formulation that was approved for the oral dosage form
30 Comparative analysis and pharmaceutical equivalency with international brand(s) or Indian brands that have been approved, if relevant
31 The insert of the packaging must include all of the generic names of the active ingredients, as well as the dosage form(s), dose, applications, and route of administration of a certain medication. Furthermore, it is imperative to include information regarding contraindications, cautions, safety measures, interactions between drugs, adverse consequences, use in special populations, an accidental overdose, pharmacodynamics and pharmacokinetic characteristics, duration of shelf life, incompatibilities, packaging details, storage conditions, and instructions for handling
32 An example of the drafting for the label and the carton
33 The regulatory environment across multiple other nations
34 The current status of approval for the proposed dosage form or novel mode of administration in other countries, as well as copies of approval in relevant countries
35 In the event that the drugs or such combinations of drugs are removed off the market for whatever reason
36 A Free Sale Certificate (FSC) or a Certificate of Pharmaceutical Product (COPP) is necessary for the importation of pharmaceuticals
37 Bioequivalence or bioavailability study protocol

17.31 APPROVAL PROCESS AS A NEW DRUG USE IN NEW DOSAGE FORMS (WITHOUT FIXED DOSAGE) AND THE INDIVIDUAL COMPONENT ALREADY APPROVED UNDER THE RULE 21 OF THE DRUG AND COSMETICS RULES

An approved drug that will be used in new dosage forms to treat a disease is also known as the new drug. This is, according to Clause (c) of Rule 122 E, a new drug, and as was mentioned earlier, a separate application is required for approvals from licensing authorities as per Clause (b) of Rule 21, described in Form 44. This information is required in Appendix VI of Schedule Y. The approval of Form 45/46 is similar to the approval of a new medicine in that it allows production or import. The following information (Table 17.12) is necessary in order to take into consideration the approval, as follows:

TABLE 17.12
The Following Information Is Necessary in Order to Take into Consideration the Approval, As Follows

1	The application must make clear whether it is being submitted for the purpose of manufacturing or importing
2	List of the applicant's name and address
3	The new drug's name, as well as the names of all the components of the drug
4	The dosage form and indication that are to be applied with the new drug or combination formulation
5	Therapeutic rationale for the proposed dosage form
6	Specifics of the particular new drug's approval process in the country
7	The dosage form of the individual new drug that has been approved for use in the country
8	The composition of the individual new drug that has been approved for use in the country and the approved dosage
9	Application on Form 26 by the competent authority
10	Fees that are prescribed and come in the form of challans from the treasury
11	Include Form 25/28/26 for a valid manufacturing license
12	Included the Form 29 for a valid test licence
13	Enclosed are the Forms 46A and 45A, the source of the bulk medications, and the current regulatory status
14	Also included are copies of the manufacturing licence form, the supplier's letter of approval, Form 46A/45A, and the source of the bulk drugs
15	Information on the main ingredients, including the amount present
16	Brief information about chemicals and drugs
17	Specification of API and including impurity profile
18	The report's methodology for analytical testing and validation
19	Certification of compliance with analysis for three consecutive batches
20	Formulation-related data
21	Master forms of the method to manufacture
22	Manufacturing process/factory standard operating procedure record analysis of excipient compatibility and degradation of force in new product development report. Specifications of the finished product, including a profile of any impurities

23	Analysis of the finished product
24	Method for analytical testing and a validation report on the finished products
25	Conformity of the analysis reports for three batches/three validation batches with finished product certificate
26	Check the specifications and perform quality control checks during the procedure
27	Data on the stability of three separate lots in accordance with Schedule Y of the rules regulating drugs and cosmetics, including information about the batch number, the batch size, the date of manufacturing, the date of initiation, and details about the packaging
28	Detailed analysis of the dissolution and release of the oral dose form
29	A comparison of the dissolution and release profiles using the formulation that was approved for the oral dose form
30	Comparative analysis and pharmaceutical equivalency with overseas brand(s) or Indian brands already on the market, if relevant
31	On the insert of the package, all of the generic names of the active components, the composition, the dosage form or forms, the dose, the indications, and the method of administration must be mentioned. In addition, the contraindications, warnings, precautions, drug interactions, undesirable effects, use in special populations, overdose, details of pharmacodynamic and pharmacokinetic properties, shelf life, incompatibilities, packaging details, storage conditions, and instructions for handling are to be mentioned
32	A sample of the draft for the label and the carton
33	Status of regulations in other countries
34	The status of approval for the other countries of the proposed dosage form or new route of administration, as well as copies of approval in key countries
35	In the event that the medications or similar combinations of drugs are removed from the market for any reason at all
36	There is a need for a Certificate of Pharmaceutical Product (COPP) or a Free Sale Certificate (FSC) when importing pharmaceuticals
37	Bio- equivalence or bioavailability study protocol
38	An overview of the research
39	investigators carrying out the tasks outlined in appendix VII of schedule Y in conjunction with the biodata
40	In the event of a clinical trial, the volunteer must be provided with an informed consent form in accordance with schedule Y. This document must include the subjects' addresses, qualifications, occupations, and annual incomes, as well as audio-visual recordings
41	Agreement or guarantee by the sponsor in accordance with the pay clause set forth in Rule 122 DAB
42	Copies of letters of permission from the "Ethics Committee" together with registration information for the Ethics Committee
43	Waiver of the need for a bioequivalence study if justifiable
44	In the event that parenteral are used, statistics on the substance's sub-acute toxicity are required
45	Included are 11 sets of technical literature (where relevant), namely ten soft copies and one hard copy for the experts' review. Each attachment must have a size that is less than or equal to 20 megabytes (MB) and must be correctly indexed

17.32 APPROVAL PROCESS AS A NEW DRUG USE IN ADDITIONAL STRENGTH AND THE INDIVIDUAL COMPONENT ALREADY APPROVED UNDER THE RULE 21 OF THE DRUG AND COSMETICS RULES

According to Clause (c) of Rule 122 E, as a new drug, additional strength of the active ingredient for use in treatment of different purposes or use in treatment of the same disease is known as a "new drug," and, as was mentioned before, a separate application is required for approvals of licensing authorities as per Clause (b) of Rule 21, described in Form 44 as is required in Appendix VI of Schedule Y. Form 45 or 46 is used to grant authority for the manufacturing or import of a drug, which is analogous to the approval of a new drug. For this category of novel medications, the following documents (Table 17.13) are mandatory:

TABLE 17.13
For This Category of Novel Medications, The Following Documents Are Mandatory

1	The application must make clear whether it is being submitted for the purpose of manufacturing or importing
2	Applicants' names and addresses in full
3	The new drug's name, as well as the name of each component of the drug
4	The dosage form and indication that are to be employed for the newly developed medication or combination formulation
5	Therapeutic rationale for proposed dosage form
6	Specifics regarding the approval of the individual new drug in the country
7	Approved dosage form of the individual new drug in the country
8	Approved composition of the individual new drug in the country as well as approved indications
9	Submission of the application on Form 26 by the competent authority
10	Fees that are prescribed and come in the form of challans from the Treasury
11	Enclosed the Form 25/28/26 for a legal manufacturing licence
12	Please enclose the Form 29 for a valid test licence
13	Please enclose the Form 46A/45A as well as the source of bulk pharmaceuticals and current regulatory status
14	A copy of the manufacturing licence forms the bulk medicine supplier must have, together with a consent letter for supply
15	Specifics regarding the active components, including the amount present in percentage
16	Some nformation regarding chemicals and pharmaceuticals
20	Description of the API, including the impurity profile
17	The approach taken for the analytical work and validation on the report
20	Conformity of the certificate analysis for three batches that have come before it three times in a row
21	Information pertaining to the formulation
22	The manufacturing formula in its master forms
23	Procedures for manufacture and the master manufacturing record report on product development, including an analysis of excipient compatibility and a study of force degradation. Specification of the finished product, including a profile of any impurities

24	Procedure for finished product analysis
25	Report on the validation of the analytical method and the completed products
26	Conformity of the analysis reports for three batches/three validation batches together with the finished product certificate
27	Check for quality control throughout production and adherence to the standards
28	Data on the stability of three separate lots in accordance with Schedule Y of the rules governing drugs and cosmetics, including information on the batch number, the batch size, the date of manufacturing, the date of initiation, and the package details.
29	Characterisation of the dissolution and release of the oral dose form
30	A comparison of the dissolution and release kinetics with approved oral formulation.
31	Comparative analysis and formulation equivalency with approved international brand(s) or approved Indian brand(s), if appropriate
32	On the insert of the package, all of the generic names of the active components, the composition, the dosage form or forms, the dose, the indications, and the method of administration must be mentioned. In addition, the following should be mentioned: contraindications, warnings, precautions, drug interactions, undesirable effects, use in special populations, overdose, pharmacodynamic and pharmacokinetic properties, shelf life, incompatibilities if any, details of packaging, storage conditions, and details for handling
33	An example of the design for the label and the carton
34	Therapeutic Rationale and justification for the proposed in additional strength
35	The regulatory environment in various other countries
36	The current status of permission to additional countries of the proposed dosage form or novel mode of administration and/or copies of approval in important countries
37	If the drugs or such combinations of pharmaceuticals are removed, any and all reasons must be provided
38	In order to import medications, it's necessary to have either a Free Sale Certificate (FSC) or a Certificate of Pharmaceutical Product (COPP)
39	Protocol for the study of bioequivalence or bioavailability
40	An overview of the research
41	Investigators that are carrying out research in accordance with Appendix VII of Schedule Y in addition to the biodata
42	Inform consent form of the volunteer as per Schedule Y in the event of a clinical trial, with the stating of address, qualification, occupation, annual income of subjects, and providing audio-video recordings
43	Any published report that indicates the use of greater strength
44	Conformity or undertaking on the part of the sponsor for the compensation clause in accordance with Rule 122 DAB
45	A copy of the "Instituted Ethics Committee" permission letters, along with the data of the Ethics Committee registration
46	Exemption from the bioequivalence study, if necessary and supported by justification
47	In the event that parenteral are used, data on the substance's sub-acute toxicity must be provided
48	Enclosed 11 sets of technical literature (where relevant), namely ten soft copies and one hard copy to be new CDSCO for the experts' opinion. Each attachment must have a maximum size of one megabyte (MB) and must be correctly indexed

BIBLIOGRAPHY

Bhaduri S, Kipgen T. New Drugs' approvals in India: An institutional perspective. *Science, Technology & Society* 2017, 23(3): 444–462.

Chakraborty R, Yadav K. Drug approval process in US, Europe and India and its regulatory requirements: A review 2008, 6: 31–39.

Chakraborty K, Yadav K. Drug approval process in US, Europe and India and its regulatory requirements: A review. *International Journal of Drug Regulatory Affairs* 2017, 6(3): 31–39.

G.S.R.227(E). New drugs and clinical trials rules, 2019. Ministry of Health and Family Welfare, India. March 2019. http://www.egazette.nic.in/WriteReadData/2019/200759.pdf. Accessed 19 July 2019.

Jain P, Chauhan R. India's new drugs and clinical trials rules: An industry perspective. *Regulatory Focus.* July 2019. Regulatory Affairs Professionals Society. https://www.raps.org/news-and-articles/news-articles/2019/7/indias-new-drugs-and-clinical-trials-rules-an-in.

Jawahar N, Lakshmi V. Regulatory requirements for the drug approval process in US, Europe and India. *Journal of Pharmaceutical Sciences and Research* 2017, 9: 1943–1952.

Jawahar N, Shrivastava N, Ramachandran A, Priyadharshini BR. Procedures and applications for marketing authorisation of medicinal products in European Union. *Journal of Pharmaceutical Sciences and Research* 2015, 7(4): 219–225.

Morulaa Health Tech Pvt Ltd, online https://morulaa.com. Accessed 3 October 2023.

Patel J, Parikh K, Shah D. New drug approval procedure in India. Pharmatutorhttps://www.pharmatutor.org/articles/new-drug-approval-procedure-india.

Sawant AM, Mali DP, Bhagwat DA. Regulatory requirements and drug approval process in India, Europe and US. *Pharmaceut Reg Affairs* 2017, 7: 2. Schedule y at URL Schedule%20Y(ammended%20version)%20-%20CDSCO.htm. Accessed 26 December 2020.

The drug development and approval process. Available at: www.mhsource.com/resource/process.html. Accessed 26 December 2020.

U.S. Food and Drug Administration. CFR—code of federal regulations title 21. Chapter I, Sec 312.21, phases of an investigation. Available at: http://www.accessdata.fda.gov/scripts/cdrh/cfdocs/cfcfr/CFRSearch.cfm?fr=312.21. Accessed 26 December 2020.

U.S. Food and Drug Administration. Guidance documents for drug applications. Available http://www.fda.gov/Drugs/DevelopmentApprovalProcess/ucm090361.htm. Accessed 26 December 2020.

U.S. Food and Drug Administration. Pre-IND consultation program. Available at: http://www.fda.gov/Drugs/DevelopmentApprovalProcess/HowDrugsareDevelopedandApproved/ApprovalApplications/InvestigationalNewDrugINDApplication/Overview/default.htm.

18 Medical Device Rules and Enforcement

18.1 INTRODUCTION

Medical devices are critical components of modern medical care. The use of medical devices makes diagnosis and treatment more efficient, reliable, and effective, increasing the quality of care. The range of medical devices is quite broad, ranging from a spatula to a heart valve to a high-end computer-controlled device. The common items that fall under the purview of the Medical Device Act include any device or apparatus, instruments, appliances, implants, or combinations of instruments used for disease diagnosis, treatment, prevention, or mitigation. India is the largest importer of medical devices from other countries, and medical instruments are required for better health care. Manufacturing of and research into medical devices necessitate an understanding of Indian regulations for selling and marketing medical devices in India. The CDSCO, which operates within the boundaries of the Drug Controller General of India (DCGI), Ministry of Health and Family Welfare, regulates the marketing of medical devices in India.

18.2 REGULATION ENFORCEMENT

The Government of India issued a Gazette identifying sterile devices as drugs (Form No. 11014/2/2005—DMS and PFA; Gazette No. 1077 dated October 6, 2005), and the Medical Device Rule was recently implemented via Gazette Notification on January 31, 2017. GSR 78 (E) (E). The newly implemented Act improved regulatory standards, simplified them, and compared the provision of responses to adverse situations with global guidelines.

18.3 THE CENTRAL LICENSING APPROVAL AUTHORITY (CLA)

Excise power has been entrusted to a constituted committee for controls on the manufacture of medical devices in accordance with the provisions of Sub-rule (1) of Rule 68A of Part VII of the Drugs and Cosmetics Rule, 1845. This was notified in GSR 127 (E) dated October 7, 2005, and GSR 78 (E) on December 31, 2017.

1. The CLA is enforced by the GSR 78 (E), which came into effect on December 31, 2017, as Chapter III of the Government Notification.
2. The CLA is a notified and specialised authority that was established by the CDSCO. Its primary responsibility is to deal with regulatory issues pertaining to medical devices.

DOI: 10.1201/9781003397854-2

3. The CLA ensured that medical devices adhered to safety standards and conformed to norms for uniformity across the country of India.
4. The CLA is also responsible for post-market surveillance, the investigation of adverse reactions, and the issuance of warnings.

After confirming the safety and effectiveness of the medical device and ensuring that it complies with the standards set forth by the Bureau of Indian Statistics (BIS) and/or the International Organization for Standardization (ISO), the device will be considered approved.

18.4 CHAPTER I: TITLES, APPLICATIONS, AND DEFINITIONS

In this chapter, the titles, applications, and definitions are described in detail and the regulation's boundaries and its scope are also defined.

In addition, medical devices, experimental medical devices, invasive devices, custom-made medical devices, active diagnostic medical devices, active therapeutic medical devices, and other medical devices are also described.

18.5 CHAPTER II: REGULATION OF MEDICAL DEVICES

Classification of medical devices can be performed according to their use, level of invasiveness, utility, design, potential risk, manufacturing process, applicative body system, length of contact, and systemic effects.

In this chapter, the classification of medical devices is based on the level of risk that is associated with the device, as outlined in Part I of the First Schedule.

Low risk, which corresponds to Class A; low to moderate risk, which corresponds to Class B; moderate-to-high risk, which corresponds to Class C; and high risk, which corresponds to Class D.

In addition, devices are classified as *in vitro* diagnostic medical devices within Part II of the First Schedule.

According to the first Sub-rule, Class A medical devices are not required to have any licence, and the quality of the product is controlled according to the applicable standards that have been established.

When a manufacturer of a Class A medical device, as defined in Sub-rule (1), voluntarily submits an application for a licence to comply with the regulatory requirements specified in these rules, the application must undergo evaluation by the Notified Body. The purpose of this evaluation is to determine conformity with the applicable section of the Quality Management System, in accordance with the procedure outlined in the regulations.

The companies that import medical devices for the purpose of selling or distributing them; that manufacture medical devices for the purpose of selling or distributing them; or sell, stock, exhibit, or offer medical devices for sale, are required to obtain a licence for medical devices in accordance with the guidelines that will be issued from time to time by the CLA.

In addition to this, manufacturers of medical devices should be concerned about both the performance and the safety of their products.

This chapter is also designed to obtain an understanding of the uniform product standards that were recognised by the BIS, which was established in accordance with Section 3 of the Bureau of Indian Standards Rule, 1885 (63 of 1885), the International Electro-Technical Commission (EC), any relevant pharmacopoeia standards, and the ISO standard.

This chapter outlines the requirements for the different types of licences that must be obtained before a medical device can be manufactured, exhibited, distributed, or sold in a retail setting in India.

18.6 CHAPTER III: AUTHORITIES, OFFICERS, AND BODIES

CLA is authorised to rule as the competent authority for the purpose of enforcing these regulations. In addition, the CLA is responsible as the enforcing agency for the approval of medical devices and other functions that are related, such as the manufacture and import of Class C and Class D medical devices, clinical trials, and clinical performance evaluation. Only products that fall under Classes C or D are permitted to be licensed by the State Licensing Authority, whereas the CLA is licensed as the competent authority for Classes A and B products. In this situation, the CLA is considered to be the competent authority, and a separate state licence is not necessary for manufacturing or selling of Classes A and B products. At the manufacturing site, the Quality Management System (QMS) and any other applicable standards for Class A and Class B products are subjected to inspection by the notified agency. This chapter also included a provision that allows for the delegation of powers from the CLA to the State Licensing Authority, provided that the State Government gave its approval.

In addition, in this section, provisions are delegated by the Central Government to institutes, government organisations, or government-aided establishments in the capacity of a National Accreditation Body by notification. Under Sub-rule (1) of this section, the National Accreditation Body is authorised to access the firms to set standards and issue certification. Furthermore, it is the responsibility of the National Accreditation Body to conduct periodic reviews of the quality, norms, and guidelines that have been established. Listed accredited establishments must register with the CLA to become a Notified Body for auditing manufacturing sites, assessing, and verifying specified categories of medical devices for compliance with standards and other requirements. This Act includes a description of the functionary in Part II of the Third Schedule.

This section also describes the appointment of a Government Analyst under Section 20 of the Act and referred to as the Medical Device Testing Officer, as well as the appointment of Inspector and Government in Section 21 of the same Act, which is declared in the official Gazette. Both of these appointments are described in this section.

Provisions for the establishment of a laboratory by the central government by notification, to be known as the Medical Device Testing Centre, are included in this Act. This laboratory will have defined functions for testing and evaluating medical devices, as well as serving as an appellate centre for the laboratory.

The State Government has given permission for the establishment of a testing centre or laboratory specifically dedicated to testing and evaluating medical devices. The chapter related to this establishment holds legal significance, indicating that there are specific legal provisions governing the creation and operation of such testing facilities. The chapter grants authorization for the delegation of power related to the issuance of licenses. This suggests that the State Government may have the authority to delegate certain powers, potentially related to regulatory approvals, licensing, or oversight of medical devices, to specific entities. The delegation of power may involve the transfer of authority from the Central Drugs Standard Control Organization (CDSCO) to the Central Licensing Approval (CLA) and State Licensing Authorities.

The chapter likely addresses the role of the National Accreditation Body. National accreditation bodies are organizations that assess and accredit conformity assessment bodies, ensuring they meet specific standards.

The chapter may also describe the role and functions of a Notified Body. Notified Bodies are entities designated by regulatory authorities to assess the conformity of certain products, including medical devices, with applicable regulations. The chapter is said to empower medical devices, suggesting that it provides legal authority or support for the development, testing, and regulation of medical devices within the state.

18.7 CHAPTER IV: MANUFACTURE OF MEDICAL DEVICES FOR SALE OR DISTRIBUTION

This chapter has the most content concerning the rules and defines the application to the approval procedure for the manufacturing process.

18.7.1 Application for Manufacture for Sale and Distribution of Medical Devices

As described earlier, the State Licensing Approval Authority (SLA) is the competent authority for approval of manufacture for selling and distribution of products of Class A or Class B medical devices, whereas the CLA is the competent authority for approval of manufacture for selling and distribution of products of Class C or Class D devices. Furthermore, the CLA is the competent authority for the approval of the manufacture of Class C or Class D medical devices, along with Class A or Class B medical devices. Application should be made through the specified form, Form No. MD 3 for Class A or Class B, and Form No. MD 4 for Class C or D devices, with the fees specified as described in the Second Schedule, along with documents as specified in Clause (ii) of Part II of the Fourth Schedule. The authorities and functions stipulated in this regulation shall be executed by the CLA for inspection to confirm the requisite technical competence of the manufacturer.

18.7.2 Loan Licence to Manufacture for Sale and Distribution

The classification of medical devices into different classes is common in regulatory frameworks. In this context, Class A and Class B are mentioned as categories for medical devices. The characteristics, risks, and regulatory requirements for Class A devices are likely different from those for Class B devices. The specific criteria for classifying devices into different classes are typically outlined in relevant regulations. The mention of an application for approval of a loan indicates that there is a financial aspect involved, and a loan is being sought for the manufacture of a Class A medical device. This suggests that the regulatory authorities may be involved in approving or overseeing financial transactions related to the manufacturing of medical devices.

Rule 5 and the Second Schedule is referenced as parts of the regulatory framework or legislation. Rule 5 likely contains specific provisions related to Class A medical devices, while the Second Schedule may provide details about Class B medical devices. The application for loan approval may require regulatory scrutiny to ensure that the funds are being used appropriately for the manufacture of Class A medical devices in compliance with the rules and regulations.

The loan application should be submitted in Form No. MD 6 along with the required documents as specified in Clauses (i) and (ii) of Part II of the Fourth Schedule. The manufacturing and testing processes should be monitored by someone who has a degree in engineering (in a relevant branch), pharmacy, or science in an appropriate subject from a recognised university, and the individual should possess a minimum of two years of work experience in the production or testing of medical devices. Alternatively, they should hold a diploma in engineering (in a related field) or pharmacy from a recognised university and have a minimum of four years of experience in the manufacturing or testing of medical devices. The manufacturing process must adhere to the rules as described in the Fifth Schedule.

Provision of auditing of the manufactured device, in accordance with Rule 18, to the CLA, via the Central Government's online portal as referred to in Rule 15. Class A and B medical devices should be audited by the Notified Body, whereas Class C or Class D medical devices should be inspected for suitability and the assessment of appropriateness by the medical device inspector and may be conducted with or without the involvement of an expert in the relevant subject. Under the Drugs and Cosmetics Rules, 1845, the SLA or the CLA issued a licence to manufacture the medical device in Form No. MD 7 or a loan licence in Form No. MD 8 after the inspection report was approved.

The licence owner is obligated to abide by certain guidelines, such as storing the licence within the manufacturing premises, informing the authority of any untoward incidences, and adhering to the Sixth Schedule of the Act with regard to the modification of product specifications and the technical personnel staff. In addition, quality control should be carried out in order to guarantee that the requirements are met. In the event of a failure to meet the quantitative requirements, the licensing authority has the authority to re-validate the product in accordance with the specifications, with the seizure of the entire production lot resulting from such a failure. In addition to an auditable or inspection book in the form of Form No. MD 9, the holder of the licence is required to keep a minimum of one unit of the medical device from each batch of the process. The person who holds the licence is responsible for informing either the CLA or the State Licensing Authority when the manufruleuring process has been completed.

In accordance with Rule 15, an appeal can be lodged against the granting of a licence in accordance with Section 20 if the licence's terms and conditions are altered. After an appeal, the licence is acceptable for another ninety days, or until a new license is issued, whichever comes first. The Second Schedule of the Rule specifies that a license or loan license shall be valid until suspended or cancelled. This suggests that the license is granted for a certain duration and remains in effect unless specific actions, such as suspension or cancellation, are taken. The license holder is required to deposit a license retention fee. This fee is likely intended to be paid at regular intervals to retain the validity of the license. The information suggests that the license retention fee must be deposited every five years from the date the license was issued. This indicates a periodic payment requirement to ensure the continued validity of the license. The validity of the license is contingent on the payment of the retention fee. If the fee is not paid or if there are other reasons, the licensing authority may suspend or cancel the license.

In addition, the Act stated that a licence or loan licence shall stay valid for a period of time equal to the length of the loan.

An appeal can be submitted within sixty days of receiving a copy of the order if a licence is revoked by the SLA or the CLA, and there is a possibility that the order will be confirmed, reversed, or modified. The deadline for submitting an appeal is sixty days after receiving the order. If the terms of the licence or the loan licence are not satisfied, either the SLA or the CLA has the authority to order the destruction of the stock.

This Act is also considered in accord with Section 3 of the Bureau of Indian Standards Rule, which was passed in 1885 (Rule No. 63 of 1885) and has been revised on numerous occasions by the Central Government. In the absence of the Indian Standards Rule, 1885, other international organisations such as the ISO or the International Electrotechnical Commission, or any pharmacopeia standard, are recognised and approved.

In addition, in the event that neither national nor international standards are available, the item in question must conform to the standards set by the manufacturer. In order to conduct clinical studies, testing, assessment, examination, demonstration, or training, a limited quantity of any class of medical device must be submitted to the CLA along with the designated Form No. MD 10 as outlined in the Second Schedule of the Act.

18.8 CHAPTER V: IMPORT OF MEDICAL DEVICES

According to the provisions outlined in Sub-rules (1) and (2) of Rule 5, the CLA can issue a licence allowing for the importation of medical devices. The authorised agent who possesses a licence to manufacture for sale or a licence to sell is qualified to submit an application for the import of a medical device using the MD 12 form. This application must be accompanied by the required documentation listed in Parts I, II, and III of the Fourth Schedule as well as the appropriate fees that are outlined in the Second Schedule. If any more medical instruments are manufactured or sold, the seller or manufacturer of those instruments is obliged to get a licence and pay a fee, as described in Sub-rule (3) of the Second Schedule. In addition to this, the CLA is responsible for ensuring quality control and conducting routine testing and inspections at overseas manufacturing sites. If the particular seller or manufacturer is selling the particular instruments in Australia, Canada, Japan, European Union countries, or the United States of America with the approval of the regulatory authorities, an equivalency licence certificate may be issued in accordance with Sub-rule (1).

The clinical study is mandatory for Class A and Class B medical devices in accordance with the regulation included in Chapter VII, but only if the devices are being imported from a country that is not Australia, Canada, Japan, a member state of the European Union, or the United States of America.

The granting of the licence is contingent on the recipient's fulfilment of a number of predetermined requirements. The licence should be kept in the fruleory, and any administrative decision should be conveyed to the licensing authority. This includes any adverse reactions, regulatory restrictions, market withdrawals, non-regulatory compliance with the other country, or any medical devices that have not been sold or distributed.

Any modifications that are made to the organisational structure of a licensee, in accordance with Rule 32, authorised agents are required to submit an application for a new licence in accordance with Rule 30 within ninety days of receiving the notices. After submitting an application with Form No. MD 14 and the necessary fees, the CLA may authorise the sale of a medical device or an *in-vitro* diagnostic medical device in a limited quantity. This authorisation comes in the form of a test licence, which is applied for using Form No. MD 15. The licence is only for the purposes of clinical investigation, testing, evaluation, demonstration, or training, depending on the circumstances, as well as such clinical investigations, testing, evaluation, or training. It is imperative that every record be kept, and the standard validity period for a licence is three years.

Under exceptional circumstances, a medical device that is not approved in India can be imported from another country. However, the instrument must be approved in the country of origin before it can be used in India in the treatment of a patient suffering from a disease that poses a risk of death, a disease that causes serious permanent disability, or a disease that requires therapy for an unmet medical need. In this particular scenario, the application needs to be submitted using Form No. MD 16, along with the required fees that are outlined in the Second Schedule. It is required that the application is submitted to the Medical Officer via the medical superintendent of a government hospital or statutory medical institution in order to receive approval, and this approval will be issued in the form of Form No. MD 17. The imported instrument needs to be used for the specific patient, and the full address information for the consignment needs to be provided.

Tourists are required to make a declaration to customs authorities. This declaration is likely related to the contents of their personal baggage, including items they are bringing into the country. Section 10 of the relevant Rule specifies the legal basis or authority for the declaration requirement. The details of Section 10, including its provisions and requirements, would be outlined in the legislative or regulatory document.

If the tourist complies with the declaration requirement as specified in Section 10, customs authorities will permit the passenger to bring their personal baggage into the country. There is a condition that the personal baggage should not exceed a certain limit. This limit could be in terms of quantity, value, weight, or other relevant criteria, and it would be defined by the regulations or laws governing customs procedures. The application must be submitted using Form No. MD 18, and, if the CLA is satisfied with it, they will issue a licence using Form No, MD 18 if the application is granted.

18.9 CHAPTER VI: LABELLING OF MEDICAL DEVICES

The Legal Metrology (Packaged Commodities) Rules, 2011, must be complied with to sell or distribute notified medical devices in India. The name of the medical device, a description of its net contents (measured or weighed), the date of manufacture, the expiration date, the manufacturer's name and address, the location where the notified medical device was made, the batch number, and the manufacturing licence number (if made in India) should all be listed on the label.

Imported products are mandated to display specific information, including the import license number and the expiration date. This information is likely required for regulatory compliance and consumer safety. Each imported product is expected to prominently display its import license number. This number serves as a unique identifier and is likely issued by the regulatory authorities in the importing country.

The expiration date of the product is also a critical pece of information that must be displayed. This is particularly important for products with a limited shelf life, such as pharmaceuticals and certain medical devices. Re-labelling is necessary to ensure that the imported products comply with the labelling requirements of the country. This process may involve updating or modifying labels to meet local standards and regulations. The re-labelling process can occur in the warehouse of the customs house. This is a common practice, ensuring that products are appropriately labelled before entering the local market. Re-labelling may also need to adhere to specific requirements approved by the Central Drugs Standard Control Organization (CDSCO), particularly if the products fall within the purview of pharmaceuticals or medical devices in India.

The label must be printed with a type of ink that cannot be removed and must be clearly visible on the packaging of the medical device's innermost pack. The date that a sterile device was sterilised should be stated on the device. It is not necessary to include an expiration date on medical devices composed of stainless steel, titanium, or other inert materials. The criteria also mandate that the device's use, which can either be a single use or several uses, must be specified. If the equipment is meant for use in clinical investigations, it must also include a mandatory disclaimer, such as "CLINICAL INVESTIGATION ONLY." The label ought to carry precise information about its intended use, such as "Physician's Sample—Not to be Sold," so that it can be given away free of charge to medical professionals. The sample should only be used within the hospital and should not be sold to individual patients; it should instead be marked with the information "Hospital supply only," using an additional label or sticker on the outer shelf pack. These days, a one-of-a-kind device identification or QR bar code is included as a standard feature for improved identity. The information about the manufacturer, as well as any symbols that are approved by the BIS or the ISO, should be included on imported devices. The shelf life of the medical equipment must not be less than sixty months from the date of production or the date of import, whichever comes first. Additionally, the shelf life must not be less than three months.

18.10 CHAPTER VII: CLINICAL INVESTIGATION OF MEDICAL DEVICES AND CLINICAL TRIAL EVALUATION OF NEW *IN-VITRO* DIAGNOSTIC MEDICAL DEVICES

The clinical investigation of an experimental medical device involving a human subject is not allowed until the CLA gives its authorised permission for the investigation to take place. The responsibilities and obligations outlined in these rules are to be carried out by the Ethics Committee, which was established in accordance with Rule 122DD of the Drugs and Cosmetics Rules, 1945. As stated earlier, any clinical research must be approved by the CLA, and the sponsor must apply for approval along with Form No. MD 20 and the pre-requisite information that is outlined in the Seventh Schedule.

The Second Schedule holds importance in the context of clinical trials, and it likely contains specific details, guidelines, or regulations related to the conduct of clinical trials. These details could include procedural requirements, ethical considerations, and other relevant information. The mention of a pilot clinical trial suggests a preliminary or small-scale trial conducted to assess the feasibility, safety, and efficacy of a particular intervention before a full-scale clinical trial. Parenthetical references in the Second Schedule likely provide additional information or explanations for specific clauses or sections. They may offer clarification or guidance on the interpretation of the content. The statement indicates that there is no provision for mandated costs when a clinical trial is carried out in a hospital supported by the central or state government. This suggests that certain costs associated with the clinical trial may not be mandated or required in such cases, possibly as an incentive for conducting trials in government-supported healthcare institutions.

Before conducting any clinical study, especially those involving medical devices or interventions, it is crucial to seek and obtain approval from an Ethics Committee. The Ethics Committee ensures that the study adheres to ethical principles and safeguards the rights, safety, and well-being of study participants. Substantial equivalence is a concept often used in the evaluation of medical devices, particularly in regulatory processes. When a new device is being compared to a standard device, it must demonstrate substantial equivalence in terms of safety and effectiveness.

For a clinical study to establish substantial equivalence, it must demonstrate not only the safety but also the clinical efficacy of the device. Clinical efficacy refers to the ability of the device to produce the desired therapeutic effect under specific conditions. Ethics Committee approval is essential because it ensures that the study design and conduct meet ethical standards. This includes considerations such as informed consent, fair participant selection, and appropriate risk-benefit assessments.

After an in-depth investigation into the safety of the standard device efficiency itself, the CLA is the authority that is ultimately recommended for determining substantial equivalence. According to the Seventh Schedule of this Act, if it seems to the CLA that the clinical data are inadequate, the requisite trial should be concluded within thirty days and no more than ninety days. After the period of ninety days, during which the applicant's sponsor has failed to comply with the requirements, the application is at jeopardy of being rejected. It is imperative that the Seventh Schedule of this Act be adhered to, in addition to maintaining stringent compliance on clinical trials in the following areas:

1. Very trial must be approved by the CLA and monitored by an ethics committee that is registered with either the CDSCO or the Act of the jurisdiction.
2. As a standard operating procedure, the investigator's brochure needs to include information on all aspects of the experiment, including the protocol, compensation, procedure of data analysis, and conclusion of the endpoint.
3. The guideline known as Good Clinical Practices has to be followed for every single trial.
4. Before the first patient is investigated for a clinical trial, the trial must first be registered with the Clinical Trial Registry of India (CTRI).
5. Any trial that is terminated or non-compliant should be informed to the CLA within thirty days with comprehensive reasons for the termination, and any suspected unanticipated major adverse event should be informed to the CLA within 15 days of the occurrence of the event.
6. If a fatality or other adverse event takes place during the trial, the sponsoring organisation must compensate and reimburse all related medical expenses.
7. In this chapter, provision was also made for the delegate to empower the CLA to investigate a clinical trial by confirming the premise behind a clinical trial that the sponsor had declared, including their subsidiaries' register/data, employees, and branches, as well as their agents, contractors, subcontractors, and clinical trial locations.
8. Once authorisation has been granted, a clinical trial should begin as soon as possible by enrolling the first patient in the study. This should be done within one year of receiving approval.

The CLA has the authority to revoke permission after being informed of specific deficiencies with respect to compliance with the requirements. In addition, the CLA has the authority to deny the investigator and the sponsor permission to carry out any clinical investigations in the future. This includes the investigator and the sponsor's employees, subsidiaries, and branches, as well as their agents. The CLA was also given the authority to disqualify anyone from participating in any trial or to partially terminate the trial. There are also provisions for the investigator to appeal to the CLA within thirty days of receiving such an order and to have the case reinvestigated.

According to Section 45 of this Rule, if any volunteer suffers an injury that can be attributed to the testing of the experimental medical device, the sponsor is responsible for providing all necessary medical care. This responsibility is outlined in Rule 122DAB of the Drugs and Cosmetics Rules, 1945, and it shall be applicable in the same manner for the purpose of medical management.

The Medical Devices Officer is authorized by the rule to conduct searches for, seize, and record any medical devices. This authority extends to both marketed medical devices and experimental medical devices. The officer has the right to enter premises where a clinical trial is being conducted. This implies that the officer can visit locations where medical research is taking place, including hospitals or research facilities.

The officer has the authority to validate registers related to the clinical trial. This likely involves reviewing and confirming the accuracy of records and registers maintained during the trial. The officer is empowered to review any documents related to the clinical trial without prior notice. This includes but is not limited to, documents such as protocols, informed consent forms, adverse event reports, and other trial-related records.The mention of "without prior notice" suggests that the officer has the right to conduct these activities without informing the involved parties in advance. This is common in regulatory enforcement actions to ensure that inspections are unannounced, providing a more accurate representation of the situation.

According to Regulation 49 of this Act, the sponsor is required to keep all of the data, records, and other materials connected to the clinical study for a period of twenty years. However, in accordance with the instruction from the CLA, the specifics of individuals need to be disclosed. The confidentiality of all trials will be preserved.

It is against the law to collect tissues or blood for the purpose of evaluation of any *in vitro* diagnostics if the CLA has not given its clearance. The CLA should be applied to by the sponsoring body using Form No. MD 22 and paying the prescribed fees as outlined in the Second Schedule.

Before beginning a clinical trial of an *in vitro* diagnostic device, ethical permission must first be obtained, and the Ethics Committee overseeing the trial must be registered with the CLA, in accordance with the requirements outlined in Appendix VII of Schedule Y of the Drugs and Cosmetics Rules, 1945, which are referred to in the Seventh Schedule. It is necessary, when requesting the CLA for permission for a clinical trial, that details of the origin and quantity of all types of samples are required, as is a description of the device that includes the specifications of both the raw material and the final product, data that allow for the identification of the device, and suggested instructions for use, labelling, and information regarding the regulatory status in other countries. Before commencing a clinical trial for any *in vitro* diagnostic, it is necessary to include many forms of supplementary data, including but not limited to in-house performance evaluation data. These additional data points are crucial for establishing key factors such as its stability, specificity, sensitivity, consistency, and reproducibility. Also required is the scope of the trial, its purpose, medical requirements, and the case report disclosed as per the Seventh Schedule. Before the start of the trial, the investigator should ensure that the investigation is carried out in accordance with the Seventh Schedule. The investigator should also make a declaration that complies with safety measurements during the trial in order to protect the volunteer's health and safety as well as their best interests.

The Central Licensing Approval (CLA) holds the authority in the context of granting authorization for the manufacture or import of new medical equipment. This authority is likely associated with regulatory oversight related to the introduction of such equipment into the market. The CLA has the power to make decisions that may include shortening the duration of a clinical trial, postponing it, or even completely waiving the need for a clinical trial. These decisions are made in the interest of the general public.

The reference to shortening, postponing, or waiving clinical trials indicates that, under certain circumstances, the CLA may determine that traditional, lengthy clinical trial processes can be modified or bypassed. The decisions made by the CLA are explicitly stated to be in the interest of the general public. This implies that the CLA takes into consideration factors such as public health, urgent medical needs, or other compelling reasons that may warrant expedited approval processes.

The approval of the licence is contingent on a review of the necessary reports, which are outlined in the Second Schedule of this Act. If the review reveals any missing or inadequate data, the applicant is obliged to resubmit the information within ninety days of submitting the first application and within thirty days of the first extension.

18.11 CHAPTER VIII: PERMISSION TO IMPORT OR MANUFACTURE OF A MEDICAL DEVICE WHICH DOES NOT HAVE A PREDICATE MEDICAL DEVICE

In order to import or manufacture a medical device that does not have a predicate device or one which has been subjected to clinical trial, approval must be obtained from an authorised agent recognised by the CLA or the manufacturer him/herself. The details of this process are outlined in Chapter VII. In addition to the information that is provided in Part IV of the Fourth Schedule, the necessary fees that are mentioned in the Second Schedule must also be submitted. The provision is only authorised to indicate that it may be used in treatment of serious diseases or diseases that have a unique significance to the current state of the Indian health scenario, as well as in times of great national urgency, emergencies, and epidemics. Also, it is necessary to mention those ailments or diseases for which there is no treatment; in such a scenario, the requirements for pre-clinical or clinical data can be abbreviated, postponed, or avoided entirely, depending on which route the CLA considers to be the most appropriate course of ruleion.

It is possible to relax the standards for emergency situations involving medical devices that pertain to animal toxicity, reproductive studies, teratogenic studies, perinatal studies, mutagenicity, and carcinogenicity. After the establishment has been granted approval, a periodic safety update report must be submitted to the CLA every six months. This report must include all relevant safety information. In addition, any suspected unanticipated serious adverse event must be reported to the CLA within fifteen days of its occurrence.

18.12 CHAPTER IX: DUTIES AND POWER OF THE MEDICAL DEVICE OFFICER, MEDICAL DEVICE TESTING, AND THE NOTIFIED BODY

The Medical Device Officer has been given the authority to make (and to delegate other authorities to make) seizures of medical devices, including the inspection of factory premises or stored medical devices. In accordance with the provisions of Chapters IV, V, and VII of these Rules, every sample should be sent in its original packaging to the responsible authority. In accordance with the requirements of Section 26 of this Act, a triplicate sealed packet, together with a specimen of the reference sample, should be submitted for examination.

The Medical Device Officer has been given the authority to conduct an annual inspection of any establishment that is licensed by either the CLA or the State Licensing Authority within the jurisdiction that has been assigned to him/her. Also, medical device officers are given the authority to take samples from medical devices that are manufruleured or imported for sale, as well as those that are stored or exhibited for sale. It is the responsibility of the Medical Device Officer to keep a record of all inspections, as well as to exercise and perform their duties, and to provide copies of this record to either the CLA or the State Licensing Authority, where it should be noted whether any seizures were made. Where it is not physically practical to test large instruments in this situation, the Medical Device Officer can observe, evaluate, test, and report on them with or without expert support. Any suspicious contravention or any investigation into any report of a violation of any provision of the Act, as well as any seizure of stocks or action taken by the Medical Device Officer, is informed to the CLA or the SLA. In the presence of the prosecutor, the Medical Device Officer is obligated to obtain permission in writing from his office before disclosing to any individual any information that he/she obtained while performing such official duties.

In accordance with Clause (c) of Subsection (1) of Section 22 of the Act, the Medical Device Officer has to grant permission before any individual can possess a medical device for marketing or business purposes. Under Paragraph (c) of Subsection (1) of Section 22 of the Rule, a Medical Device Officer must provide a written order before selling or distribution of the device. Any stock of medical devices or records, registers, documents, or other tangible items confiscated by a Medical Device Officer pursuant to Paragraph (c) or Clause (c) of Sub-section (1) of Section 22 of the Act must be returned within twenty days of the date of the seizure. In the event that a Medical Device Officer obtains a sample of a medical device other than those listed in the provision to Rule 63's Sub-rule (iii) for the purpose of testing or evaluating, the Medical Device Officer shall notify the person from whom the sample was obtained of the reason for doing so in writing on Form No. MD 32 and shall provide the fair market value of the medical device in exchange for a signed acknowledgement. The Medical Device Officer must provide a receipt in the form of Form No. MD 33 to the individual from whom the sample was taken if they refuse the reasonable price offered under Sub-section (1) of Section 23 of the Act for the purposes of testing or assessment.

Sub-section (4) of Section 23 of the Act says that information about mode of shipment must be sent to CLA by registered mail or by hand in a sealed packet with a memorandum on Form No. MD 34. A copy of the memorandum must be sent to the manufacturer and whoever is found guilty of breaking any of the Act's acts will have their consignment seized. The confiscation provision also encompasses the production of any medical device specified in Sub-clause (iv) of Clause (b) of Section 3 of the legislation, which is deemed to be misbranded, adulterated, or counterfeit, for the purposes of selling, stocking, presenting for sale, or distributing without a valid licence or authorisation. This regulation is relevant to all tools or equipment utilised in the production, trade, or dissemination of said medical device, as well as any container, package, or enclosure in which the device is placed, vehicles, or other confiscated medical devices which the Medical Device Officer been given the power to seize. After approval of the CLA or SLA has been granted, the report can be sent to the Court for further prosecution. The direction of the Court is that all of these medical device seizures should be done under the supervision of the Medical Device Officer in the presence of the relevant authority, if any, as the Court may direct the order accordingly as deemed appropriate.

Once it has been determined by the Court that the requirements for the seized medical devices that have been confiscated have been fulfilled, the Court may decide to return them to the legitimate owners who were previously in possession of them. In the event that ownership cannot be established, the seized medical devices in question may be given to a charitable organisation as a donation; alternatively, they may be given to a health care institution operated by the government or one of the health care institutions subsidised by the government.

The Notified Body is required to carry out its responsibilities and functions either by itself or by any other competent person acting on their behalf in accordance with the prescribed method that is referenced in Part II of the Third Schedule of the Act. A "Notified Body," which is referred to in Rule 12, is required to carry out its responsibilities and functions with regard to Class A or Class B medical devices in accordance with Part II of the Third Schedule.

At the very least once every two years, the Notified Body must submit to an evaluation and audit conducted by the CLA in accordance with the provisions that are found in Part II of the Third Schedule. In compliance with the legislation, any irregularity constitutes grounds for the CLA to send a notification calling for the cancellation of the registration.

18.13 CHAPTER X OF THE MEDICAL DEVICE RULE, 2017, WHICH IS TITLED "REGISTRATION OF LABORATORY FOR CARRYING OUT TEST OR EVALUATION"

18.13.1 Responsibilities of the Medical Device Officer

The Medical Device Officer (MDO) has the power and purpose to visit the manufacturing sites of the assigned circles at least once per year of any company that has been licensed by either the CLA or SLA in order to guarantee that they are in proper order with the conditions under which the licence has been issued.

The MDO is authorised to withdraw the samples for validation purposes. The medical officer is responsible for keeping every record of the inspection, including any samples that were taken or any seizures that were made, and this information must be provided to either the CLA or SLA. The MDO has the authority to enforce the rule and take the necessary actions in response to any violations that may occur. In addition, the MDO has the authority to investigate any complaint relating to medical equipment, as well as to review technical dossiers or institutional prosecutions.

It is against the law for the MDO to reveal any information that is connected to the performance of his duties, except for when the court or his superior gives him a written order to do so. In addition to this, the MDO is entrusted with the powers shown in the following clauses.

- Preventing or having an injunction implemented to prevent the disposal of stocks of medical devices
- Prohibition or compelled order for the sale of the inventory of medical devices

This rule also provides a clear and comprehensive definition of the seizure procedure. The all-sized papers and materials details and receipt Form ND 35 are to be provided to the person from whom they were recovered, and the same are to be returned as soon as possible, no more than 19 days after the seizures. The medical device is collected by the MDO, and the reason for the seizures must be mentioned in writing using Form 36. The samples were sent to the Medical Device Testing Officer in a sealed packet together with a memo in accordance with Form 38. In addition, the specifics of the device imprint of the memoranda should be sent separately by registered mail or handed over to the Medical Device Testing Officer.

18.13.2 The Confiscation of Medical Equipment, Machinery, and Other Types of Property

If a person or an entire company is responsible for stocking, distributing, or exhibiting a medical device without the appropriate licence, or if they manufacture a misbranded or spurious medical device that is in violation of any of the rule's provisions, then that person or company is subject to having the item confiscated. After the court has received the real report from the Medical Device Testing Officer, stating that the device does not conform to the standard, the court will then command the supply and disposal of the medical device that was confiscated. The appropriate steps are taken to dispose of the confiscated medical equipment in accordance with the court's order and the instructions of the CLA or the state licensing authority. If it is discovered that the quality of the seized medical devices is up to standard, and that no violation of the rule provisions could be shown, the

CLA or the SLA would report the case to the court as appropriate. The court may order the confiscated gadgets to be returned to the legitimate owner or to the inviolability of the owner. Alternatively, the court may require that the equipment be returned to a hospital or charitable dispensary.

18.13.3 Delegated Responsibilities to the Medical Device Testing Officer and Notified the Appropriate Agencies

The Medical Device Testing Officer is responsible for collecting samples in accordance with the regulation, which is stated in Chapters IV, V, VII, and XI of the Medical Device Rule, 2017. The results of any tests or evaluations must be reported in accordance with these rules. In the name of the Director of the Central Medical Device Testing Laboratory, the appropriate dispatch items, along with the memorandum included on Form MD-30, are to be sent. In addition, a specimen impression memorandum written on Form MD-30 and sent in a separate package to the Direc tor of the Central Medical Device Testing Laboratory is necessary. The results are written down using MD 32 Forms in triplicate, and a detailed description of the testing process is provided.

18.14 CHAPTER XI: SALE OF MEDICAL DEVICES

This chapter details the marketing of medical devices, the provision of supplies to health care facilities, and the withdrawal of instruments that have been supplied if they breach any laws. Additionally, any laws that have been broken are also discussed in this chapter. The portion of the Drugs and Cosmetics Rules, 1845, known as Part VI, that deals with the "Sale of Drugs Other than Homoeopathic Medicines" applies to medical devices that are for sale, stocked, exhibited, or offered for sale or distribution by retail or wholesale channels. In addition, the document relating to any surgical intervention that used any medical device must be kept in accordance with the requirements of Sub-clause (1) of the Act. This chapter also defines any defective medical device or instrument that has been replaced by the manufacturer or distributor, along with providing the appropriate information to the competent authority in order to prevent, reduce, or eliminate any risk.

18.15 CHAPTER XII: MISCELLANEOUS

This chapter describes the provision of exemptions of this Act and the medical devices specified in the Eighth Schedule that were considered in exemption of this Act or the conditions specified in that schedule. In addition, this chapter outlined the conditions that must be met in order to qualify for the exemption. In order to import medical equipment, the country of origin must issue a certificate attesting to the product's quality, safety, and performance. The certificate, along with the applicable fees, must then be submitted to either the CLA or the State Licensing Authority.

BIBLIOGRAPHY

Apporva Agrawal New to Medical Device Rules 2017, India? Here Are the 8 Schedules to Know. Available from: https://www.linkedin.com/pulse/new-medical-device-rules-2017-india-here-8-schedules-know-agarwal [Accessed on 24 July 2020].

Device Advice: Investigational Device Exemption (IDE) Available from: https://www.fda.gov/medicaldevices/deviceregulationandguidance/howtomarketyourdevice/investigationaldeviceexemptionide/default.htm [Accessed on 24 Dec 2020].

Nitin Desai Associates. New Delhi. Available from https://nishithdesai.com. [Accessed on Jan 20, 2020].

Premarket Notification 510(k). US FDA. Available from: https://www.fda.gov/medicaldevices/deviceregulationandguidance/howtomarketyourdevice/premarketsubmissions/premarketnotification510k/default.htm [Accessed on 15 Dec 2020].

Singh and Associates A Brief Overview of Regulatory Framework for Medical Devices in India. Available from: https://www.lexology.com/library/detail.aspx?g=e39ba922-f7c6-4568-a7e0-9b753769ada6 [Accessed on 15 Dec 2020].

The Gazette of India. Notification, 31 Janurary, 2017. G.S.R. 78 (E) New Delhi: Ministry of Health and Family Welfare [Accessed on 20 Jan 2020]. Available from: http://www.cdsco.nic.in/writereaddata/Medical%20Device%20Rule%20gsr78E.pdf [Accessed on 15 Dec 2020].

World Health Organization Medical Device Regulations. Global Overview and Guiding Principles. Geneva. Available from: http://www.who.int/medical_devices/publications/en/MD_Regulations.pdf [Accessed on 15 Dec 2020].

19 Schedule of Medical Device and Minimum Requirement of Approval

19.1 INTRODUCTION

The Government of India (GOI) implemented regulatory requirements for the registration and approval of medical devices, aiming to foster an efficient regulatory system that enables the Indian medical industry to produce high-quality, reliable, and cost-effective equipment. The government's initiatives supporting small-scale industries, coupled with the increased demand for medical devices, have significantly expanded the scope of the medical device industry in India. Consequently, many successful indigenous medical instruments have been developed, replacing expensive foreign alternatives, such as the affordable cardiac valve Chitra.

Prior to 1905, the Indian medical device industry operated without regulation due to the absence of legislation or regulatory standards for ensuring safety, quality, and standards. To address this gap, the Central Drugs Standard Control Organisation (CDSCO), a regulatory agency operating under the Ministry of Health and Family Welfare, assumed control over the implementation of the Medical Device Rules, which were announced in 1917 and enforced in January 1918.

Under the regulatory framework, devices falling under the category of "Notified Medical Devices" are considered "drugs" and are subject to regulation under the Drugs and Cosmetics Rules, 1945 (D & C Rules). Manufacturers of such devices do not require separate registration but must obtain approval from the CDSCO before introducing their medical devices onto the Indian market, as per the Gazette Notification SO 1468 (1905). Additionally, certain categories of medical devices are regulated by the Bureau of Indian Standards (BIS) and the Nuclear Medicine Board of the Bhabha Atomic Regulatory Commission (BARC) under the purview of the CDSCO.

The classification of medical devices is categorised into different classes based on the risk associated with their use. Class A comprises medical devices with low risk at the time of use, such as thermometers, audible forks, and tongue depressors. Class B consists of medical devices with low to moderate risk, including hypodermic needles, disposable syringes, and catheters. Class C encompasses high- to moderate-risk medical devices like lung ventilators, artificial lungs, and heart machines. Finally, Class D includes high-risk medical devices, such as implantable devices and heart valves.

DOI: 10.1201/9781003397854-3

19.2 LEGITIMATE MEDICAL DEVICE AS DRUG CATEGORISATION AND ENFORCED DRUGS CONTROLLER GENERAL OF INDIA

The Central Drugs Standard Control Organisation (CDSCO), which operates under the administration of the Drugs Controller General of India (DCGI), is responsible for ensuring consistent implementation of regulations across the country in collaboration with state drug licensing authorities. The DCGI holds authority over the approval process for new medical devices, encompassing specification, standards, clinical trials, sales licences, and import licences. The inclusion of notified medical devices as drugs under the purview of the Food and Drugs Act of 1940 was established through Section 3(b)(iv) of the Act, defining the substances in detail. This encompasses devices intended for internal or external use in the diagnosis, treatment, mitigation, or prevention of diseases or disorders in human beings or animals, as specified by the Central Government through notifications published in the Official Gazette, following consultation with the Board.

Under the Drugs and Cosmetics Rules, 1945, Section 22 delegates the power to issue licenses or registration certificates to authorised persons or designated officials, as stated in written delegations of excise power by the states. Additionally, Rule 109A outlines the requirement for labelling medical devices in accordance with the norms set by the BIS. Both of these directives are applicable concurrently, ensuring compliance with licensing procedures and labelling standards for medical devices.

19.3 SCHEDULE OF MEDICAL DEVICE

In understanding the licensing process, device categorisation, and study requirements for registering a medical device, schedules play a crucial role. The Medical Device Rules of 2017 introduced eight different schedules, each serving a specific purpose within the regulatory framework. These schedules provide detailed guidelines and requirements for various aspects of the licensing and registration process for medical devices.

19.4 FIRST SCHEDULE OF MEDICAL DEVICE (CLASSIFICATION OF MEDICAL DEVICES AND *IN VITRO* DIAGNOSTIC MEDICAL DEVICES)

The parameters for the classification of medical equipment and medical devices used for *in vitro* diagnostics are included in this schedule. Part I focuses on non-*in vitro* diagnostic devices and Part II on *in vitro* diagnostic devices.

19.4.1 Part I of First Schedule

Rule 5(1) and 5(2) and any associated regulations to obtain specific details on the criteria used for the classification of devices, including how accessories and usage characteristics, are taken into consideration. Compliance with these rules is crucial for regulatory approval and ensuring the safety and effectiveness of medical devices.

19.4.1.1 Non-invasive Medical Devices for Application to Injured Skin

Class A covers situations in which a non-invasive medical device meets wounded skin. Class B applies to situations in which a device is employed with a mechanical barrier and expedites the healing of a wound without breaking the skin. Any equipment that causes an injury to the skin is a class "C" instrument.

19.4.1.2 Non-invasive Medical Devices for Channelling or Storing Substances

Any non-invasive medical equipment that is used for the purpose of infusion, or introduction of any types of body liquids or tissues, as well as liquids or gases, is considered to fall within the classification of Class A.

Class B instruments are primarily non-invasive and are utilized either in conjunction with an active medical device belonging to Classes B, C, or D, or for the purpose of directing blood flow or storing organs, organ parts, or body tissues. In addition, there is a direct correlation between the safety problem of category A instruments and this kind of device. Class C medical devices are those that do not fall within the A or B categories and include all of the other products.

19.4.1.3 Compositions of Substances are Modified in Non-invasive Medical Devices

Any medical equipment that is not invasive and is used for modifying the biological or chemical composition of any body fluids, including the enrichment of blood, and that is thereafter used for infusion into the body, is under the category of Class C. The apparatus that is used for any modification by methods, such as centrifuging or any exchange of gas or heat or filtration, but that is not directly used to infusion, is classified as a Class B medical equipment.

19.4.1.4 Other Non-invasive Medical Devices

Other than instruments as described above, that do not use direct contact or are limited to using human skin, are classified as Class A.

19.4.1.5 Medical Devices Containing Body Orifices: Invasive Uses for Transient Use

This category is divided into mainly Class A, where most devices are used transiently or connected to medical devices, while Class B is limited to use externally, like on the surface of the eyeball or mucus membrane.

19.4.1.6 Medical Devices Containing Body Orifices for Short-term Uses

In this clause, medical devices are divided into two categories. Class A medical devices are designated for limited use in the oral cavity up to the pharynx, the ear canal up to the ear drum, or the nasal cavity, and not to be adsorbed, whereas Class B devices are limited to use for a short time, not connected directly to an active medical device, or limited to connecting Class A category devices.

19.4.1.7 Medical Devices Containing Body Orifices: Long-term Uses

Class C is not particularly directly conduct to an active medical device or indirectly attached to a Class A medical device only, whereas Class B in this category is designated for limited use in the oral cavity up to the pharynx, the ear canals up to the ear drum, or the nasal cavity and not to be adsorbed through mucous membranes.

19.4.1.8 Medical Devices Contain Body Orifices Connected to Active Medical Devices

Designated under Class B, they are used irrespective of the duration of use and are directly connected to an active medical device of Class B, C, or D.

19.4.1.9 Medical Devices Used for Invasive Surgery for Transient Use

In this category, classifications are based on A to D. Briefly, Class A medical devices are transiently used in invasive surgical methods and are reusable, whereas Class B medical devices in this category are not reusable. Class C medical devices are surgically invasive medical devices that produce or supply the energy from ionising radiation and are absorbed through the human body to produce biological effects. Class C is not limited to ionising radiation but extends to any surgically transient delivery of medicinal products that are considered hazardous and assigned to Class C. Class D devices of this category are mainly surgically invasive medical devices used for diagnosis, treatment, or correction through direct contact with the heart, central circulatory system, or central nervous system.

19.4.1.10 Medical Devices Used for Invasive Surgery for Short-term Use

A surgically invasive medical device used short-term or placed in a tooth is assigned to Class B. Class C differs from Class B in that chemical change reactions take place in Class C medical devices.

19.4.1.11 Implantable Medical Devices Used for Invasive Surgery for Long-term Use

A surgically invasive medical device used long-term is categorized as Class C, and its application to the limit of dentistry is categorized as Class D, whereas the medical device is intended to use the heart, central circulatory system, or central nervous system, which may be absorbed or undergo chemical changes after implantation in the body. These types of medical devices are like life-support systems or sustaining and active medical devices.

19.4.1.12 Medical Devices That are Used for Treatment Therapeutically or for Energy Exchange

Any medical device that, following treatment, exchanges energy with the human body is placed in the Class B category. On the other hand, the same medical device that exchanges energy that is regarded as potentially hazardous, such as radiation or ionizing radiation, is placed in the Class C category.

19.4.1.13 Medical Gadgets That are Utilized Actively in Diagnostic Procedures

A Class B medical device is a type of medical equipment that either generates energy that is absorbed by the human body, is used for image analysis, diagnostics, or for monitoring physiological processes using radiopharmaceuticals, and falls into one of the following three categories.

Class A medical devices are quite like Class B medical devices; however, rather than using ionized radiation to illuminate the human body, Class A medical devices make use of visible or infrared spectrum light. Monitoring physiological parameters in critically ill patients, such as cardiac, respiratory, or central nervous system performance, are the responsibility of medical devices classified as Class C. In addition, medical devices that are utilized for the diagnosis of disease while the patient is in a critical condition, as well as any equipment that emits ionizing radiation and is used for interventional radiology or diagnosing in a clinical setting, are both considered to be Class C medical devices. In addition, Class C medical devices are considered if they are utilized for the elimination of bodily fluids or if they are provided, either of which is regarded as having the potential to cause harm to the patient.

19.4.1.14 Other Categories of Active Medical Devices

Class A medical devices are those that do not satisfy the requirements of Sub-clauses (xii) and (xiii) of the definition of medical devices.

19.4.1.15 Medical Items and Equipment That Incorporate Pharmaceuticals

Class B medical devices are those that either have a medicinal product that is incorporated into an integral part of the device itself, have an action that is confined to an auxiliary action on the human body, or have a medicinal substance that is exempted under the preview of licensing provisions.

19.4.1.16 Medical Devices That Have Been Incorporated with Derivatives of Animal or Human Cells, Tissues, or Organs

A Class D medical device is one that contains non-viable tissues or cell derivatives or combinations of animal, human, microbial, or recombinant origin, and that is utilized as a single component or in combination with other components. Class A is quite like Class D in the sense that a Class A medical device can only be used on the skin and cannot be inserted into the body.

19.4.1.17 Medical Devices That are Utilized in the Process of Sterilization or Disinfection

Class C medical devices are those that are utilized in the processes of sterilization, the determination of the endpoint disinfection of medical equipment, or the cleaning, raising, and disinfection of contact lenses. Class B medical equipment that falls into this category are those that are put through sterilization or endpoint disinfection detection processes before being utilized on patients.

19.4.1.18 Contraceptive Medical Devices

The medical device, which has been assigned the Class C designation, is designed to protect users from contracting sexually transmitted diseases. Implantable or otherwise intrusive medical devices that are intended for long-term usage fall under the category of Class D medical devices.

19.4.2 Part II (*In Vitro* Diagnostic Medical Devices)

Part II regulates *in vitro* diagnostic medical devices.

19.4.2.1 General Guidelines for the Classification of Medical Devices Used for *In Vitro Diagnostics*

The uses of *in vitro* diagnostic medical devices are what determine their category status in the medical device industry. The combinations of the two different types of devices are placed into the appropriate classifications according to their individual characteristics. The class of the equipment determines how accessories such as software for operation or stand-alone software that has control over, impacts, or is used for analysis of the results are categorized. It is generally accepted that the usage of the calibrators for standardizing the device fall under the same category as the device itself. When a great number of classification rules are relevant to the making of the device, that gadget is placed in the more stringent category of classification rules.

19.4.3 The Fundamental Principles behind the Categorization of *In Vitro* Diagnostic Medical Devices

No matter whether it transmits blood or a blood component, a derivative of blood, a cell, an organ, or tissue for transfusion or transplantation, any device that is employed as an *in vitro* diagnostic for the detection of transmissible agents is regarded to be a Class D device.

19.4.4 The Utilization of a Medical Device for the Diagnosis of Several Life-Threatening Conditions That Have a High Risk

Most *in vitro* medical diagnostics that fall into this category are classified as Class C, primarily aimed at detecting sexually transmitted diseases and infectious agents in blood or cerebrospinal fluid, that have the potential to spread, such as Infections caused by *Neisseria meningitidis* or *Cryptococcus neoformans*. Furthermore, this categorisation considers the risk associated with erroneous detection, which could lead to severe disability or even death, such as the diagnosis of swine flu infection, dengue, *Chlamydia pneumoniae*, and methicillin-resistant *Staphylococcus aureus*. These examples represent diseases encompassed by this category. *In vitro* diagnostics related to prenatal screening for transmissible agents and assessing immunological status against Infections like HIV, rubella, or toxoplasmosis also fall under Class C *in vitro* medical diagnostics.

It is important to note that the conditions and methods utilised for diagnosing infectious diseases or immune status, as well as any potential incorrect results, can potentially pose urgent life-threatening risks to patients. For instance, the diagnosis of Enteroviruses or Cytomegaloviruses falls within Class C, as does the identification of herpes simplex virus in transplant patients or the detection of malignancies. Class C also encompasses diagnostic methods used for identifying hereditary diseases like cystic fibrosis or Huntington's disease, as well as diseases, ailments, or drug levels in blood, such as cardiac indicators, prothrombin time tests, and cyclosporin content. Furthermore, foetal diagnosis procedures for congenital abnormalities like Down syndrome or spina bifida are included in this category.

Class D comprises blood, blood products, blood cell derivatives, and tissue and organ typing for transplantation purposes, and *in vitro* diagnostic medical devices used for blood grouping, tissue typing, or immunological compatibility. On the other hand, in Class C, we find *in vitro* diagnostic medical devices used for blood grouping based on the principles of the ABO, Duffy, Kell, Kidd, or Rhesus systems. Class C medical devices are those capable of conducting self-testing, while Class C medical devices are involved in preliminary testing and require confirmation if the results are unrelated to the patient's critical condition. Results that do not impact the patient's critical condition do not require validation. Additionally, medical devices used for patient monitoring, such as blood gas analysis, anticoagulant surveillance, online diabetes monitoring, and C-reactive protein determination, are also categorised as Class C devices.

19.5 SECOND SCHEDULE OF MEDICAL DEVICE (FEES PAYABLE FOR LICENSE)

Fee payable for license, permission, and registration certificate as mentioned in Table 19.1.

19.6 THIRD SCHEDULE OF MEDICAL DEVICE (REGISTRATION PROCEDURE AND THE MINIMUM DOCUMENTS REQUIRED)

The registration process, the requisite documentation, and the allocation of responsibilities are all laid forth in this chapter. The schedule is broken down into two different chapters. Part I of this chapter outlines the Specifics of the documents that need to be submitted, together with the required format form MD 1 in order to be granted registration. Part II of the chapter, meanwhile, explains the responsibilities and roles of the notified body.

TABLE 19.1
Class of the Medical Devices and the Regulatory Authority

	Class of Instrument	Functions: Manufacture	Sale	Import	Permission of Clinical Trial	Quality Management System (QMS) Verification
1	Class A	SLA	SLA (State Licensing Authority))	CLA	CLA (Central Licensing Authority)	Notified Body
2	Class B	SLA				Notified Body
3	Class C	CLA				CLA
4	Class D	CLA				CLA

Notified body shall be registered to CLA (SLAs).

19.6.1 Part I

The following Records are necessary for registration to submit a duly certified copy to the Central Licensing Authority

1. The establishment of the notified body's constitution
2. The Current Accreditation Status, as granted by the National Accreditation Body, as mentioned in Rule 10.
3. The responsibility of individuals and the submission structure of the notified body

The following commitment is to be made to the Central Licensing Authority

1. The important members of the notified body, including the directors, executives, and personnel, are the ones who are in charge of assessing and verifying the operations that are related to the production of the product.
2. The personnel of the notified body are responsible for the procedures involved in the manufacturing and testing of the product; the product's producer is not to be involved in any consultations.

19.6.2 Part II

Duties and functions of the notified body

19.6.2.1 Duties

In accordance with the first paragraph of Subrule 15 of Rule 15, a notified body is responsible for conducting the audit of the manufacturer. This rule is applicable to

Class A or Class B medical devices that are produced at a domestic manufacturing site. The notified body is responsible for the maintenance of the standard operating procedure as well as the records, which includes the identification, review, and resolution of any and all cases in which a conflict of interest is established or suspected.

19.6.2.2 Functions

The development of high-quality personnel requires activities such as evaluation and verification in order to train staff members effectively.

1. Evaluation and verification of any activities with professional integrity, independently, and in accordance with technical parameters.
2. The location of the manufacture and the products themselves must be following the requirements that have been specified.
3. Appointment: Appropriate auditors are selected who possess the necessary skills and are a good fit for the manufacturing facility and the medical device.
4. Steps are taken to ensure that all of the procedures and documents are kept up to date in accordance with the quality management system's requirement.
5. The Process of Auditing

The audit verifies that the quality management system of the manufacturer is in agreement with the results of an evidence-based investigation, and it can only be performed on-site.

19.7 FOURTH SCHEDULE OF MEDICAL DEVICES (DOCUMENTATION REQUIREMENTS FOR THE GRANTING OF PERMISSION, LICENCE, AND IMPORT OF MEDICAL DEVICES)

The directive found in the Fourth Schedule is predicated on the document criteria that must be met in order to get a licence, distribute medical equipment, or import them.

19.7.1 Power of Attorney

Exercise of power of attorney is divided into two distinct parts. The first part of this document furnishes details pertaining to the requisite documentation that must be submitted alongside an application for the issuance of an import or manufacture licence, specifically for the purpose of selling or distributing a medical device classified as Class A whereas, in the Second part, the focus shifts to medical devices that fall under Class B, Class C, or Class D.

The application must be submitted by the manufacturer through CDSCO's online application portal known as "Sugam," together with the required documentation as outlined in the Fourth Schedule and the costs indicated in the Second Schedule.

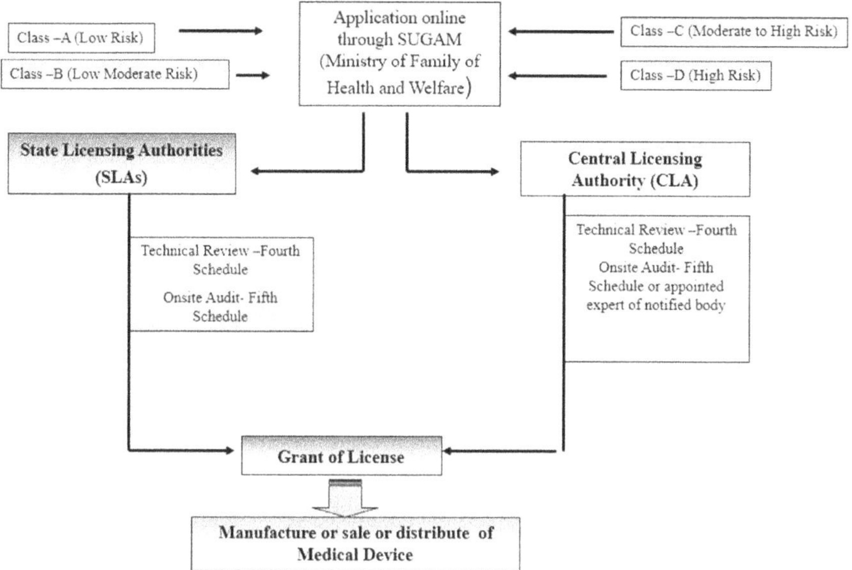

FIGURE 19.1 Procedures for granting a licence of the manufacture, sale, or distribution of the medical device.

When it comes to Class A devices, an audit is not required prior to the granting of a licence; instead, the licence is provided in a manner that is self-regulated and in conformity with the standard. The audit is carried out by the notified body within one hundred and twenty days of the licence being granted. In the process of providing licences for Class C and D devices, the CLA is responsible for conducting the inspection or audit. However, any expert from the notified body could finish the examination within a period of sixty days from the date of application. It is not necessary to submit to an audit or inspection in order to acquire a loan licence because it is presumptively understood that the manufacturer already obtains an authorised licence for the devices in question. Within a period of thirty days, the notified entity is required to submit its report to the SLA. Additionally, according to these rules, SLAs are granted the authority to grant licences and regulate lower-risk medical devices. On the other hand, the CLA is the only competent authority for enforcement in relation to the import and manufacture of higher-risk medical devices (Class C and Class D) (Figure 19.1; Table 19.1)

19.8 GUIDELINES FOR THE ISSUANCE OF REGULATORY LICENCES REGARDING THE IMPORTATION OF MEDICAL DEVICES IN INDIA

1. The Form MD12 licence is issued by CDSCO to the Indian authorised agent of medical device companies for manufacture for sale or wholesale

operations, while the Form MD13 licence and necessary documentation are issued to the manufacturing site for import.

2. It is necessary to get a Free Sale Certificate (FSC) in order to sell to India from any country/region outside of India, such as the European Union, Australia, Canada, Japan, or the United States of America. The national regulatory authority or any other qualified entity must provide this certificate. The Free Sale Certificate received CDSCO's approval, and an extra licence to sell products in India was obtained.
3. The Central Drugs Standard Control Organization (CDSCO) in India also conducted safety and effectiveness trials by clinical study as indicated in the Fifth Schedule in India for Class C and Class D medically imported devices, and it provided permission to sell in India with a Free Sale Certificate (FSC) from the place of origin. Imported medical devices that fall under Class A or Class B have not been required to undergo any further testing; the CDSCO is able to give the licence based on the public data on the device's efficiency and safety.
4. The issued licence has a validity period of five years beginning on the date it was issued, and a deposit is required for the payments. If the required fees are not deposited within six months, the contract will be considered to have been terminated. Changes that are significant or include changes to authorised agents need to be approved in advance by CLA (Figure 19.2, Table 19.2).

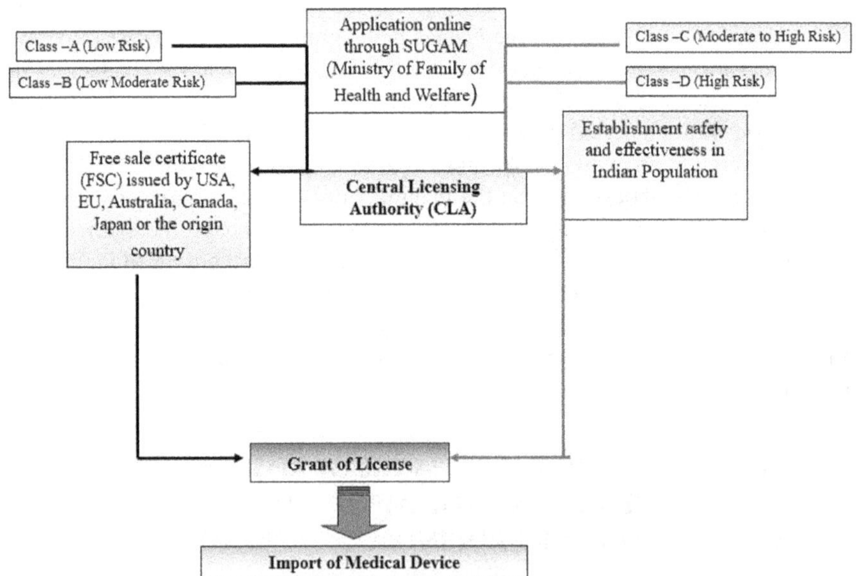

FIGURE 19.2 Regulatory requirement of medical devices in India.

TABLE 19.2
Different Forms Are Required for the Approval of the Medical Device

Sl no.	Information and Applications Regarding	Forms No.
1	Submission of an application to a notified body for the issuance of a certificate of registration	Form MD1
2	Submission of an application for a licence to manufacture medical devices in either (i) Class A or Class B for the purpose of sale and distribution, for Class C or D, or (ii) Class A or B, and Class C or D	Form MD3, Form MD4
3	Application for the provision of a loan Licence to manufacture, for the purpose of sale or distribution, a medical device classified as either (i) Class A or Class B For C or D Class, or (ii) A or B Class, and C or D Class	Form MD5, Form MD6
4	Submission of an application for a licence to manufacture medical equipment in either Class C or Class D, or both Classes A or B and Class C or Class D, for the purpose of sale and distribution, regarding medical equipment classified as Class A, Class B, Class C, or Class D	Form MD7, Form MD8
5	Form used to keep track of inspections or audits	Form MD9
6	A request for the issuance of a manufacturing licence for medical devices for the purposes of clinical research, assessment, examination, testing, demonstration, or training.	Form MD10
7	Submission of an application for the authorisation to import medical devices	Form MD12
8	Submission of an application for the granting of a licence to import medical devices for the purposes of clinical research, testing, evaluating, demonstrating, or training	Form MD14
9	Submission of an application for the issuance of a licence to import medical instruments for the purpose of patient care at a statutory medical institution or a government hospital.	Form MD16
10	Submission of an application for the issuance of a licence to import, for personal use, a limited quantity of medical devices	Form MD18
11	Submission of an application for the authorisation to import personal-use quantities of medical devices in small quantities.	Form MD19
12	Submission of a request for authorisation to carry out clinical performance evaluation	Form MD22
13	Application for permission to manufacture or import a medical device in the absence of a comparable reference product	Form MD24
14	Submission of an application for the authorisation to either import or manufacture a novel *in vitro* diagnostic medical device	Form MD26

19.9 APPENDIX I: SITE OR PLANT MASTER FILE

According to the Industrial Act, the layout and pertinent certificates require access to the plant master file. In addition, they include information from the site master file and plan, such as water supplies, ways to recycle waste, or reduce effluent discharge, etc. The company must provide the defined obligations together with a documented pledge or agreement.

19.10 APPENDICES II AND III: DEVICE MASTER FILE FOR *IN VITRO* MEDICAL DEVICES OTHER THAN *IN VITRO* DIAGNOSTIC MEDICAL DEVICES

This master file requires a significant number of documents in accordance with the classification of the instrument types.

1. Requirements for *in vitro* medical devices of the Class A type and all other types of *in vitro* medical devices
    - Details about the apparatus device including the description
    - Details about the device including the description
    - Use for which it was intended
    - Details about the device, including the specification
    - The guiding principle of the device
    - Packaging and labelling as per Indian Standard (IS) format
    - Instructional manual
    - Any adverse drug reactions that have been reported, if any
    - Control of quality and analytical performance
2. Requirement for Class B, C, and D *in vitro* medical devices and other *in vitro* medical devices
    - Information about the producer or authorised representative
    - Master file for the plant (including land contract, construction site, blueprints, etc.)
    - Checklist for conformity for safety and performance
    - Device master file includes details of component, design, etc.
    - Specifics of quality assurance
    - Undertaking agreement stating that manufacturing site is compliant with schedule
    - *In vivo* device evaluation report
    - *In vitro* device evaluation report
3. Part IV: The following documentation must be provided in order to import or manufacture medical device in India that are not predicate devices
    - Data assessment and interpretation
    - Documents for input and output, along with related design
    - Results of any applicable tests, including electrical or mechanical
    - Test results and quality and safety
    - Software and the validation process
    - Performance reliability and dependability
    - Data confirming the biocompatibility of the material
    - Risk management procedure
    - Confirmation data regarding the performance of the animals
    - Clinical trial—pilot and pivotal
    - Specifics of the data gathered throughout the study
    - The product's current regulatory status and any potential safety concerns
    - Instructions for use

19.11 FIFTH SCHEDULE OF MEDICAL DEVICE (QUALITY CONTROL OF THE MEDICAL DEVICE)

In this separate schedule, the quality management of medical devices as well as *in vitro* diagnostic medical devices are as follows:

19.11.1 Medical Device Validation, Verification, and Documentation

When the medical equipment was being produced, the quality check was carried out, and it met all the quality requirements for the claim. It is essential to have product verification and validation documentation to comprehend the characteristics of the medical equipment. The documentation is necessary in many different elements, such as the verification of engineering tests, laboratory testing, and simulated tests, and such tests shall be presented for feasibility tests in the animal model as proof of the concept of the product that was created. In addition, investigators are obliged to provide statements that they conform to the acceptance criteria for standard data and a summary of the data if there are no acceptance criteria that are supported by the explanation. The confirmatory declaration is necessary to express the adherence to established norms of industry techniques, an in-house test, a description of the method employed, and sufficient data for evaluation. This is a mandatory requirement. In addition, the published literature created by other people also contributes to the assessment of the instrument's or device's long-term viability. The investigator additionally provided biocompatibility, biological safety, sterilization, software validation, pre-clinical data, and clinical data.

19.12 COMPATIBILITY OF MEDICAL DEVICES

It is recommended that the application dossier be written using materials that are either directly or indirectly in contact with the patient. The mandatory biocompatibility report must be submitted along with all of the relevant data, which must include the physical, chemical, biological, and toxicological reactions or compatibilities, as well as the testing technique.

19.13 STUDIES OF A MEDICAL DEVICE IN PRE-CLINICAL SETTINGS

It is necessary to establish both animal studies and a dossier before proceeding with the principles of functional safety. In the study, you are required to discuss the methodology, results, and analysis, as well as the justification for choosing animals, and to document your compliance with Good Laboratory Practices.

19.14 STERILIZATION OF MEDICAL EQUIPMENT AND SUPPLIES

Sterile devices, particularly implanted materials, must comply with the sterility requirement, and specific details such as validation of sterilization, pyrogen testing, bioburden testing, and sterility residues, if any, must be disclosed. In addition, the sterility of the conditions in which the packaging is being held as well as the validation criteria must be mentioned. In addition to that, the processes of sterilization and revalidation need to be mentioned.

19.15 BIOLOGICAL SAFETY OF MEDICAL DEVICES

Any medical device that contains any component derived from animal or human origin is required to comply with safety norms and disclose any donors, sources, or procedures that were used in the harvesting, preservation, processing, testing, and handling of tissues, cells, and substances of such origin. It is important to take notice of the process validation and the procedure for lowering the biological risks. The confirmatory statement demanded that the medical device be free of any transmissible illnesses, such as bovine spongiform encephalopathy (BSE) or transmissible spongiform encephalopathies (TSE), among others. To demonstrate compliance with the GLP requirement, a quality-control, record-keeping, and data-retrieval system are also necessary. The majority of the biological safety data evaluation conforms to the International Organization Standard, ISO-10993, and CDSCO has approved this standard.

19.16 INFORMATION REGARDING THE SHELF LIFE OR STABILITY

It is necessary to collect data on the accelerated stability of the medical device as well as its real-time stability before it is possible to establish ideal stability conditions, effectiveness of a medical device and how long it will continue to be effective in the absence of environmental influences.

To verify the stated shelf life, it is necessary to conduct tests on three separate lots that were all manufactured in the same way. Additionally, accelerated stability data are required to conduct an analysis of the expected shelf life or expiration date of a product. The data on the product's stability must be included in the required dossier, together with a statement of the number of lots that were tested, conditions that were reproduced, acceptance criteria, testing intervals, and validating procedures for rapid studies that use real-time data.

Analyses of the actual environments and data validation of the device's stability and life duration are both essential when the device is being used for its intended purpose. Some examples of such devices include pacemakers and implant devices. The evaluation is required to conclude that the factor effectiveness of transportation, packaging, and climate stability considers both real and simulated environments.

19.17 POST-MARKETING SURVEILLANCE OR VIGILANCE REPORTING

The government organization or regulatory authority is accountable for post-marketing surveillance, and the dossier is compiled based on the re-addressed complaints that were received and the responses to these complaints. Considering post-marketing strategies, it is important information for assessing the status of the medical device, including the number of adverse event reports, an understanding of the safety performance of this *in vitro* medical device, and the status of the device in the other country.

19.18 SIXTH SCHEDULE (LABELLING OF MEDICAL DEVICES)

Every label needs to be printed in permanent ink on the medical device's shelf pack, outside of the medical device, or on the outside of the medical device.

- Name of medical device
- Identifying criteria of the medical device and discuss any potential applications it may have
- Name of the manufacturer and address
- The net quantity expressed using the metric system
- Both the date of manufacture and the date of expiration, or an equivalent date, must be included on the product's label. After the manufacturer has provided satisfactory results and CLA has approved the product, it must have a shelf life of at least one year before it may be imported
- Sterile Devices: The sterilization date and manufacture date are required to be mentioned when the device is constructed of material such as stainless steel or titanium and supplied non-sterile, or in the case of medical equipment, instruments, or apparatus, the date of expiry may not be required if the device is constructed of any active material.
- The specific use of the medical device is required to be mentioned on the label, like for a physician sample, "Physician's Sample—Not to be sold," whereas, for clinical investigation, "For Clinical Investigation Only." Medical devices or *in vitro* diagnostics are sold for use by hospitals or diagnostic labs that only mention "Not to be sold individually."
- The unique device identification of the medical device will become effective after the first day of January 1922 and will disclose both the device identifier and the production identifier. Although the production identification reveals information about the lot or batch number, software version used for the medical device, manufacturing date, and expiration date, the device identification includes the worldwide trade identifier number.

19.19 SEVENTH SCHEDULE OF MEDICAL DEVICES (CLINICAL INVESTIGATION)

The Seventh Schedule makes clinical investigation a prerequisite for getting the licence and performing clinical trials. Sections 45(1), 45(6), 46(ii), 46(v), and 52(3) of the Food, Drug, and Cosmetic Act, 1940 grant the clause and requirements for approval to perform clinical tests of medical devices regardless of whether they are imported or made locally.

19.19.1 Required Application for Participation in a Clinical Trial of a Medical Device

The CLA accepts applications via the form MD19; this application requires the planned layout of the trial, the results of biocompatibility testing, a brochure from the lead investigator, a case report form, an informed consent form, a statement from the lead investigator, and approval from the ethics committee. All data must be submitted to the CLA, and a pilot clinical trial to establish safety for humans is required for any developed medical devices. On the other hand, any foreign medical device imported into India must also have safety and regulatory approval status in other countries. In the case of an investigational medical device, it is necessary to notify the CLA about its regulatory status in other countries, adverse effects, and whether it is withdrawn from the market. This information must be provided in accordance with the unique design of the medical prescription.

Labelling of the medical equipment in accordance with the medical equipment Rule 1916, with particular mandatory instructions, usage, and information regarding any deviation is required to alert the CLA until the completion of the pivotal clinical studies in India, without which any investigational medical device from another country is prohibited from being imported. According to the legislation, the necessary forms are MD14 or MD10, and according to the Act, the specifics of clinical data from a foreign nation, the purpose of the study, the status, side effects, directions, etc. are required to be informed through these forms of the CLA. In addition, the Act mandates that these forms of the CLA be completed. Considering this, the CLA decided to grant authorization after conducting an analysis of the objectives for the clinical study, which included specifics regarding the number of volunteers, sites, and other relevant information.

CLA has the authority to abbreviate, omit, or differ from any clinical data where it appears that medical devices are useful for any emergency data, life-threatening disease, national priority, etc. CLA also has the authority to change any clinical data where it appears that medical devices are useful for any emergency data.

19.19.2 Clinical Trial of Medical Devices

The Ethics Committee for Medical and Health Research will be responsible for the following:

According to the draft of the New Drugs and Clinical Trials Rules, 1918, which was published in the Gazette of India, Extraordinary, Part II, Section 3, Sub-section (i), dated February 1, 1918, subsequent to the published GSR 227(E), dated March 19, 1919, in order to exercise the powers conferred by Sub-section (1) of section 12 and Sub-section (1) of Section 33 of the Drugs and Cosmetics Act, 1940 (23 of 1940), the Government of India has mentioned. The rule mandates that any institution or organization engaged in health or medical research must establish an institutional ethics committee in order to conduct medical research on human subjects.

In accordance with Directive 15 of the National Ethical Guidelines for Medical and Health Research, the Ethics Committee has been formally established. In addition to that, Rule 16 stipulates that registration on the Ethics Committee is necessary. Any clinical trial, bioequivalence study, or bioavailability study conducted by the institute is subject to CDSCO registration per regulations 8 and 17. Registration is awarded for five periods until it is either cancelled or revoked. Approval from the Ethics Committee is subject to an initial approval period of two years and is known as provisional registration. Registration is granted after applying through CT-03 and having the application reviewed. An appeal against the authority's decision is allowed if made within 60 days following the rejection or disapproval of any subject. Rule No. 17 includes provisions for the termination of registration on any committee after observing the procedure in a manner that is not in accordance with the law; under such circumstances, an appeal can be made to the Ministry of Health and Family Welfare within the Indian government. There is a possibility that the government will take more action regarding the investigation.

19.19.2.1 Approval for a Clinical Trial

Before beginning any kind of clinical trial investigation, researchers must first obtain authorisation from the CLA and approval from the Ethics Committee that has been registered in accordance with the requirements of Section 122 DD of the Drug and Cosmetics Rules, 1945. It is recommended to monitor any clinical trial by enrolling through the Clinical Trial Registry of India (CTRI) and acquiring the trial number for the purpose of further communication and validation of the trial. When a clinical trial is first initiated, it is essential to maintain certain quality requirements, such as having a competent individual with experience, an investigation plan, appropriate laboratory practice, the sites of the study, and other such needs. A foreign trial partner is now permitted, but CLA must first review the study, the specific service, the foreign partner's information, and the specimen sample to ensure it meets their standards. CLA is not allowed to make any changes to the clinical trial plan or to deviate in any way from the original plan.

Ideally, any approved protocols cannot be adjusted, and any alterations in the approved trial protocol are changed in view of safety issues that must be notified to the CLA and Ethics Committee within thirty days of the occurrence of the alterations.

19.19.2.2 Sponsor Responsibilities

Sponsored clinical trials have the responsibility to adhere to all applicable standards, such as those pertaining to quality and good clinical practices for medical devices, which are outlined by the CDSCO and the Director General of Health Services. The sponsor is also obligated to provide CLA with an overview of the ongoing clinical study, during which they must note both the participants' safety and any significant departures from the protocol. Furthermore, the chairman of the Ethics Committee must be notified within 14 days of any adverse effects discovered during the experiment. In addition, the act includes a provision that will compensate the volunteer for any injuries or deaths that occur because of their participation in the clinical trial in accordance with the Drugs and Cosmetics Rules, 1945, and the published gazette GSR 227 (E) that was issued on March 19, 1919, by the Department of Health and Family Welfare within thirty days of the order of CLA. Any clinical experiment that is cancelled or terminated must provide an explanation along with a detailed report that describes the number of patients who were affected, any adverse effects, and any compensation that was offered.

19.19.2.3 Investigator Responsibilities

The investigator is the one who needs to be accountable for enforcing the GCP guidelines to guarantee the best possible level of patient safety and compliance. After getting permission within 14 days, the clinical trial must begin immediately, and any delays must be reported to the CLA. The investigator is responsible for ensuring that the standard operating procedures are followed. If an adverse reaction is discovered, the subject will be treated with the highest possible standard of medical care. Following the receipt of approval from the CLA, the clinical investigations must begin the clinical trial within forty-eight hours, and any delay must be explained to the CLA. Any major adverse event that is noticed during the study is required to be reported to the CLA within fourteen calendar days of the occurrence of the serious adverse event.

19.19.2.4 Clinical Investigation: Pilot Scale

A pilot clinical trial is an exploratory study with a small number of participants designed to get insight into the performance and safety of medical technology.

19.20 CLINICAL INVESTIGATION: PIVOTAL SCALE

This kind of clinical study is carried out with the participation of many patients with the purpose of conducting confirmatory research to reach a conclusion regarding the efficacy and any adverse reactions. The unapproved medical device in India, but the approved medical device outside of India, was required to undergo the pilot clinical trial with approval from the CLA. The clinical trials for a new medical device often involve multiple centres and patients and thus require the blessing of a centralised licensing authority.

19.21 CLINICAL RESEARCH ON CERTAIN POPULATIONS

It is considered a special case when a clinical investigation involves pregnant women, children, nursing mothers, elderly patients, or patients who suffer organ system failure. Patients in their senior years, often known as geriatric or elderly patients, are categorised as a distinct subset of the population due to the metabolic changes that accompany advancing age. In the case of diseases affecting the elderly, investigations must specify their justifications, and a statistically significant sample size must be recruited for trials.

When it comes to the research of the pediatric, the members of the Ethics Committee need to have a solid understanding of the ethical, psychological, and clinical issues involved. If the medical equipment in question is intended for use by both adults and children, then sufficient safety data, including information on post-marketing surveillance, must be compiled before it may be approved for use. After that, children are recruited for the clinical trial in a phased manner and for the appropriate reason. The legal guardian's written informed consent is requested, and it specifically mentions the treatment research for serious or life-threatening diseases as well as the consideration of the children's participants' requests to withdraw from the study.

In the establishment of clinical data, pregnant or breastfeeding women are also considered a distinctive segment of the population. If the safety data are established independently and the medical equipment is exclusively intended for utilization by either fetuses or nursing infants. Alternatively, if the medical device is specifically designed for usage solely by pregnant or nursing women and has obtained approval for a clinical investigation, a restricted trial may be authorised.

19.22 SURVEILLANCE AFTER PRODUCT RELEASE AND DISTRIBUTION

After receiving approval for an investigational medical device, the manufacturer is obligated to provide the CLA with periodic safety update reports (PSURs). The PSUR must be presented within the first thirty days of each calendar month at a frequency of once every six months for the first two years. After each year has passed, the PUSR is required to be submitted, and the CLA may, for the benefit of the public, extend the time schedule. Any major adverse event involving a medical device is required to be reported within 15 days of the incident, and any delay in the sale of medical equipment after it has been approved by CLA is required to be included in the PSUR on a periodic basis.

19.23 AUTHORISATION OF THE IMPORT OR PRODUCTION OF NEWLY DEVELOPED *IN VITRO* DIAGNOSTIC MEDICAL DEVICES

In vitro diagnostic devices play a crucial role in disease diagnosis and management, especially in the context of deadly diseases. The concept of orphan drugs or medical devices is mentioned, indicating a focus on conditions or diseases for which there are no available alternative diagnostic methods. The Central Licensing Authority (CLA) is involved in granting approval for the importation or manufacture of new in vitro diagnostic medical devices. Form MD-28 is used for granting approval to an approved agent, applicant for importation, or the manufacturer themselves.

In critical situations, such as epidemics or when there are no alternative diagnostic methods, the CLA may expedite the approval process. The CLA has the authority to shorten, postpone, or eliminate the necessary clinical trial based on the circumstances.

The new in vitro diagnostic medical device is mentioned to be placed in Class A. This classification suggests that, in certain instances, clinical investigation data may be withheld, except in exceptional cases. The CLA is required to decide on the approval of an application within 119 calendar days. Additionally, the approval period should not exceed 30 days from the date the application was submitted.

If deficiencies are found in the application, the applicant is informed in a written format. The applicant is then given a period of ninety days to address and correct the identified deficiencies. The approval decision is communicated using Form MD-29. This regulatory process ensures a streamlined and expedited approval pathway for new in vitro diagnostic medical devices, especially in situations where prompt access to such devices is critical. The classification of Class A and the ability to withhold clinical investigation data in exceptional instances highlight the flexibility in the regulatory approach to address urgent healthcare needs.

19.24 AUTHORISATION FOR THE IMPORT OR MANUFACTURE OF A NEW *IN VITRO* DIAGNOSTIC MEDICAL DEVICE AS WELL AS A MEDICAL DEVICE THAT HAS NOT YET BEEN PREDICATED

Permission under Regulations 63 in Form MD-27 and Rule 64 in Form MD-29 for new *in vitro* diagnostic kits may be obtained from the CLA for the production or import of medical devices. It is required that medical devices correspond to the specifications that have been submitted to the CLA, and after they have been on the market for two years, the safety data must be reported once every six months. In addition, the terms of Form 27 apply to the holder of the license, and they provide that any adverse reaction that was unanticipated must be submitted within 15 days of the incident in question. Figure 19.3

The Medical Devices Rules, 1917, are all-encompassing regulations that were put into effect beginning in January 1918 for the purpose of medical device registration. This current legislative framework is comprehensive, including the US Food and Drug Administration and the EU Biological Guidelines. In addition to that, the rule mandates government auditing, regulation through a single window, and application via the internet. The entire process was also tracked using an online system, beginning with the pre-market clinical trial and continuing through marketing authorisation. In addition to that, this rule adopted the clinical trial, made provisions for remuneration, and fostered the production of new goods related to medical devices. The government has demonstrated its dedication to meeting the time frame, and additional time has been saved by streamlining the review processes. Because of government scrutiny and the implementation of new regulations for the research and development of novel medical equipment, a significant number of international businesses are focusing their attention on the Indian market. As a result of this, many new creative items and multinational corporations are anticipated to enter the Indian market. It is anticipated that the streamlined laws will

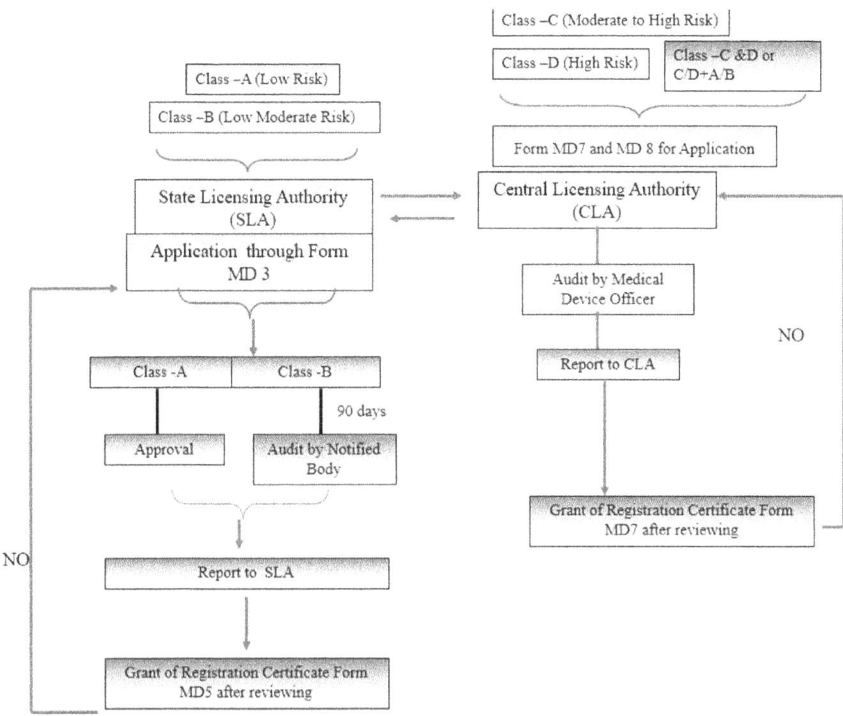

FIGURE 19.3 Process for obtaining a licence or registration of a medical device.

attract investors from all over the world. Additionally, because of the streamlined rules and increased government control, the quality and range of products and services will improve, which will allow for better service to be provided to the residents of India.

BIBLIOGRAPHY

Brolin, S. Global Regulatory Requirements for Medical Devices. http://docshare01.docshare.tips/files/19017/190178428. pdf. Accessed 13 November 1917.

Chadha, K., Goswami, K., Bhatoa, R., Jaggi, P. and Thakkar, A.R. A Review of in Vitro Diagnostic Kits and Their Regulation in the Indian Market, 2021, 8: 3–11. 10.2174/2213476X07999201029212448.

Charu, S. and Anjan, B. Medical Devices: Making in India - A Leap for Indian Healthcare. March 1916. https://www2. deloitte.com/content/dam/Deloitte/de/Documents/life-sciences-health are/Medical-Devices-Making-in-India.pdf. Accessed 13 November 1917.

Classification of Medical Devices and In Vitro Diagnostic Medical Devices Under the Provisions of the Medical Devices Rules, 1917. http://www.cdsco.nic.in/writereaddata/Classification%19wise%19list%19of%19MD%19and%19IVDs17.pdf.

Ghosh, S., Shah, D., More, N., Choppadandi, M., Ranglani, D. and Kapusetti, G. Clinical Validation of the Medical Devices: A General Prospective. In *BioSensing, Theranostics, and Medical Devices*, Springer, Singapore, 2021, pp. 265–297. 10.1007/978-981-16-2782-8_11.

Herold, D. and Vardahn, V. Make in India Mittelstand! Opportunities in the Medical Equipment Market India. 7 April 1917. http://www.makeinindiamittelstand.de/wp-content/uploads/1915/09/Opportunities-in-the-Medical-Equipment-Market-India.pdf.

https://morulaa.com/cdsco/regulatory-india-medical-device-rules.

https://www.raps.org/regulatory-focus%E2%84%A2/news-articles/1916/9/cdsco-advances-draft-medical-device-rules,-outlines-fees.

Kumar, D., Yadav, V. and Mathewson, M. A New Regulatory Paradigm for Medical Devices in India. *Regulatory Focus*, 1917. Regulatory Affairs Professionals Society, pp. 1–15.

Medical Devices: Guidance Document – Classification of Medical Devices. MEDDEV 2.4/1 Rev. 9 June 1910. http://EC.europa. eu/consumers/sectors/medical devices/files/meddev/2_4_1_rev_9_classification_en.pdf. Accessed 13 November 1917.

Nishith Desai Associates. The Indian Medical Device Industry: Regulatory, Legal and Tax Overview. August 1917. http://www.nishithdesai.com/fileadmin/user_upload/pdfs/Research_Papers/The_Indian_Medical_Device_Industry.pdf.

Pacifici, E. and Bain, S. Introduction to FDA Regulated Products. In Pacifici, E. and Bain S (Eds) *An Overview FDA Regulated Products: From Drugs and Cosmetics and Tobacoo*. Academic Press, 2018, pp. 1–11.

Radhadevi, N., Balamuralidhara, V. and Kumar, T. Regulatory Guidelines for Medical Devices in India: An Overview. *Asian Journal of Pharmaceutics*, 1912, 6: 10. https://www.asiapharmaceutics.info/index.php/ajp/article/download/68/34.

Sethi, R., Popli, H. and Sethi, S. Medical Devices Regulation in United States of America, European Union and India: A Comparative Study. *Pharmaceutical Regulatory Affairs*, 1917, 6: 1. https://www.omicsonline.org/open-access/medical-devices-regulationin-united-states-of-america-european-unionand-india-a-comparative-study-2167-7689-1000179.pdf.

20 Approval and Registration Process of a Medical Device

20.1 INTRODUCTION

The Drugs and Cosmetics Act of 1940 and the Rules of 1945 govern the import, manufacturing, sale, distribution, and export of medical equipment. These activities are regulated by the Central Drug Standard Controlled Organization (CDSCO), which is a component of the Ministry of Health and Family Welfare.

In addition, the CDSCO, Ministry of Health and Family Welfare (MoHFW), Government of India, published the proposal of the Medical Devices Rules, 2017 through a Gazette notification (No. 724) published on October 17, 2017, and enacted the rule beginning January 1, 2018.

Regulations for medical devices were created with the intention of guaranteeing that these products meet the highest possible safety and quality standards.

The Indian market is a lucrative and extensive one for the sale of medical equipment.

A notified device that has already been approved in the United States, the European Union, or Japan may be marketed in India.

According to the level of safety offered by the medical equipment, defined as belonging to Classes A, B, C, or D, was discussed in Chapter 18.

According to Section 3 (b) (iv) of the Drugs and Cosmetics Act, 1940, medical devices are considered as being drugs. Medical devices refer to equipment or apparatus that are intended for either internal or exterior application in order to diagnose, treat, alleviate, or prevent diseases or disorders in either humans or animals.

In February 2020, by the Gazette notification SO 648(E), it was notified that, in agreement with Sub-paragraph (iv) of Clause (b) of Section 3 of the Drugs and Cosmetics Act, 1940, this was done to comply with the provisions of the Act (23 of Drugs and Cosmetics Act, 1940).

The notification states that "All devices including an instrument, apparatus, appliance, implant, material, or other article, whether used alone or in combination, including software or an accessory, intended by its manufacturer to be used specially for human beings or animals which does not achieve the primary intended action in or on the human body or animals by any pharmacological or immunological or metabolic means, but which may assist in its intended function by such means" are subject to the regulation. This regulation applies to "all devices including an instrument, apparatus, appliance, implant."

DOI: 10.1201/9781003397854-4

20.2 INDIGENOUS MANUFACTURING OF A MEDICAL DEVICE

The indigenous product or any product developed in India has to have clearance from the CLA and to be registered with the government. Only once CLA has given its approval will it be acceptable to import or manufacture a novel medical device and determine its marketability. The CDSCO is the regulating body, while the CLA is the approval authority. Both authorities are under the purview of the Ministry of Health and Family Welfare, which is part of the Government of India. In accordance with the safety category ranging from least to maximum risk, medical devices are divided into four distinct groups. Class A and Class B medical equipment were granted permission by the State Licensing Approval Authority for marketing while Class C and Class D medical devices were granted permission by the Central Licensing Approval Authority (CLA).

A medical device is considered new if there is no equivalent on the market, if it has been modified for a new use, or if the design has been altered. A new medical device needs to be registered before a clinical study can be conducted to assess its safety. Medical devices in Classes A and B may not be required to undergo clinical investigation, while Class C and D devices typically require clinical trials. Clinical testing of medical devices involving human subjects is governed by the Central Drugs Standard Control Organization (CDSCO). Consent from willing human subjects is obtained from the Central Licensing Approval (CLA) using Form MD-23.

The new medical equipment must be approved by the CLA, which has the jurisdiction in this regard. The "Sugam" portal, managed by CDSCO, along with Form MD-26 and the required fees, is used to request licensing approval. Seven Medical Device Advisory (MDA) groups are mentioned, focusing on specific areas such as cardiovascular, dentistry, reproductive, urology, orthopaedic, ophthalmology, and miscellaneous. Twelve New Drug Advisory Committees (NDACs) are established to assess clinical trials and approve new drugs. The MDA claims to have received and examined all supporting documentation for the new medical device. Based on the MDA's suggestion, the CLA approves a new medical device, using Form MA-27.

20.3 MEDICAL DEVICE AND THE REQUISITE FORMS

Medical devices have a few distinctive qualities, such as biocompatibility, ISO symbol standards, clinical evaluation (feasibility or pivotal), safety and performance, accuracy, and clinical performance. Good Manufacturing Practice (GMP) is required by Schedule M III, Rule 109-A, and medical device labelling by Rule 125-A, where a medical device falls within the drug clause.

It is evident that there are two different forms of applications for licences and registrations. First, there are two categories of medical devices, medical and new, the latter of which will be used in India for the first time. Current technology wants to be offered in India. Importer and manufacturing licences are of two types, and their regulations and scope of application vary (Tables 20.1, 20.2, and 20.3)

TABLE 20.1
Documents Necessary for the Approval of a Medical Device that Was Developed Indigenously

S. No.	Administrative	
1.	Authorisation letter	The letter is issued to the admitted individual by the responsible authority in their capacity as either the director, company secretary, or partner of the Indian agent firm, and it is attested by them in their individual names. The authorised person bears the responsibility of further complying with the product.
2.	Covering letter	Submission of an application for approval to manufacture, import, or conduct clinical trials involving a new medical device or technology. It is important to make clear both the use and the purpose of the thing being indexed.
3.	Application	In order to get permission for a novel biomedical equipment, the applicable Form 44 needs to be filled out in a way that is clear and includes the appropriate signatures and stamps from the authorised person.
4.	Fess	A Treasury Challan (TR-6), together with the applicable fees, must be submitted.
5.	Drugs and Clinical Trials Rules, 2019 (the protocol for the clinical study), is effective from September 20, 2019. Applications can be submitted to the CLA in the required format of Form CT-4A. The CLA is responsible for approving any clinical trials that are conducted. The documents that are included on the Form CT 4A are significant and will be noted. According to Rule No. 20, no individual, establishment, or organisation was permitted to carry out any sort of clinical experiment unless given authorisation to do so by CLA. After reviewing the Form CT-4A, the CLA gave its approval to the issuance of the Form CT-06, which is necessary to obtain authorisation for conducting a clinical trial of a medical device within ninety days. The registration of clinical trial sites and registration by CLA is another essential component of the clinical study.	
6.	The title page as well as the table of contents	Explanations are required for both the individual table descriptions and the specifics of the study.
7.	Research aim(s)	In addition to including primary and secondary data that have a logical relation to the study design, it is necessary to provide a justification for the study's purpose and demonstrate why it became necessary to conduct the research in its initial stages.
8.	Design of study	There are a variety of possible study designs, such as stratified randomisation, blinded open-label, cross-over design, randomisation by body halves or paired organs (split body trials), cluster randomisation, etc., all of which should be mentioned explicitly in order to comprehend the importance of the statistics.

(*Continued*)

TABLE 20.1 (CONTINUED)
Documents Necessary for the Approval of a Medical Device that Was Developed Indigenously

S. No.	Administrative	
9.	Subjects in research	It is necessary to make note of the population in the area where the trial was carried out. Mention needs to be made of a description of the disease, including the stage, indication, or circumstances, as well as the diagnostic criteria for selecting members of the population. It is unethical for some groups of people, including pregnant women, children, members of the military services, prisoners in custody, and geographically placed ethnic people, to participate in the trial without special permission.
10.	Eligibility requirements, including both inclusion criteria and exclusion criteria for the subject	The criteria that will be used to decide which patients will be allowed to take part in the planned clinical trial and which will be disqualified from participating in the clinical trial.
11.	Research the evaluation.	It is important to provide a comprehensive description of a clinical study, which may involve exploratory or confirmatory characterisation of the safety or efficacy of a treatment.
12.	Study treatment	Both the treatment and its results must be documented.
13.	Adverse events	Any adverse reaction that is discovered must be reported within the first twenty-four hours, and any delay in reporting must be properly justified. The nature of any major reactions, as well as a description of the incident, its severity, and any reactions to the occurrence, must be communicated. In addition, a report regarding the signs and symptoms, as well as the exact diagnosis of the occurrence, is required to be submitted.
14.	Ethical factors to consider	The following documents are required Risk/benefit evaluation. Ethical review and dissemination of information. Giving consent after being informed. A statement regarding the confidentiality of the data, ownership of the data, and the processes that have been established for maintaining confidentiality, such as coding procedures.
15.	Investigate both monitoring and supervision.	It is necessary to use a case record form, also known as a CRF, in order to properly complete and assess the case record corrections. The procedure of data handling and the identification of errors are going to be included.

TABLE 20.1 (CONTINUED)
Documents Necessary for the Approval of a Medical Device that Was Developed Indigenously

S. No.	Administrative	
16.	Management of the investigational product	The investigational product description and packaging must be specified, in addition to the specifics of the instruments and deliverable drugs. Placebos that were utilised in the trial. The exact dose, if it is supplied by the medical device, as well as the precision with which the medical device operates, are both things that need to be noted. It is important to address the methods by which the study was packaged, labelled, and conducted in a blind fashion. The procedure for assigning test subjects and recognising test subjects should include a discussion of the instrument retrieval code numbering scheme. Accountability of the investigational medical device, including both the technique and the retrieval system that was utilised. Summarise the policy and procedure governing the disposal of unused investigational products.
17.	Analysis of data	This should include all of the statistical analysis, including the sample size of recruitment, the selection of sample sizes, assumptions, and efficacy (primary as well as secondary), and safety outcomes, along with a description of the statistical tests that were performed. Describe the level of significance as well as the approaches that were employed for the information that was found to be absent. Additionally, the method of analysis of the data for treatment failures, compared with the data, patient withdrawals, and intermediate analysis to be mentioned.
18.	Commitment on the part of the investigator.	This is to include all of the particulars and components that are specified in Section 15 of the New Drugs and Clinical Trials Rules, 2019.
19.	Legal forms of consent	Every participant in a clinical trial is obliged to provide their free, informed permission in writing before the experiment may begin. According to Rule 2019 of the New Drugs and Clinical Trials Rules, Section 2 of the Rules. A recording, either audio or video, documenting the process of obtaining informed permission from vulnerable patients participating in clinical trials of a novel medical device is necessary to ensure that the patient has a complete understanding of the experiment and the procedures by providing them with the necessary facts and walking them through the facts. The investigator is responsible for keeping track of all records and obtaining formal consent. It is required in the declaration that any enquiries be directed to the investigator. In the event that a participant sustains an injury while participating in the clinical trial, the associated hospitalisation and treatment costs are their responsibility. According to Rule No. 39 of the aforementioned rules, the participant is entitled to receive monetary compensation in the event that they experience any mortality or co-morbidity.

(Continued)

TABLE 20.1 (CONTINUED)
Documents Necessary for the Approval of a Medical Device that Was Developed Indigenously

S. No.	Administrative	
21.	Case report template	Case Record Forms are extremely significant, and they will be filled out in accordance with any incident that was observed to involve death or life-threatening adverse event instances. Record forms, informed consent, and trial subjects are used according to Table 3 of the Third Schedule.
22	The justification behind carrying out the research in India	The necessity of conducting research in India needs to be backed up by evidence that it is feasible, and both the pilot study and the pivotal study stages need to be described.
23.	Specifics regarding the pre-clinical study	It is required that a report be made outlining the particulars of the test battery in accordance with the toxicity testing for Tiers 1 through 3, including the selection of species and the number of subjects. The nature, frequency, and intensity of pharmacological or toxic effects are some of the things that can be determined as a consequence of post-exposure research. It is necessary to note the amount of time required for the effects to become noticeable, as well as their duration, any reversibility, and dose response. Reports on non-clinical pharmacology, also known as Tier 3 toxicity, are required to include a summary of the pharmacological elements of carcinogenicity, irritancy, and sensitisation, reproductive toxicity, and genotoxicity (mutagenicity) investigations. This is one of the requirements of the Food and Drug Administration (FDA).
24.	Specifics of any previous clinical tests that have been carried out in regard to the said product in other countries	Approval Status to the other country, including the clinical trial or the clinical trial that was terminated, if there was one, shall be mentioned.
25.	Literature reviews and clinical evaluations that have been previously published	Any published material on medical devices, their underlying principles, their functions, or their applications, as well as any relevant clinical studies, should be mentioned.

TABLE 20.1 (CONTINUED)
Documents Necessary for the Approval of a Medical Device that Was Developed Indigenously

S. No.	Administrative	
26.	Approval Status of the proposed study and any participating nations if any	If any of the proposed investigations require approval from the other nations.
27.	Ethics Committee clearances that may be available (the Ethics Committee should be from the same region as the location of the clinical trial site).	Clinical trial Ethics Committees (EC), which are constituted under Rule 7 and registered under Rule 8; medical and health research Ethics Committees, which are constituted under Rule 16 and registered under Rule 17; clinical trial sites that do not have their own EC may use the registered EC of another trial site; or a (registered) independent EC that is located within the same city or within a radius of 50 kilometres of the clinical trial site as per Rule 25 (ii).
28.	Brochure for the investigators	On the basis of previous experiences with the product under research and with related medications, the Investigators Brochure (IB) should give a summary of the potential hazards and adverse drug responses that should be anticipated as a result of these experiences. As part of the exploratory use of the items, there should also be a description provided of any particular precautions to be taken or monitoring that is to be performed in addition to the standard monitoring.
29.	Documents pertaining to technology:	Sample copies of Labels, Instructions for Use, and Inserts into Packages: (if the product is being sold in any nation)

TABLE 20.2
Documents Required for Authorisation to Sell and Distribute (Forms MD-14 and MD-15: for Import Licence

1	Covering letter	Along with the page number and index, it is imperative that the objective of the import or test licence be made very apparent.
2	The letter of authorisation	Authorisation letter from an Indian agent firm that is self-attested and can be signed by a director, company secretary, or partner
3	Properly completed Form 12	Completed, signed, and dated by an authorised signatory of the applicant; includes manufacturer's name and address or testing facility's name and address. Mention must be made of both the product's name and the pack size, or the number of tests included in each package.
4	Challan	The TR-6 Challan along with the required payments
5	Utilisation	Justification of the suggested quantity for import and a breakdown of its intended use
6	Inserts for the proposed product and labels for the proposed product	In accordance with the provisions of Rule 109 A of the Drug and Cosmetics Rules, notarisation of any and all specimen labels, including any accompanying product inserts, is obligatory.
7	Procedures for testing	The testing methodology and protocol for the product under consideration
8	An authenticated copy of the manufacturing licence	Manufacturing requires either a manufacturing licence or a wholesale distribution licence.
9	Committing to refrain from using for commercial purposes	An undertaking is necessary, and within it, it must be declared that these kits will not be utilised for any kind of commercial activity.

20.4 CLINICAL INVESTIGATION IN ORDER TO OBTAIN CLEARANCE TO USE AN INVESTIGATIVE MEDICAL DEVICE

Clinical research is necessary for Class C and Class D devices, and such groups of medical devices are required to be examined for safety and efficacy in human volunteers; these types of medical devices are referred to as "Investigative Medical Devices." Clinical research is required for Class C and Class D devices. Clinical trial applications for Investigative Medical Devices are submitted via Form MD 22 to the CLA and approval is given via Form MD 23. The clinical research can be submitted for any type of medical device by the investigator.

20.5 CLINICAL INVESTIGATION PRIOR TO THE IMPORTATION OR PRODUCTION OF MEDICAL DEVICES

SLA have control over the licensing of Class A (low risk) and Class B (low to moderate risk) devices. Applications are made by the MD-26, CLA while MD-27 is in

TABLE 20.3
The Approval of the Medical Device must be Contingent upon the Submission of the Following Documentation

		Part A (Administrative)
1	Covering letter	The import or test licence's stated purpose, as well as the page number and index, should be written out in full.
2	Authorisation letter	An application that has been duly filled out and signed, together with an official letter of authorisation from an Indian agent firm
3	Form- MD 16/22	Application duly filled out and signed
4	Prescribed Fee	The necessary payments are made concurrently with the submission of the TR6 challan.
5	Schedule DII	Indemnity by Indian agent or manufacturer with properly completed, signed, stamped, and dated, along with the name and identity of the manufacturer.
		Regulatory Certificates
1	Free Sale Certificate (FSC)	Free-of-Charge Sales of Marketing participation of foreign medical devices requires a copy of the product's authorisation from the national regulatory authority in the country of origin, along with an apostille or notary seal, and is required before the product can be sold in a foreign market.
2	Certificate required	Valid copies of the certificate that have been duly notarised and that pertain to the legal and real manufacturing site(s) are necessary in the following situations: Quality Management System Completion of All Quality Assurance Requirements European Community Quality Assurance for Products CE Product Quality Assurance CE Design Certificate Public Declaration of Conformity
3	Notarised labels	All specimen labels that have been notarised, as required by Rule 109 A of the Food, Drug, and Cosmetics Rules.
4	Instructions for use that have been notarised	Copies of the certificate's accompanying usage instructions that have been properly notarised and are currently valid
		Part B (Plant details)
1	Plant Master File	The manufacturer is obligated to provide a Plant Master File that has been notarised and contains the employee, area, production area, and other information as specified before. In the event of re-registration, a notarised assurance from the manufacturer, confirming that no change in the Plant Master File is necessary, is required to be submitted.
2	Device Master File	Authenticated copy of the Device Master File provided by the manufacturer, and an undertaking from the manufacturer, duly notarised, that there will be no changes made to the Device Master File (in the event of re-registration).

(Continued)

TABLE 20.3 (CONTINUED)
The Approval of the Medical Device must be Contingent upon the Submission of the Following Documentation

3	Undertaking	Notarised undertaking about complaints received during the course of the past three years in relation to the proposed products being "Not of Standard Quality" (in the event that re-registration is required).
4	PMS study report	In the event that the registration needs to be renewed, a report on the most recent Post-marketing Surveillance (PMS) research must be submitted.
5	Specifics regarding any adverse reaction, extremely harmful adverse reaction	It is necessary to file reports of any adverse reactions, including major adverse reactions, deaths, recalls, and complaints. The manufacturer has conducted an investigation into the underlying cause, and they have taken corrective action to prevent further incidents (CAPI).

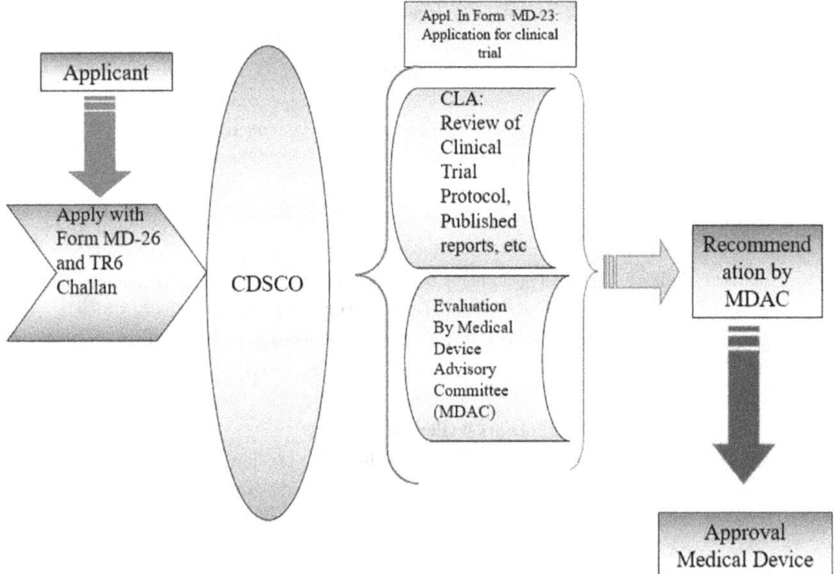

FIGURE 20.1 Procedure for registration of the medical device.

charge of granting approval. Class A devices pose a low risk, while Class B devices pose a low to moderate danger. Approval is necessary in order to import medical products or other medical devices comparable to those already on the Indian market (Figure 20.1)

20.6 PERMISSION FOR MANUFACTURING ON LOAN LICENCE TO MANUFACTURE MEDICAL DEVICES IN CLASSES A AND B IN INDIA

The SLA grants licences to manufacture Class A and Class B devices, which are low- and moderate-risk devices, using Form MD-3, whereas permission is provided using Form MD-6. Licences can be issued for the manufacture, sale, and distribution of medical devices, and any firm can apply for a loan licence to produce medical devices. Form MD-4 is to be used for manufacturing and sale or distribution under loan licence applications, and Form MD-6 is to be used for granting authorisation for Class A and Class B medical devices. The application form itself, along with the necessary supporting documentation, is required. Authorities take measures to verify that medical devices are risk-free for use on humans and demand the submission of a test medical device that is substantially identical to the device that served as the basis for the evaluation.

20.7 CERTIFICATIONS FOR QUALITY AND COMPLIANCE WITH REGULATIONS

Countries that are part of the Global Harmonisation Task Force (GHTF), such as the United States of America, Canada, Australia, and Japan, exempt biomedical equipment from the need to undergo clinical testing. It is necessary for the nation of origin to provide a Regulatory Certificate Free Sales Certificate that has been notarised. It is necessary to provide the Quality Certificates (ISO 13485), the Conformities Europe (CE) Certificate for Quality Assurance (CQA), design, and the Declaration of Conformity, and identify the manufacturing warehouse site and the manufacturing site. Understanding the risk assessment clause and the risks that are linked to it requires the Declaration of Conformity (DOC). A similar document signed by the appropriate personnel should be printed on the manufacturer's letterhead.

20.8 ESTABLISH A MASTER PLANT FILE FOR ALL MEDICAL DEVICES IN INDIA

It is required that you provide a Plant Master File (PMF) with all of the appendices, as well as information regarding the layout of the premises, manufacturing activities, total employees, organization chart, details about quality control, and important instruments. In addition, other documents such as an organization chart, a certificate of plant registration, or an authorization certificate issued by a national regulatory body, are also necessary. These certificates must be issued by a national regulatory authority. A diagram of the process flow and the manufacturing process, a quality control system, a conformity document, and the manufacturing process all need to have condensed versions of their respective details submitted.

20.9 MEDICAL DEVICES IN INDIA THAT HAVE A DEVICE MASTER FILE (DMF)

The DMF is an essential document that must be understood in order to gain knowledge regarding the device description, the specifications, and the comparable type of the device that has been approved in India or elsewhere. In addition, DMF includes the necessary quality control measures for the raw components as well as the end product. Additionally, the clinical trial reports, reports on biocompatibility, physiochemical testing, method testing, batch release, analysis of results, draft labels, stability data for accelerated and real-time testing, instructions, and packaging specifications are all included in the DMF file.

20.10 CONCERNING THE LABELLING OF MEDICAL DEVICES (RULE 109A)

The following information needs to be printed on the label or sticker that is attached to the outer covering layer of every medical device, in accordance with the guidelines provided by CDSCO for the registration of medical devices in India.

1. Mention must be made of the correct name of the medical device, as well as its details, identification, and how it is to be used.
2. The manufacturer's name and address, as well as the location of the actual manufacturing facility, should be included.
3. Statement in the metric system that is accurate with regard to the net content of medical devices.
4. Dates of production and expiration are required for most medical devices; however, dates of manufacturing and expiration are not required for medical devices constructed of stable materials such as stainless steel or titanium, bio ceramic, and supplied as non-sterile.
5. If the item is sterile, the date it was sterilised as well as the procedure used to sterilise it should be indicated.
6. If the medicinal or biological material is contained within the medical device, for example, a medicated cardiac stent, it needs to be mentioned on the label.

7. It is necessary to include a description of any unique requirements for the device's storage or handling, if there are any.
8. On the label, it should specify whether the medical device is designed for a single use or several uses.
9. Medical device is only meant to be used for clinical research, it should be indicated by the possible inclusion of the phrase "FOR CLINICAL INVESTIGATION ONLY" on the packaging.
10. In the case of medical equipment that has been brought into the country from another nation, the address of the importer must be disclosed.
11. *In-vitro* medical devices are not allowed to be sold directly to customers. Instead, they must be sold by affixing an additional label or sticker to the outer shelf pack, and this must only be provided to medical facilities or diagnostic laboratories.
12. On the exterior label are printed the following details: the distinctive batch number, the lot number, the date of manufacturing, the expiration date (if there is one), the manufacturing licence number, and the location of the manufacturer or importer.
13. A mark from the International Organisation for Standardisation (ISO) or the Bureau of Indian Standards (BIS) could be placed on the product's exterior label to guarantee its quality and safety.

20.11 PERMISSION FOR MANUFACTURE ON LOAN LICENCE TO MANUFACTURE CLASS A AND B MEDICAL DEVICES IN INDIA

The Central Licensing Authority is the organization that has the jurisdiction to grant permission for high-risk and extremely high-risk medical equipment. These devices fall under Classes C and D. Extensive amounts of information will be needed for the application procedure. Form MD-7 is to be used to submit the application to CDSCO and Form MD-9 is to be used in order to approve the application.

The principle that guides CDSCO's examination is to identify any hazards that are foreseeable or already recognized and then quantify the risks that relate to using the medical device. In addition to this, CDSCO assesses risks connected with the implementation of novel medical technologies. Attached to the application is the Device Master File, which defines the technical, clinical, and safety facts, as well as the Plant Master File, which outlines the manufacturing-related information.

20.12 AUTHORISATION TO APPLY FOR A TESTING LICENCE IN ORDER TO PRODUCE A MEDICAL DEVICE

A test licence can be obtained from CLA after filling out Form 12 and submitting the necessary documentation for approval in Form 13. This licence can then be used for training, testing, clinical evaluation, or demonstrations. In addition to the application and the purpose statement, a cover letter is included in the form. The application must also include an explanation of the necessary risk-benefit ratio, or how it will improve the quality of the patient's life, as well as a description of similar-type devices that already exist so that the related risk can be understood.

20.13 AUTHORISATION TO SELL AND DISTRIBUTE (FORMS MD-14 AND MD-15); REQUIRED FOR IMPORT LICENCE

In Chapter 5 of the Medical Device Rules 2017, laws were outlined regarding the distribution and sale of medical devices that were brought into India from other countries. According to the first paragraph of Sub-rule 36 of Rule 36 of the Medical Device Rule 2017, any authorised agency that possesses a licence to manufacture medical devices for sale or distribution may apply for an import licence. Additionally, any wholesaler may apply for an import licence for the purpose of sale and distribution of the medical device. The application is submitted to the CLA using Form MD-14, and registration is confirmed using Form MD-15. If the application comes from an international supplier, the supplier must be in possession of a wholesale licence in order to be allowed to distribute or sell the medical device in India. The Indian agents that the foreign vendor hires are required to have manufacturing or wholesale licences in India. The foreign vendor has the option to recruit Indian agents. In addition to being essential, the Free Sale Certificate (FSC) must also be presented, and it must be understood that the medical devices that are being imported are permitted for unrestricted sale on the open market in the nation that is exporting them and that they have been granted approval for export and trade liberalisation. The following documents are required as follows (Figure 20.2):

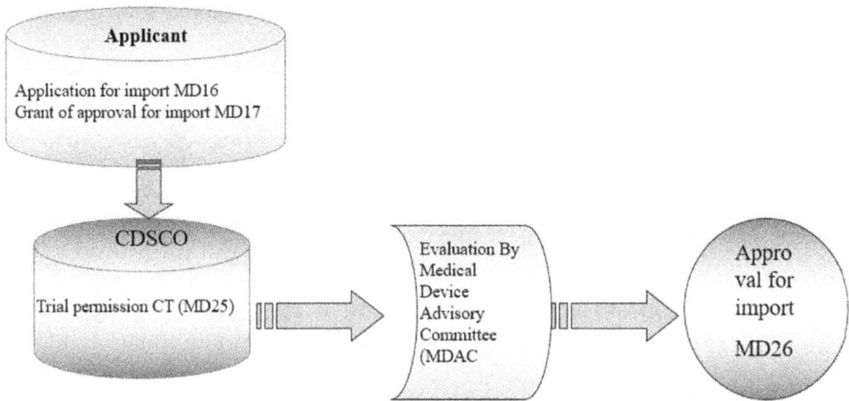

FIGURE 20.2 Approval process of manufacturing/import of medical devices.

TABLE 20.4
Types of Medical Device and Forms Required for Registration of Import and Manufacturing

Class of Medical Device		Form No.
		Import
1	A, B, C, D	Application must be made using Form MD-14, and authorisation must be granted using Form MD-15.
		Manufacturing
1	A, B	Application shall made through Form MD-3 and the permission granted through Form MD-5
2	C, D	Permission requests and renewals must be submitted using Forms MD-3 and MD-5, respectively.
		Manufacturing under loan
1	A, B	Form MD-4 is to be used for submitting the application, and Form MD-6 is to be used for granting approval.
2	C, D	Form MD-8 is to be used for submitting the application, and Form MD-9 is to be used for granting approval.

TABLE 20.5
Type of Medical Device and the Forms Required for Registration for Clinical Investigation Permission, Import, and Manufacturing

Class of Medical Device		Form No.
		Importing and manufacturing
1	A, B, C, D	Permission is requested on Form MD-26 and granted on Form MD-27.
		Clinical investigation permission by import and manufacturing
1	A, B, C, D	Form MD-22 must be used for the application process, and Form MD-23 must be used for the approval process.
		Test Licence by import and manufacturing
1	A, B, C, D	Form MD-16 is to be used for making applications, and Form MD-17 is to be used for granting approval.

20.14 DOCUMENTS NECESSARY FOR THE MANUFACTURING AND IMPORTATION OF MEDICAL DEVICES

Records, such as those pertaining to administration, regulation, and production facilities, are necessary.

TABLE 20.6
Different Forms Required for Registration of the Licence of the Medical Device

	Form number	Application
1	MD-1	Under the Medical Devices Rules, 2016, you are required to submit an application for registration as well as approval of a notified body registration certificate.
2	MD-2	Submission of an application for registration and approval of a licence to manufacture medical devices of either Class A or Class B in order to be sold and distributed.
3	MD-3	Application for registration and approval of a licence to produce Class C or Class D medical devices for sale and distribution, as well as Class A or Class B medical devices.
4	MD-4	Submission of an application for approval of a loan licence to manufacture Class A or Class B medical devices for the purpose of sale and distribution.
5	MD-5	Submission of an application for approval of a loan licence to manufacture Class A or Class B medical devices for the purpose of sale and distribution.
6	MD-6	Application for the approval of a loan licence to manufacture Class C or Class D medical devices for sale and distribution, as well as Class A or Class B medical devices.
7	MD-7	The granting of a licence or approval for the production of medical devices classified as Class C or Class D, as well as Class A or Class B, for the purpose of sale and distribution.
8	MD-8	The provision of a loan licence, an operating licence, or an approval for the production, sale, and distribution of a medical device classified as Class C or Class D, or Class A or Class B is requested.
9	MD-9	A book containing the necessary forms for the adopted procedures for maintaining an audit or inspection book.
10	MD-10	Documents required for the grant of a licence to manufacture a restricted amount of a medical device for the purposes of experimentation, which may include clinical studies, examinations, demonstrations, or training.
11	MD-11	Application forms for obtaining a licence to manufacture medical equipment for the purpose of conducting clinical research, testing, evaluating, demonstrating, or training.
12	MD-12	Submission of an application for the issuance of a licence to import medical equipment.
13	MD-13	Licence to import medical devices
14	MD-14	The submission of an application for the issuance of a licence to import medical devices is restricted to any usage for the purpose of clinical investigations, testing, demonstration, assessment, or training.
15	MD-15	The provision of a licence for the importation of medical devices is restricted to the use of those devices in clinical studies conducted by any government hospital or statutory medical institution for the purpose of treating patients.

(Continued)

TABLE 20.6 (CONTINUED)
Different Forms Required for Registration of the Licence of the Medical Device

	Form number	Application
16	MD-16	A request for permission to import medical devices for the treatment of patients at a government-run hospital or other medical institution.
17	MD-17	Provision of a licence for the use of the medical equipment in the treatment of patients by a medical institution or a government hospital.
18	MD-18	Submission of an application for permission to import a medical device solely for personal use.
19	MD-19	The authorisation to import medical gadgets for one's own personal use, in limited quantities.
20	MD-20	Request for authorisation to carry out clinical research as part of a clinical trial.
21	MD-21	The request for authorisation to perform clinical inquiry has been granted.
22	MD-22	Submission of a request for authorisation to carry out clinical performance evaluation
23	MD-23	Provision of authorisation to carry out clinical performance evaluations
24	MD-24	A precedent medical device is not included in the application for the granting of authorisation to import or manufacture medical devices.
25	MD-25	A prerequisite medical device is not required in order to obtain permission to import or manufacture a medical device.
26	MD-26	A formal petition requesting authorisation for the importation or production of a novel *in vitro* diagnostic medical device.
27	MD-27	Authorisation for the importation or production of a newly developed *in vitro* diagnostic medical device
28	MD-28	After assessing the medical device, the Medical Device Testing Officer wrote an evaluation report.
29	MD-29	Submittal of a request by the purchaser for the testing of a medical device in accordance with Section 26 of the Drugs and Cosmetics Act of 1940.
30	MD-30	In accordance with Sub-section (c) of Section 22 of the Drugs and Cosmetics Act of 1940, a warrant is thus issued prohibiting the disposal of any stock currently held by any individual.
31	MD-31	In accordance with Sub-section 22(1)(c) or (cc) of the Drugs and Cosmetics Act of 1940, the receipt of a medical device that was confiscated.
32	MD-32	Specific information pertaining to the individual regarding the sized samples that were in possession.
33	MD-33	The sample receipt for custody of medical device(s) that is required by Sub-section (1) of Section 23 of the Drugs and Cosmetics Act, 1940 is not permitted.
34	MD-34	Memorandum to the Medical Device Testing Officer for medical devices

BIBLIOGRAPHY

Buch B. FDA medical device approval: Things you didn't learn in medical school or residency. *Am. J. Orthop. (Belle Mead, NJ)* 2007; 36: 407–412.

Central Drugs Standard Control Organization https://cdsco.gov.in/opencms/opencms/en/Medical-Device-Diagnostics/Medical-Device-Diagnostics/(Accessed on 2020).

CliniExperts. Available from: https://cliniexperts.com (Accessed on 3 October 2023).

Food, Administration D, Health UDo, and Services H. Medical device reporting: Manufacturer reporting, importer reporting, user facility reporting, distributor reporting. *Fed Regist* 2000; 65: 4112–4120.

Guidelines for import and manufacture of medical devices [Internet]. India. CDSCO; February. Available from: http://cdsco. nic.in/medical%20device%20A42.html (Accessed on 2020).

Kapoor V. Kaushik D. A comparative study of regulatory prospects for drug-device combination products in major pharmaceutical jurisdictions. *J Generic Med: The Business Journal for the Generic Medicines Sector* 2013; 10: 86–96.

Morula Health Tech (P) Ltd. https://morulaa.com/medical-device-registration-in-india/things-to-remember-while-preparing-your-regulatory-dossier/ (Accessed on 10 July 2020).

Radhadevi N, Balamuralidhara V, Pramod Kumar TM, Ravi V. Regulatory guidelines for medical devices in India: An overview. *Asian J Pharm* 2012; 6: 10–17.

Rathi VK, Krumholz HM, Masoudi FA, Ross JS. Characteristics of clinical studies conducted over the total product life cycle of high-risk therapeutic medical devices receiving FDA premarket approval in 2010 and 2011. *JAMA* 2015; 314: 604–612.

Sanjana P, Kirti H, Begum S. Medical devices and their approval procedure in India. *Int J Drug Regul Affairs* 2016; 4(3): 19–29.

Shah AR, Goyal RK. Status of the regulation for medical devices. *Indian J Pharmal Sci* 2008; 70: 695–700.

21 Quality Assurance of Medical Devices Central Drugs Standard Control Organization (CDSCO), the United States Food and Drug Administration (US FDA), and European Union (EU) Regulations

21.1 INTRODUCTION

A stringent regulatory framework has been incorporated into medical devices in order to guarantee the quality, safety, and efficacy of medical equipment. The Government of India is responsible for the implementation of an effective regulatory framework that is targeted not only at the development of India's domestic industry but also at the improvement of the healthcare sector. The majority of medical devices are required to comply with particular legislation, safety standards, and quality requirements in order to be sold in the United States. According to a report by the Ministry of Health and Family Welfare (MoHFW), India, there was a total of 2,868 deaths of participants in clinical trials that took place between 2005 and 2012. However, only 89 of those deaths were deemed to be attributable to the experiment, and 82 of those victims received compensation.

The Central Drugs Standard Control Organization (CDSCO) under MoHFW regulates the manufacture, distribution, import, and sale of medical devices for the purpose of ensuring the availability of standard quality to the consumer authorities, whereas the Drug Controller Government of India (DCGI) is the responsible authority for product approval, framing standards, clinical trials, the introduction of

DOI: 10.1201/9781003397854-5

new medical devices, and import licences. However, the authority that is principally responsible for regulating medical devices in India is the CDSCO. In accordance with Gazette Notification SO 1468 (2005), all businesses are required to be registered with the CDSCO before they are allowed to put any of their products on the Indian market.

Sterile medical devices, including cannulae, bone cements, heart valves, scalp vein set, orthopaedic implants, and internal prosthetic replacement, are to be considered as pharmaceuticals in accordance with Section 3 (b) (iv) of the Drugs and Cosmetics Act (DCA), and registration is necessary for them. Over 160 different medical devices are currently included on the list.

21.2 COMPARISON OF THE STANDARDS FOR MEDICAL DEVICES ESTABLISHED BY THE FDA AND THE CDSCO

The United States Food and Drug Administration (FDA) was initially established by the Federal Food, Drug, and Cosmetic Act on May 28, 1976. In light of this, the Act brings to a close the title of 21 CFR (Code for Federal Regulations), which had parts 800–1299 that defined the requirements for medical devices and IVDs. The Good Manufacturing Practices (GMP) are specified in 21 CFR Part 820, although ISO 13485:2003 also describes GMP, but with minor differences. The former ISO 9001 (2000) standard, which was primarily generic, has been replaced by the newer ISO 13485 (2003) standard, which is extremely particular to medical devices. The standard for the ISO 9000 group was produced in the notion of the selling of product as the standard of quality control; however, the standard for the ISO 10000 family is more practical, and this family's guidelines are more accepted throughout the world and industries. The International Organization for Standardization (ISO) holds a legal position in Europe, and the European Commission publishes annual updates to the various ISO criteria for the certification of conformity. A post-marketing surveillance programme for medical products was also initiated by the DCGI, in a manner analogous to that of the FDA. Products that have either the CE mark or the FDA's approval can be sold in India, and the Bureau of Indian Standards (BIS) recognises either the global standard ISO 13485: 2003 or the Indian Standard (IS) 15579: 2005 as the Indian National Standard. Rule 125A of the Medical Devices Act, 2017, identifies the articles as being the Sterile Disposable Perfusion Sets for single use only, with IS 9824:1981 for Single-Use Perfusion Set, IS 10258:1982 for Sterile Disposable Hypodermic Syringes, and IS 10654:199 for Sterile Disposable Hypodermic Needles.

21.3 REGULATION AND QUALITY CONTROL OF MEDICAL DEVICES IN THE US

21.3.1 Changing the Medical Devices and Updating the Laws

The USA began the process of setting guidelines for medical devices quite a while earlier. Edward M. Kennedy presided over the Senate Committee that drafted the medical device legislation that was ultimately enacted between 1970 and 1976. Industry has accepted the clearance of individual types of medical instruments by class only, thus 510(k) is only used for pre-marketing and post-marketing approval, and the FDA has no jurisdiction to be stringent or enforce them. Section 513 of the Federal Food, Drug, and Cosmetic Act classified the instrument on the basis of most likely risks and benefits into Class I, II, or III, whereas Section 510(k) notified the government of the start of the pre-marketing of medical devices. The statute was changed in 1990 to make it so that submitting a 510(k) report to the FDA is necessary for any medical device prior to it being marketed. The US Food and Drug Administration is given opportunities to examine the instrument's types and determine whether or not their classification is acceptable.

21.3.2 The FDA Modernization Act of 1997

Because of the greater sensitivity and risk associated with Classes II and III instruments, the FDA had a difficult time classifying all medical instruments and establishing regulatory control over those instruments for a long time. The Food and Drug Administration (FDA) is currently in the process of putting into effect substantial legislation that includes regulations for patient access to experimental medications and medical devices, clinical trials, safety, and labelling. The legislation that is put into effect to restrict manufacturers from disseminating information about unapproved medical devices. Publication of the first information on a medical device in peer-reviewed journals is contingent upon filing for approval having been made within the allotted time frame.

21.3.3 The Medical Device User Fee and Modernization Act (MDUFMA)

This Act was initially enacted in 2002, and it was revised a total of four times during the course of 2017. As of October 1, 2017, it was renamed the Medical Device User Fee Amendments to the FDA Reauthorization Act (MDUFA IV), and it went into effect on that day. According to the legislation, the corporation is required to pay the registration fees for the instrument or medical device in order to obtain the best and most expedient review possible in order to investigate the availability of a reliable and efficient medical device on the US market. The Food and Drug Administration Amendments Act of 2007 (H.R. 3580) was signed into law by President George W. Bush on March 27, 2007, making it into law. The implementation of the Prescription Drug User Fee Act (PDUFA) and the Medical Device User Fee and Modernization Act (MDUFMA) brings the amendment into effect and raises more resources for FDA. The Paediatric Research Equity Act (PREA) and the Best Pharmaceuticals for Children Act (BPCA) were both put into effect as a result of this modification, which furthered the advancement of research pertaining to the field of paediatric medicine. In this amendment to the FDA clause of Section 801, 42 U.S.C. 282(j)(5)(B) was enforced to require the certificate from industry for human drugs, biological devices, and biomedical equipment that fulfilled the standards of Section 402(j), including the required human clinical trial. The certificate that is necessary for the drugs in accordance with the provisions of sections 21 U.S.C. 355, 360e, or 360j(m), 351 (21 U.S.C. 262) of the Public Health Service Act (PHS Act), and 510(k) of the Food and Drug Administration and Control Act (21 U.S.C. 360(k)).

21.3.4 Food and Drug Administration Safety and Innovation Act (FDASIA)

This legislation was signed into law on July 9, 2012, and it gives the FDA the authority to collect the required fees from the innovator in order to conduct evaluations of medical devices, biosimilar biologics, generic medicines, and other products. The act promoted increased research for the development of paediatric drugs. The Food and Drug Administration Modernization Act places a strong emphasis on the research and development of novel medications, and the Act itself is referred to as "breakthrough therapy." In addition, the FDA has been given an edge by this Act, both financially and in terms of the amount of funds available to conduct accelerated clinical studies and reassess the claims made about various products.

21.3.5 The Cures Act of the 21st Century

The FDA has been given more power as a result of the implementation of the FDASIA Act, and the FDA has investigated ways in which the drug discovery process can be accelerated to combat life-threatening diseases. If the FDA's early examination of a drug shows that it has the potential to improve the treatment of a potentially fatal illness more effectively than current treatments, the agency votes in favour of the measure and encourages the development of the drug at a faster pace. The proposed regulation that was released by the FDA, which was given the acronym "Cures" for the accelerated programme for the discovery of drugs and biological treatments for critical illnesses, was ultimately approved by both houses of Congress. On December 13, 2017, former US President George W. Bush's "Expedited Programmes for Serious Conditions—Drug and Biological" bill was approved by Congress and signed into law by US President Barack Obama. The bill is critical, as is the process of tailoring drug research to the needs of individual patients, often known as patient-focused drug development.

21.3.6 The Food and Drug Administration (FDA) Reauthorization Act of 2017 (FDARA)

As a result of the modification to the Federal Food, Drug, and Cosmetic Act that was approved and signed into law on August 18th, 2017, the FDA is authorised to collect user fees, which are then utilised for post-marketing surveillance of brand-name medications, medical equipment, and generic versions of those medicines. The primary objective is to maintain a continuous market analysis of medical devices and to either improve or create existing medical technology in response to feedback from end users.

21.3.7 Federal Regulations

Title 21 of the Code of Federal Regulations (CFR) is where regulations related to food and drugs, including medical devices, are codified in the United States. Subchapter H within Title 21 is specifically designated for regulations related to medical devices. Subchapter H is further divided into eight major sections, and each of these sections contains its own subsections. This organizational structure is designed to address different aspects of the regulation of medical devices. It is emphasized that having a fundamental understanding of these regulations is essential for those involved in the development, manufacturing, distribution, and regulation of medical devices. The regulations outlined in Title 21, Subchapter H, cover a wide range of topics related to medical devices, including classification, premarket approval, labelling, good manufacturing practices, post-market surveillance, and more. Medical device manufacturers are required to comply with these regulations to ensure the safety and effectiveness of their products. The FDA enforces these regulations through inspections, reviews, and other regulatory activities. Each of the eight major sections within Subchapter H likely focuses on specific aspects of medical device regulation, such as premarket requirements, post-market surveillance, quality system regulations, and more.

In accordance with the federal regulations, Title 21 of Subchapter H is designated for medical devices. It is essential to have a fundamental understanding of the regulation of medical devices. The subsection is broken up into eight major sections, and each of those sections has its own subsection. The following are the subparts and subsections that are mentioned:

21.3.7.1 Subpart A—General Provisions

- Sec. 812.2: Applicability
- Sec. 812.2 (b): Abbreviated Requirements
- Sec. 812.2 (c): Exempted Investigations.
- 812.3: Definitions
- 812.5: Investigational Device Labelling
- 812.7: Promotion and Other Practices are Prohibited
- 812.19: Address for IDE Correspondence
- Subpart B—Application and Administrative Action
- Sec. 812.20: Applications
- Sec. 812.25: Investigational Plan
- Sec. 812.27: Report of Prior Investigations
- Sec. 812.30: FDA Action on Applications
- Sec. 812.35: Supplemental Applications
- Responsibilities of Sponsors
- Sec. 812.40: General Responsibilities of Sponsors
- Sec. 812.42: FDA and IRB Approval
- Sec. 812.46: Monitoring Investigations
- IRB Review and Approval

- Sec. 812.62: IRB Approval
- Sec. 812.66: Significant Risk Device Determinations
- Subpart E—Responsibilities of Investigators
- Sec. 812.100: General Responsibilities of Investigators
- Sec. 812.110: Specific Responsibilities of Investigators
- Therapeutic Devices
- Records and Reports
- Sec. 812.140: Records
- Sec. 812.150: Reports

21.3.7.2 The Clinical Trial and Post Marketing Surveillance of Medical Device

Section 21 Code of Federal Regulations (CFR) is also defined as follows:

- 21 CFR Part 50: Protection of Human Subjects
- 21 CFR Part 56: Institutional Review Boards
- 21 CFR Part 54: Financial Disclosure by Clinical Investigators
- 21 CFR Part 801: Labelling (Devices)
- 21 CFR Part 58: Good Laboratory Practice for Non-clinical Laboratory Studies
- 21 CFR Part 803: Medical Device Reporting
- 21 CFR Part 809: *In Vitro* Diagnostic Products for Human Use
- 21 CFR Part 814: Pre-market Approval of Medical Devices
- 21 CFR Part 820: Quality System Regulation
- 21 CFR Part 821: Post-market Surveillance

According to the act, the medical devices were classified into different classes according to the safety and effectiveness of the device (Table 21.1).

Canada, Australia, Japan, and the European Union have formed the Global Harmonization Task Force (GHTF) to coordinate their respective regulatory inspection and certification processes.

21.4 PART 807 OF 21 CFR SUBPART E: 510(K) OR 510(K) CLAUSE OF MEDICAL DEVICE PRE-MARKET NOTIFICATION

Medical devices that were on the market before May 28, 1976, before the amendments entered effect, are called "pre-amendments devices," whereas those introduced on or after that date must undergo the 510(k) process for clearance. A 510(k) is a document that is solely technical in nature and is required to be submitted to the FDA in order to receive clearance and authorisation for the commercialisation of a medical device or IVD in that country. There are instances when this provision is significant, and, in the context of law, it is known as a notification of pre-market. This notification makes sure that the medical device meets the quality standards for

TABLE 21.1
Classification of Medical Devices as per 21 CFR

Classification	Examples	Safety/Effectiveness Controls
Class I (low risk)	Cannula, examination gloves, elastic bandages, hand-held surgical instruments, disposable syringes, and syringes, as well as other medical supplies.	The majority of class I devices do not need any approval in order to be sold, although they do need to maintain their specifications in accordance with government notifications and adhere to general control criteria. In most cases, the formatted 510(k) will not be appropriate. The exemption for investigational devices has been formed as a clause that is subject to consideration.
Class II (medium risk)	Infusion pumps, syringes, surgical drapes, and other medical equipment	Demand that a marketing clearance be obtained through the 510(k) process. The manufacturer is obliged to submit to the FDA information supporting the claim that the proposed device exhibits substantial equivalence to items already available on the American market.
Class III (high risk)	Devices for the heart and the cerebellum have been inserted. Metal-on-metal hip joint, some dental implants, silicone gel-filled breast implants, etc.	The specifics of PMA, PDP, and investigational device exemptions will depend on the regulatory framework in place. It's crucial for manufacturers to be familiar with and adhere to the regulatory requirements in the relevant jurisdiction.

its performances as well as the technical and safety standards. The limitation does not apply to any classified medical devices from Class I to Class III, and all medical devices that are intended for use on humans must first receive clearance from their respective pre-market applications. No risk-associated biomedical equipment is exempt from the clause of 510(k) in most cases; however, the FDA may provide an exemption under the clause of 513(g) after an application has been submitted. Additionally, in accordance with the provisions of 21 CFR 807.92(a), the FDA made certain that the medical devices that were subject to the 510(K) notifications were substantially identical to one another and were risk-free. The notion of equivalency, sometimes known as the "predicate" medical device, is one that assures that medical devices are equivalent to those that can be legally marketed. According to Subsection 513(f)(2) of the Food and Drug Act, the applicant is required to provide substantial evidence that the proposed medical device is equivalent to one or more similar types of medical devices that are already being legally marketed. The FDA conducts a comprehensive review of the medical device to determine whether or not it satisfies the requirements of Section 510(K) for approval. Chapters 21 CFR 862.9 and 864.9 of the 21 CFR include the regulations that classify medical devices. While 21 CFR 807, Subpart E, provides the required documentation and guidelines for the filing of 510(k), there are no strict forms or formats accessible regarding the submission of

510(k). The FDA has given the medical device its substantially equivalent certificate and has ruled that it can either be marketed in the United States or researched for potential commercial distribution.

21.5 THE QUALITY AND KIND OF THE MEDICAL DEVICE'S CLEARANCE 510 (K) APPLICATION OR APPLICATION FOR CLEARANCE

US Food and Drug Administration Title 21 of the Code of Federal Regulations, part 807, or the US Food and Drug Administration, has not specified any forms and has only offered a guideline for the introduction of the device to the market in the United States. At the time of the 510(k) clearance application, the FDA required a quality system in accordance with 21 CFR 820. Having said that, in order to secure your market right here in the USA, you will need to submit an application under each of the following categories:

1. Finished Products in Accordance with the Specifications of the Domestic Producers This law also extended to the accessories of finished devices as they are used for replacement components, which means that manufacturers of finished biomedical products with their own specifications are required to submit a 510(k) prior to marketing their products in the United States. There has been no requirement placed on the indigenous manufacturer to file the 510(k) application. Foreign manufacturers and exporters, as well as their US representatives, are required to file the 510(k) application in order for equipment to be brought into the USA. Even though another company or entity is under contract to build the finished device, a specification developer is in charge of creating the specifications for it. Instead of the contract manufacturer, it is the standard developer who is responsible for submitting the requisite 510(k).
2. The 510(k) is a premarket submission made to the U.S. Food and Drug Administration (FDA) to demonstrate that the new medical device is substantially equivalent to a legally marketed predicate device. In the context of 510(k) submissions, there are specific considerations for re-labelling or re-packaging. Re-labelling or re-packaging becomes necessary if there are changes to the instructions for use, intended use, cautionary statements, contraindications, or other labelling elements. If the modifications to the labelling are considered significant or if they alter the device in any other way, re-labelling or re-packaging may be required.

   Significant labelling changes may include alterations that impact the safe and effective use of the device, or changes that affect the information provided to healthcare professionals and end-users. Changes to the intended use of the device are particularly significant, as they may influence how the device is used or the population for which it is intended.

   Ensuring that the re-labelling or re-packaging is in compliance with FDA regulations is crucial for obtaining regulatory approval under the

510(k) pathway. The FDA reviews the labelling information as part of the 510(k) submission to assess whether the modifications are appropriate and whether they impact the safety and effectiveness of the device.

At the time of the inspection, the FDA required the production of control documents in compliance with 21 CFR 820.30 under Classes II and III instruments. Additionally, the application for approval under 510(k) was to be submitted a minimum of ninety days before the examination. The documents in 21 CFR 820 are essential in order to explain the efficacy and safety of the device. This regulation is also referred to as the quality system regulation or the Master Device Record. Although the requirements for Pre-Market Approval (PMA) of the medical device were stated in 21 CFR Part 814, the rules for PMA are found in Section 515 of the Food, Drug, and Cosmetic Act (FD&C) Act. The Act is more severe due to the safety and effectiveness of medical devices and the need to establish the facts necessary to establish and approve them. In addition, establishing the facts requires lots of scientific data.

3. Investigational Device and Exemption under Clause of 510 (K) and Design Control (21 CFR 820.30) of Part 812 of the 21 CFR

   Understanding the efficacy and safety of an FDA-approved investigational medical device requires the participation of a small number of willing volunteers. Since the products are not being sold commercially, the pre-marketing information requirement of 510 (k) and the design control regulation of 21 CFR 820.30 do not apply to them. There are exemptions in the FD&C Act for the registration of establishments, the listing of medical devices, and the transportation or shipment of investigational devices. Although investigational devices are not needed to comply with the 510(k) approval process, certain Class III medical devices, such as heart valves, heart catheters, and other similar devices, must do so in order to allow interpretation of clinical data. However, the following permissions are necessary for the experimental medical device.

   Approval from an institutional review board (IRB) is necessary before conducting the experiment, and, in the event that any of them represent a major risk, authorisation from the FDA is necessary. The FDA is also very strict about the investigational drug exemption and the approval that is provided, both of which are required to follow the fundamentals of a clinical trial such as giving permission in writing, noting on the label that the drug is only for investigational use, monitoring the study, keeping records and reports, and so on.

21.6 QUALITY CONTROL OF MEDICAL DEVICES ACCORDING TO THE FDA

Quality System Regulation (QSR) set by the U.S. Food and Drug Administration (FDA). 21 CFR Part 820 outlines the Good Manufacturing Practice (GMP) requirements for medical device manufacturers in the United States. It's common for the term "Good Manufacturing Process" to be a typo or misinterpretation, as the correct term is "Good Manufacturing Practice" (GMP). GMP is a set of regulations ensuring that products are consistently produced and controlled according to quality standards.

ISO 13485:2003 is an international standard for quality management systems specifically designed for medical device manufacturers. The mention of similarities suggests that the Quality System Regulation (QSR) in 21 CFR Part 820 aligns with ISO 13485:2003 in certain aspects, emphasizing a common focus on quality management in the medical device industry. The mention of a "Voluntary Audit Report Submission Pilot Programme" is a bit unclear. It seems to be related to a pilot program for voluntarily submitting audit reports. This may be a program where manufacturers voluntarily submit audit reports to regulatory authorities. ISO 13485:2003 is often used as a reference standard for quality management systems in the medical device industry. It provides a framework for manufacturers to establish and maintain effective quality management systems. The statement refers to "quality management service where the GMP is part of the requirement." This may imply that certain quality management services are required, and compliance with GMP regulations is a component of these requirements.

21.7 RESEARCH CARRIED OUT IN THE UNITED STATES ON VARIOUS MEDICAL DEVICES

Research on medical devices has been streamlined, and each step of the process has been clearly defined, thanks to the enforcement of severe regulations, which have led to an increase in the creation of high-quality data. The following are some areas that have been highlighted here.

This clause is crucial for understanding basic requirement and processes for controlling the design of the device or ensuring that the specified design requirements are to be met.

1. Rule 21 CFR 820 Subpart C published a Rule on the design controls and quality system, and this clause is vital to grasp fundamental requirements and processes for controlling the design of the device or assuring the specified design requirements. The regulation known as 21 CFR 56 disclosed the regulation of IRB and covers the procedures and responsibilities of IRB for the approval of any clinical trial methods.
2. The regulation found in 21 CFR 812 detailed the exemptions for investigational devices. These exemptions addressed the procedures in detail, including the obligations of sponsors and investigators of applications, records, labelling, reporting, and audits.
   Disclosure of clinical investigators' financial status, insurance, and financial compensation was required by the regulation known as 21 CFR 54.
   Regulation of 21 CFR 21 is disclosed for the minimum requirement for Good Clinical Practices (GCP) and the guidelines for clinical studies involving human subjects.
3. The sponsors, manufacturers, clinical investigators, and institutional review boards are all included in the scope of these regulations' applicability. Every

single one of the clinical trials has been carried out in accordance with the CFR.

4. The regulation known as 21 CFR 50 disclosed the rights of the volunteer, in addition to the protection of the human subject. This part is essential in order to have an understanding of the rights of volunteers, including the right to withdraw from a study as a subject, the right to withdraw from the trial altogether, and the liability of the sponsoring organisation in the event of accidents, insurance, or compensation.

21.8 QUALITY ASSURANCE AND CONTROL OF MEDICAL EQUIPMENT IN EUROPE

Medical devices include any appliance, instrument, apparatus, substance, or other product used alone or in conjunction with software to diagnose, monitor, treat, alter, or mimic human physiological functions. The pharmacological, immunological, and chemical processes are not affected by the medical device, but it may contribute to the functioning of the system.

The regulations of the European Union (EU) pertaining to medical devices are primarily regulated by three directives. These directives include active implanted devices, medical devices, and *in-vitro* diagnostics.

21.9 HARMONISATION OF NEW EUROPEAN REGULATION OVER CE CERTIFICATION

21.9.1 CE Certification

For the purpose of marketing any electronic equipment within the European Economic Area (EEA), the CE certification, which was formerly known as EC conformity, was first introduced at the beginning of 1985. The acronym CE stands for "Conformité Européenne," which literally translates to "compliance with European conformity." The CE is also known as "compliance of France." CE is not a regulatory enforcement by the European Union, but it is the sole declaration of compliance between the manufacturer and the applicable regulation of the Machinery Directive, Electromagnetic Compatibility (EMC) Directive, and Low-Voltage Directive (LVD). CE is also the only regulatory enforcement by the European Union. The CE compliance is considered to be self-certification, and it may also be confirmed by a notified organisation following testing, or it may be a combination of the two. It is a declaration that the product in question satisfies the requirements laid down by EU law pertaining to issues of health, safety, and environmental protection. The legal enforcement of CE certification has not yet been created. The responsible person of the manufacturer is required to declare that the product complies with the requirements and is then labelled with the letters "CE" to indicate this compliance. Because violation of the law or making a false statement is a criminal offence under European law, the producer made certain that the product complied with the necessary documents in order to avoid legal repercussions. As soon as the product failed to comply with CE standards, it was removed from the market immediately, and the EU was informed of the product's status as soon as CE standards were violated. It is important that the letters "CE" be legible and not shorter than the 5 mm minimum height required for the product's logo.

21.10 DIRECTIVE 2014/53/EU OF THE EUROPEAN UNION FOR THE LEGALISATION OF CE CERTIFICATION

This is a directive adopted by the European Union on April 16, 2014. Directives are legislative acts that set out specific goals, and member states are required to transpose them into their national laws. The directive aims to harmonize the laws related to radio equipment within the European Union. This harmonization is intended to create a unified regulatory framework across member states. CE certification is a conformity marking indicating that a product complies with the essential requirements of relevant European Union directives. The Directive 2014/53/EU focuses on achieving more legal control over CE certification. The directive likely includes provisions for implementing restrictions to ensure that radio equipment placed on the market meets specific regulatory standards.

The new directive, Directive 2014/53/EU, is mentioned as overcoming or superseding Directive 1999/5/EC. This implies that the new directive replaces or updates the previous directive related to radio equipment. Reference is made to overcoming Directive 1999/5/EC "with the clause of particularly." The specific details of this clause would need to be examined in the text of Directive 2014/53/EU to understand its implications. The overall goal of passing the new directive is to achieve more legal control over CE certification. This may involve strengthening regulatory oversight, enhancing conformity assessment procedures, or addressing emerging challenges in the field of radio equipment.

The enforcement of Article 10(10) of Directive 2014/53/EU establishes the constraints or requirements of authorisation in geographical areas across Europe for radio equipment or medical devices. According to the Directive of Article (10 (10), it was stated that the radio equipment or medical device required authorisation or limitation from a minimum of one member state of the European Union, and that such information needed to be included on the label. Article 2 of the legislation stipulated that a categorical word must be written on the packaging, and that phrase must indicate "Restriction or requirement in" in a language of a member state that is easily identifiable as being the location where the restriction or requirement is imposed.

21.11 RADIO TELECOMMUNICATIONS (R&TTE) AND SOFTWARE DEVELOPMENT: ARTICLE 3 OF THE ACT THAT WAS APPLIED AFTER AUGUST 8, 2017, AND THE REGULATION CONFORMANCE AS PER ARTICLE 10 (10) OF DIRECTIVE 2014/53/EU

Along with the biological device, the electronic and telecommunication industries also required assurance of the product's safety. Furthermore, in accordance with the regulation Directive 2014/53/EU, radio equipment must conform prior to being put on the market. Radio equipment is required to meet the highest safety standards and essential requirements in order to establish electromagnetic compatibility, ensure the safety of health, and make logical use of the radio spectrum.

Additionally, the Rule has taken care of a few other areas, including the protection of privacy and personal data, as well as the secrecy of the data. Interoperability, administration of emergency services and compliance with the combination of radio equipment and software for biological devices were also emphasised by the legislation. The Regulation of 1999/5/EC (R&TTED), which was later updated by Directive 2014/53/EU, has been transformed into the new regulatory framework for medical devices that contain an electronic component. In the European Union, different organisations, such as the European Committee for Standardisation (CEN), the European Committee for Electrotechnical Standardisation (CENELEC), and the European Telecommunications Standards Institute (ETSI), govern the electronic equipment that is used. Harmonisation of the various standards was completed on May 21, 2014, and published in the Official Journal of the European Union (OJEU). It was scheduled to go into effect on June 12, 2017, with the inclusion of Article 48 of the R&TTED Act. This was done with the intention of enhancing the quality of market surveillance. Before being sold, radio equipment must first be pre-registered in order to demonstrate that it complies with applicable regulations. Telecommunication Conformity Assessment and Market Surveillance Committee (TCAM) is appointed by Article 45 of the R& TTD Act and implementation as per Article 10(10) of Directive 2014/53/EU. EU legislation also appointed the TCAM committee.

21.12 DIRECTIVE 90/385/EEC FOR ACTIVE IMPLANTABLE MEDICAL DEVICES

The medical devices are both the most essential prerequisite for survival and the ones that carry the greatest risk following implantation. This type of instrument is classified as Class III by both the FDA and the CDSCO when it comes to the categorisation of medical devices. Active Implanted Medical Devices, often known as AIMDs, are those that are surgically inserted into a person in order to provide medical therapy, diagnostic information, or physiological support for otherwise normal human functioning. Moreover, for the active medical device to operate, it requires supplementary electrical energy or another power source apart from the energy produced by physiological processes of humans or by gravity. AIMDs have a wide range of applications; some examples include defibrillators, infusion pumps, cochlear implants, and ventricular assist devices. In order to protect human health, all AIMDs are required to meet comprehensive safety and efficacy requirements. It is the first directive that was introduced in 1993 as Directive 2007/47/EC16, and used for devices to implant permanently in the human body, and since then, it has undergone considerable amendments (Table 21.2).

TABLE 21.2
A Concise Summary of the Names and Sources for the Harmonised Standards for Active Implanted Medical Devices under Directive 90/385/EEC

Sl No	Reference	Title of the Standard
1	EN 556-1:2001 EN 556-1:2001/AC:2006	Sterilisation requirements for medical devices as well as their definitions. Part 1: Sterilisation requirements for medical equipment that has been terminally sterilised.
2	EN 556-2:2015	Definition of sterilisation and requirements for medical devices. Part 2: Requirements for medical devices that have been aseptically processed.
3	EN 1041:2008	Specifications of various medical devices provided by their respective manufacturer.
4	EN ISO 10993-1:2009 (ISO 10993-1:2009) EN ISO 10993-1:2009/ AC:2010	Biological testing as it relates to the evaluation of medical devices. Testing and risk management are covered in the first section.
5	EN ISO 10993-3:2014 (ISO 10993-3:2014)	Biological testing as it relates to the evaluation of medical devices. Evaluation and safety testing of genotoxicity, carcinogenicity, and reproductive toxicity are included in the third section.
6	EN ISO 10993-4:2009 (ISO 10993-4:2002, including Amendment 1:2006)	Biological testing as it relates to the evaluation of medical devices. An evaluation of the interactions with blood is included in Part 4.
7	EN ISO 10993-5:2009	Biological testing as it relates to the evaluation of medical devices. Test for cytotoxicity *in vitro* (ISO 10993-5:2009) is Part 5 of the test.
8	EN ISO 10993-6:2009(ISO 10993-6:2007)	The biological evaluation procedure for medical devices, Part 6: effects after implantation and local reactions.
9	EN ISO 10993-7:2008 (ISO 10993-7:2008)	Part 7 of the biological evaluation process for medical equipment, focusing on residuals following ethylene oxide sterilisation.
10	EN ISO 10993-1:2009 (ISO 10993-1:2009) EN ISO 10993-1:2009/ AC:2010	The testing and risk management processes are the first part of the biological evaluation process for medical devices.
11	EN ISO 10993-3:2014 ISO 10993-3:2014)	Biological testing as it relates to the evaluation of medical devices. Testing for genotoxicity, carcinogenicity, and reproductive toxicity is covered in Part 3 of the "Biological Evaluation of Medical Devices" series.
12	EN ISO 10993-4:2009 (ISO 10993-4:2002, including Amendment 1:2006)	The biological evaluation procedure for medical devices, Part IV, testing to determine whether or not there are interactions with blood.
13	EN ISO 10993-5:2009 (ISO 10993-5:2009)	Part 5 of the biological evaluation process for medical devices, also known as the in vitro cytotoxicity test.

TABLE 21.2 (CONTINUED)
A Concise Summary of the Names and Sources for the Harmonised Standards for Active Implanted Medical Devices under Directive 90/385/EEC

Sl No	Reference	Title of the Standard
14	EN ISO 10993-6:2009 (ISO 10993-6:2007)	The biological evaluation procedure for medical devices, Part 6: the effects of the device on its immediate surroundings after implantation.
15	EN ISO 10993-7:2008 EN ISO 10993-7:2008/ AC:2009	Ethylene oxide sterilisation residuals (ISO 10993-7:2008) are the topic of the seventh and final part of the evaluation procedure for the biological safety of medical devices.
16	EN ISO 10993-9:2009 (ISO 10993-9:2009)	Part 9 of the biological evaluation process for medical devices includes the identification and measurement of possible degradation products.
17	EN ISO 10993-10:2009 (ISO 10993-11:2006)	Evaluation of the potential for medical devices and the constituent materials they are made of to irritate or sensitise the skin.
18	EN ISO 10993-11:2009 (ISO 10993-11:2006)	The biological evaluation process for medical devices, Part 11: tests to determine whether or not there is systemic toxicity.
19	EN ISO 10993-12:2012 (ISO 10993-12:2012)	The biological evaluation method for medical devices, Part 12: sample preparation and reference materials.
20	EN ISO 10993-13:2010 (ISO 10993-13:2010)	The biological evaluation procedure for medical devices, Part 13: the identification and quantification of degradation products from polymeric medical devices.
21	EN ISO 10993-16:2010 (ISO 10993-16:2010)	Toxicokinetic research for degradation products This is Part 16 and the final part of the biological evaluation procedure for medical devices.
22	EN ISO 10993-17:2009 (ISO 10993-17:2002)	Biological testing as it relates to the evaluation of medical devices. The establishment of acceptable limits for leachable chemicals is Part 17 of this regulation.
23	EN ISO 10993-18:2009 (ISO 10993-18:2005)	Biological testing as it relates to the evaluation of medical devices. Part 18: Analysing the materials from a chemical perspective.
24	EN ISO 11135-1:2007 (ISO 11135-1:2007)	Evaluation of the ethylene oxide sterilisation process for medical devices and other health care items, Part 1: Development, validation, and routine control of the sterilisation process.
25	EN ISO 11137-1:2015 (ISO 11137-1:2006, including Amendment1:2013)	Development, validation, and routine control of a sterilisation process for medical equipment. Part 1 of the evaluation of the radiation sterilisation process for health care products.
26	EN ISO 11137-2:2015 (ISO 11137-2:2013)	Establishing the appropriate sterilisation dosage as part of the evaluation of the radiation sterilisation procedure for medical supplies and goods (Part 2).

(*Continued*)

TABLE 21.2 (CONTINUED)

A Concise Summary of the Names and Sources for the Harmonised Standards for Active Implanted Medical Devices under Directive 90/385/EEC

Sl No	Reference	Title of the Standard
27	EN ISO 11138-2:2009 (ISO 11138-2:2006)	Biological indicators for the evaluation of the sterilisation process for health care items, Part 2: Biological indicators for ethylene oxide sterilisation.
28	EN ISO 11138-3:2009 (ISO 11138-3:2006)	Evaluation of the sterilisation process for health care goods: biological indicators. Part 3: Biological indicators for moist heat sterilisation.
29	EN ISO 11140-1:2009 (ISO 11140-1:2005)	Evaluation of the health care product sterilisation process: chemical Indicators. Part 1: General Standards.
30	EN ISO 11607-1:2009 (ISO 11607-1:2006)	Evaluation of packing for terminally sterilised medical devices. Part 1: Selection and requirements of materials, sterile barrier systems, and packaging.
31	EN ISO 11737-1:2006/ EN ISO 11737-1:2006/AC:2009 (ISO 11737-1:2006)	Part 1 of the microbiological methods for evaluating the sterilisation of medical equipment. Part 1: viable counts of the population of microorganisms.
32	EN ISO 11737-2:2009 (ISO 11737-2:2009)	Evaluation of sterilisation of medical equipment using microbiological methods. Part 2: methodology of sterility tests, approval, and maintenance of a sterilisation process.
33	EN ISO 13408-1:2015 (ISO 13408-1:2008, including Amendment: 1:2013)	Evaluation of the aseptic processing of health care goods. Part 1: requirements.
34	EN ISO 13408-2:2011 (ISO 13408-2:2003)	Evaluation of the aseptic processing of health care goods. Part 2: Filtration.
35	EN ISO 13408-3:2011 (ISO 13408-3:2006)	Part 3: Lyophilisation. Evaluation of aseptic processing of health care goods.
36	EN ISO 13408-4:2011 (ISO 13408-4:2005)	Part 4: Clean-in-place technologies This is part of an evaluation of the aseptic processing of health care goods.
37	EN ISO 13408-5:2011 (ISO 13408-5:2006)	Part 5: Sterilisation in Place Evaluation of aseptic processing of health care goods.
38	EN ISO 13408-6:2011 (ISO 13408-6:2005)	Part 6: Isolator systems. Evaluation of aseptic processing of health care goods.
39	EN ISO 13408-7:2015 (ISO 13408-7:2012)	Evaluation of aseptic processing of health care goods. Part 7: medical devices and combo products.
40	EN ISO 13485:2016; EN ISO 13485:2016/AC:2016 (ISO 13485:2016)	Quality management and requirements for regulatory reasons for medical devices.
41	EN ISO 14155:2011 EN ISO 14155:2011/AC:2011 (ISO 14155:2011)	Good clinical practice for medical equipment and clinical research on it.
42	EN ISO 15213-1:2016 (ISO 15213-1:2016, Corrected version 2016-12-15)	Part 1: General requirements. Symbols to be used on medical gadget labels and information to be given.

(*Continued*)

TABLE 21.2 (CONTINUED)
A Concise Summary of the Names and Sources for the Harmonised Standards for Active Implanted Medical Devices under Directive 90/385/EEC

Sl No	Reference	Title of the Standard
43	EN ISO 17665-1:2006 (ISO 17665-1:2006)	Evaluation of the sterilisation of health care goods. Part 1: moist heat: Procedure, validation, and routine control of a sterilisation process.
44	EN 45502-1:1997	Implantable medical devices (active). Part 1: general standards, including safety, marking, and information.
45	EN 45502-2-1:2003	Active implantable medical devices. Part 2-1: requirements for heart pacemakers used to treat bradyarrhythmia.
46	EN 45502-2-2:2008/ EN 45502-2-2:2008/AC:2009	Defibrillators for the treatment of tachyarrhythmia fall under the category of "active implantable medical devices" and, as such, must meet the requirements laid out in Part 2-2 of the guidelines for active implantable medical devices.
47	EN 45502-2-3:2010	Implantable medical devices (active). Parts 2-3: standards for cochlear and auditory brainstem implants.
48	EN 60601-1:2006/ EN 60601-1:2006/AC:2010/ EN 60601-1:2006/A1:2013IEC 60601-1:2005/A1:2012 IEC 60601-1:2005	Medical electrical equipment. Part 1: requirements and guidelines for safety and vital performance.
49	EN 60601-1-6:2010 IEC 60601-1-6:2010	Medical electrical equipment Parts 1–6: requirements, guidelines for safety, and essential performance. Collateral standard: Usability.
50	EN 62304:2006/ IEC 62304:2006/ EN 62304:2006/AC:2008	Requirements for the software of medical devices and the procedures involved in the software life cycle

21.13 THE DIRECTIVE 93/42/EEC FOR MEDICAL EQUIPMENT

An electronic assembly, instrument, or related article, material, or apparatus is considered a medical device under the directive if it is used alone or in conjunction with other components—including software—for the purpose of diagnosing, treating, monitoring, or preventing disease in humans. Also, any replacement by any device that mimics the activity of a physiological action is considered to be a medical device. This is another aspect of the concept of medical devices.

The directive guarantees the "minimisation" of risk and the provision of safety with the highest possible degree of efficacy. The regulation also assures that any member state can approve a medical device and have it enforced in any other state or country of the European Council. This will lead to an increase in the amount of trade that occurs between governments that follow the same guidelines. There are two sets of regulations for medical products and devices: one for pharmacotoxicological safety and clinical efficacy (Directive 75/318/EEC), and another for proprietary devices and products with an integral unit, usage with combinations, and no further reusability (Directive 65/65/EEC). In Directive 93/42/EEC, a harmonised guideline was definitively established. There are a total of 11 articles that are thoroughly explored in this guideline.

Article 1 detailed the definitions that were used and the scope of the directive that was being implemented. The scope of the article was further defined to include the accessories that are used with the various biomedical equipment in the article. Article 1 of Directive 65/65/EEC states that any device that is used for the diagnosis, monitoring, treatment, or alleviation of any conditions, such as the management of a disease, the contravention of differently able persons, or the replacement or substitution of the function of any physiological or anatomical process, must be governed by the device. Article 1 of the directive is quite specific in its application to the fundamentals of human physiology, pharmacology, immunology, or metabolism. Any *in-vitro* diagnostic kits, devices, or reagents used in combination or individually for the diagnosis of disease, physiological function, or congenital anomaly, or for any clinical inquiry, are also included in the preview. The definition of "Article 1" was expanded so that it included any accessories of medical devices as well as any custom-made devices that were utilised by a competent medical practitioner.

To further understand, it was also indicated that Article 1 is extended to make the producer legally binding for the responsibility of manufacturing, packaging, and labelling the product. In addition, the Act included refurbished instruments as well as products that were ready to sell after being assembled or modified. The statute is quite specific about the marketing of devices, which includes the placement on the market by the maker or any establishment regardless of the expectation of a financial return, the provision of a free product, or the distribution of promotional materials.

1. Article 1 may be extended to Directive 65/65/EEC for the device without affecting the terms of the directive. Specifically, Directive 90/385/EEC is restricted to active implantable devices, Directive 76/768/EEC to cosmetic products, Directive 89/686/EEC to personal protective devices, and Directive to transplanted tissues, grafts, or any product originating from humans like blood, plasma, cells, or blood products. The directive is also restricted to animal tissues or cells, but the Act covers any technology that employs a non-viable product that is derived from an animal.
2. Article 2: Directive to the member states for approval requirements before approval is required to safeguard the patient's safety, efficacy, and health.
3. Article 3 states that the directive was expanded to cover the essential requirements of the instruments in accordance with the requirements that were established for approval.
4. Article 4: The order described interstate communication, transportation, and uniform marketing among union members. The approval of the state assured the Directive's Article 17 and uniform conformance as per Article 11, as well as compliance with Annexure VIII of the directive for Classes

IIa, IIb, and III of medical devices. Additionally, the article granted authority to Article 15 and Annexure VIII of the directive for the clinical study of the medical device in all member states by appropriately trained medical experts. Article 4 ensured, in addition, that any instrument may be conveyed for the presentation of any function of the full council of the state, with the exception of marketing, which is restricted until the approval of compliance is met. Article 1 of Annexure 13 mandates that, for either public exhibition or official use, all instrument information must be in the national language.

5. Article 5 describes the criteria for the reference standard for medical equipment. The obligation to ensure conformity with the article in accordance with Article 3 and the norm in accordance with the European Council falls on the shoulders of the member states. In conformity with this norm, the European Communities' official journal (as defined in Article 6(2)) shall be published. In addition to this, before the draft could be made, it was necessary to take into account the European Pharmacopoeial Monograph.
6. Article 6 describes the standards and technical evaluation procedures that were established by Article 5 of Directive 83/189/EEC.
7. Article 7 presents information regarding the Committee on Medical Devices The committee established the commission in accordance with the provisions outlined in Article 6 (2) of Directive 90/385/EEC. The chairman has the authority to direct the discussion in accordance with their preferences, but they do not have the capacity to vote. The opinion held by the vast majority was taken into consideration in accordance with Article 148 (2).
8. Article 8 is known as the "safeguard section." After installation, the biomedical equipment should not jeopardise the patient's health, safety, or any other characteristics relating to the instrument's safety. The product is rigorous and relates to concerns of safety and any compromise of safety, including installation. Any passed-down problem of the instrument leads to immediate withdrawal from the market and prohibition of marketing of the instrument. In addition to this, the option for withdrawing the instrument is highlighted, as is the fact that it does not comply with Article 3 and does not support application in accordance with Standard Article 5. Before the matter is withdrawn, the members of the state are made aware of it, a collective decision is communicated to the manufacturer, and the provisions of Article 6 (1) are given, allowing two months for compliance. Article 6 specifies that the final choice about withdrawal is made by members of the state.
9. Article 9 describes the classification of devices and divides them into Classes I, IIa, IIb, and III. The classification of the device is determined based on the criteria outlined in Annexure IX, and any disagreement on the topic of classification is referred to the commission for resolution. In addition, the committee complied with the regulation that was specified in Annexure IX as well as the terms of Article 7 (2), and it notified the appropriate parties as required by Article 10.

10. Article 10 details the post-marketing surveillance procedures for medical devices, which are carried out after a product has been put on the market. In addition to this, the commission was expected to guarantee that accurate information was provided regarding any unfavourable reports regarding the device Classes I, Ila, Lib, or III. The adverse report might be a case of non-functionality, non-compliance, or insufficiency of the instruction as it relates to the usage of the device, all of which could have an effect on the functioning of the device; alternatively, it could be an instance of causality, technicality, or medical inadequacy of the functioning. In this particular instance, both the medical practitioner and the manufacturer were promptly contacted or advised regarding the adverse occurrences that had occurred. Relevant action is contemplated without prejudice as described in Article 8.
11. Article 11 describe establishes procedures that are common and consistent for the assessment of medical devices. This ensures a standardized approach across the European Union for certain categories of devices. The procedures outlined in Article 11 are applicable to medical devices categorized as Class III. Class III devices are typically high-risk devices, and their assessment and approval process involve more rigorous scrutiny. The procedures also apply to devices that are specially manufactured for clinical applications. This could include devices designed specifically for use in medical research or clinical trials. To be used in clinical settings, devices falling under Class III or those specially manufactured for clinical applications must conform to the EC declaration. This declaration may include information about the device's conformity to relevant regulations, standards, and safety requirements. The devices may also be subject to specific tests or quality control measures to ensure their safety and efficacy.

    The devices must align with the quality assurance requirements specified in IEC. This indicates a reference to specific quality assurance standards or criteria that the devices must meet. For a device to be classified as a Class II item, it must adhere to the quality assurance requirements of EC 21.13.13. This suggests that compliance with specific quality assurance standards is a determining factor in the classification of devices.
12. Article 13 describe This refers to a specific article within a regulatory or legislative framework in the European Union that addresses the classification of biomedical equipment. The term "derogative right" indicates that member states have the authority or discretion to reconsider or alter the classification of biomedical equipment. "Derogation" often refers to a temporary exemption from or modification of certain provisions.
13. Article 14 describes the authority or person responsible for the marketing of devices as being in compliance with the EC.
14. Article 15 should be disclosed by the Member States of the European Community because it establishes the protocol for clinical studies. Implantable and long-term invasive devices (Class IIa or IIb) or Class III

equipment are required to initiate the necessary clinical investigation at the end of sixty days following the notice, or else the competent authority will issue the notification, according to public health policy.

15. Article 16 defines the notified bodies according to Article 11, and the Member States notify the commission to designate notified entities. In light of this, the Commission notifies the regulated bodies and requests that the same information be published in the Official Journal of the European Commission. The regulated bodies work to bring the norms into harmony with the baseline standard.
16. Article 17 provides a description of the CE marking rules. According to the requirements outlined in Article 3, equipment that is developed specifically for clinical investigations needs to comply with CE standards. As was said before, the CE marking needs to be comprehensible and have legible, visible, and erasable components.
17. Article 18 addresses the incorrect confirmation of an affixed CE marking. The Member State that has the power to enforce Article 8 specifies that the manufacturer or authorised person must comply with the standards without infringing the laws that are enforced by the Member State. Because of the violation of the CE rule, the member states are obligated to implement a prohibition on any further sales of the product.
18. Article 19 specifies the refusal or limitation for non-compliance with the directive, and Member States have enforced the withdrawal of devices from the market. The reason for leaving the market and the changes that need to be made within a certain time frame should be stated. Members of the council also have the authority to prohibit, refuse, or place restrictions on the use of medical devices in clinical trials.
19. Article 20 is the article that describes the confidentiality of medical devices since, without prejudice, practices are done with the individual's medical information. This information and the dissemination of warnings have previously been disclosed to the Member States and notified bodies; thus, enforcement rigorously adheres to maintaining confidentiality. However, this is not a requirement for Member States and notified bodies. A criminal case could be brought as a result of the failure. The failure could be punished under criminal law.
20. Article 21 is the clause for the revocation of the amendment and the temporal basis for the alterations that are made in the articles.
21. Article 22 describes the provisions of the articles and acts that pertain to their implementation, enforcement, and transitional phases. The directive was published before July 1, 1994, and the standing committee ensured that it was sent to the Commission in accordance with the requirements of Article 7 of the Treaty. Additionally, the member is obligated to inform the member of the provisions of the national legislation and the implementation of the Directive.
22. The fundamental direction for the Member States is associated with Article 23.

21.14 THE QUALITY ASSURANCE MEASURES OF THE CENTRAL DRUGS STANDARD CONTROL ORGANISATION (CDSCO) AND THE MEDICAL EQUIPMENT AND HOSPITAL PLANNING DIVISION COUNCIL (MHDC) OF THE BUREAU OF INDIAN STANDARDS BOTH DEAL WITH MEDICAL DEVICES

As of March 1, 2012, the standards for surgical instruments, surgical dressings, medical equipment, artificial limbs, rehabilitation equipment, veterinary surgery instruments, diagnostic kits, dental equipment, laboratory instruments and equipment, etc., were specified by the Sectional Committee of Hospital Planning Division Council (MHDC) of BIS. These standards apply to the field of Medical Equipment and Hospital Planning.

BIBLIOGRAPHY

Central Drugs Standard Control Organization, Import of Drugs for Marketing in India, published 24/08/2001 Available from: http://cdsco.nic.in/html/importdrugs.htm, printed 25/02/2008 [60] Central Drugs Standard Control Organization, Guidelines for Import and Manufacture of Medical Devices, published 06/10/2005, printed 25/02/2008.

Daniel B, Kramer MD, Xu S. Regulation of Medical Devices in the United States and European Union. *J Med*, 2012 March; 366: 848–855.

European Commission, Directive 93/42/EEC, published 14/06/1993 and valid to 31/12/2008 Available from: http://eur-lex.europa.eu.

Guidelines for Import and Manufacture of Medical Devices India. CDSCO; Accessed February 2009. Available from: http://cdsco. nic.in/medical%20device%20A42.html (Accessed 23 March 2021).

Guidance Document on Application for Grant of Licence in Form-28 for Manufacture of Medical Devices in India Under CLAA Scheme. India. CDSCO; 12 August 2010. Available from: http://cdsco.nic.in/ Guidance%20document%20on%20application%20for%20grant%20of%20 Licence%20in%20Form28%20for%20manufacture%20of%20Medical%20 Devices%20in%20India%20under%20CLAA%20Scheme.PDF (Accessed 23 March 2021).

Guidance Document on Common Submission Format for Import License in10 of Medical Devices in India. CDSCO; 2 August 2010. Available from: http://cdsco.nic.in/Guidance .PDF.

Holbein ME, Berglund JP. Understanding Food and Drug Administration Regulatory Requirements for an Investigational Device Exemption for Sponsor-Investigators. *J Investig Med*, 2012 October; 60(7): 987–994. doi: 10.2310/JIM.0b013e318262df40. PMID: 22847340; PMCID: PMC3448842.

https://eur-lex.europa.eu (Accessed 23 March 2021).

Itech Standard. https://standards.iteh.ai (Accessed 23 March 2021).

Manita, DA, Vikram, RAC, Sharma PC. Regulation and Clinical Investigation of Medical Device in the European Union , Applied Clinical Research, Clinical Trials & Regulatory Affairs, 2019, 7, 1-19.

Munir K, Biesiekierski A Wen C, Li Y. Metallic Biomaterials Processing and Medical Device Manufacturing. In Cuie Wen (Ed). *Introduction to Biomedical Manufacturing*. Woodhead Publishing (2020): 3–29, eBook ISBN: 9780081029664.Shah A, Goyal RK.

Current Status of the Regulation for Medical Devices. *Indian J Pharm Sci*, 2008, 70: 695–700.

Radhadevi N, Balamuralidhara V, Pramod Kumar TM, Ravi V. Regulatory Guidelines for Medical Devices in India: An Overview. *Asian J Pharm*, 2012; 6: 10–17.

Requirements for Conducting Clinical Trial(s) of Medical Devices in India. India. CDSCO; 2010 August. Available from: http://cdsco. nic.in/Requirements%20for%20Conducting%20Clinical%20Trial(s)%20 of%20Medical%20Devices%20in%20India.PDF (Accessed 23 March 2021).

Schedule-MIII. Requirements for the Manufacture, Import and Sale of Medical Devices. Available from: http://cdsco.nic. in/Medical_Devices_Guidelines.pdf (Accessed 23 March 2021).

Sethi R, Popli H, Sethi S. Medical Devices Regulation in United States of America, European Union and India: A Comparative Study. *Pharm Regul Aff*, 2017; 6: 1–9.

The Gazette of India. Part II, Section 3(i). New Delhi: The Controller of Publication; 2005.

U.S. Food and Drug Administration, Overview of Device Regulations, updated 11/10/2007 Available from: www.fda.gov/cdrh/devadvice/overview.html (Accessed 23 March 2021).

U.S. Food and Drug Administration, Hefflin B, Kessler L. The Global Medical Device Nomenclature. Available from: http://www.ncvhs.hhs.gov/030819p2.pdf, printed 10/04/2008 (Accessed 23 March 2021).

World Health Organization Medical Device Regulations: Global Overview and Guiding Principles. Geneva. Available from: http://www.who.int/medical_devices/publications/en/MD_Regulations.pdf (Last Accessed 5 March 2006).

22 Regulation in Practising Telemedicine at the Edge of Data Confidentiality and Medical Ethics

22.1 INTRODUCTION

The World Health Organization (WHO) defines telemedicine as the utilisation of technology for communication and information exchange to provide health care services encompassing advice, medical care, and the prevention of diseases and injuries, as well as research and evaluation. Telemedicine practices refer to the exploitation of online consultations, regardless of geographical distance, or the provision of ongoing education for health care professionals, with the aim of promoting the wellbeing of individuals and their communities.

Telemedicine is also known as treatment by medicine through distance. The use of telemedicine is recognised in many countries and by the WHO, although the regulatory challenges, the protection of right to liberty, and the rule of law remain a challenge. Understanding the legitimacy of telemedicine operations involves many elements, including patient privacy, data confidentiality *per se* and *vis-à-vis* data transfer, data retention, data retrieval, personal data sharing between health professionals, health professional certification, and ultimately the medical liability of professionals involved in telemedicine services. The impressive growth of the telecommunications industry in urban areas and telemedicine systems is also increasing. The country has seen the excellent efforts of the Indian Medical Council (MCI) and the prescribed guidelines for the use of telemedicine after COVID-19 for primary and secondary health care, and protection over a distance of 5 km through Health and Wellness Centres (HWCs). Undoubtedly, this effort reduces the patient's burden on the hospital in secondary care during a temporary closure. Telemedicine or online consultations have also helped every insurance company to see more income and more non-emergency consultations. Patients also monitored their health symptoms under telemedicine consultations.

Officially, the effectiveness of telemedicine is well explained, and the practice of telemedicine is therefore legally binding. Any medical professional involved

DOI: 10.1201/9781003397854-6

with another medical professional communicates via email or via an electronic text message to patients about treatment, or a follow-up visit is explained through telemedicine. The clause corresponds to the definition of patient involvement and, by definition, the patient is a group of users while the medical professional is the service provider. In addition, the definition is also extended to the medical service or treatment of the patient by telephone and is referred to as "telemedicine."

There are many examples of litigation in the telemedicine or teleconsultation practices. The Bombay High Court dismissed a pending bail application filed by a petitioner (Dr Deepa) who was detained under Section 304 (culpable homicide) of the Indian Penal Code, 1860 for fear of her providing telephone medical advice. The esteemed Supreme Court overturned the decision. This case is known as the case of Deepa Sanjeev Pawaskar and Anr v. State of Maharashtra. In this case, Dr Deepa, a gynecologist, admitted a patient to her clinic for surgery under her supervision. The patient collapsed, later became paralysed, and suspected that Dr Deepa decided to administer the drug following the telephone consultation after discussions with hospital staff without examining the patient. The Bombay High Court ruled that the fact that Dr Deepa had prescribed medication without a diagnosis was a case of involuntary negligence. But the remarkable point is the decision of the Bombay High Court to honour the legalisation of the telemedicine practice over the telephone by Dr Deepa. Court appearances forced people to consider the process of whether telemedicine was legal in India. Any discussion, decision, or regulatory measure of any epidemic or videoconferenced public health policy is not subject to telemedicine preview. Similarly, any health information or discussion of any medical conditions published on the website may not be considered under the telemedicine clause. In telemedicine, strict compliance is required and should not violate the patient's rights and privacy.

A policy is needed to overcome the challenges and legal obligations of telemedicine with respect to confidentiality, privacy, and patient rights. Telemedicine, used wisely and appropriately, should best benefit the patient and provide the basic right of access to health services. In addition, telemedicine will be of a high moral standard with the highest service possible without distinction of language, mental ability, geographical location, gender, and education. In telemedicine, many challenges exist, such as data protection, e-commerce, medical device guidelines, distance contract, electronic signatures, competition law, guidance regarding professional qualifications, and ultimately the solution for the patient of any unwanted episode. There is no law or rule specifically dealing with the operation of telemedicine in India.

The practice of treating disease with the help of information technology is known as telemedicine, and laws and regulations governing telemedicine are interconnected between the fields of medicine and information technology. Other important issues include the legitimacy of Article 19 of the Constitution of India, which gives every citizen of India a basic right to freedom of speech and expression. Therefore, the practice of telemedicine has a legal responsibility to protect the rights of every patient. Indian laws are permitted to impose both criminal and civil penalties for improper disclosure, administration, sale, or financial gain through the disclosure of any medical information or data. The technical features of telemedicine must ensure

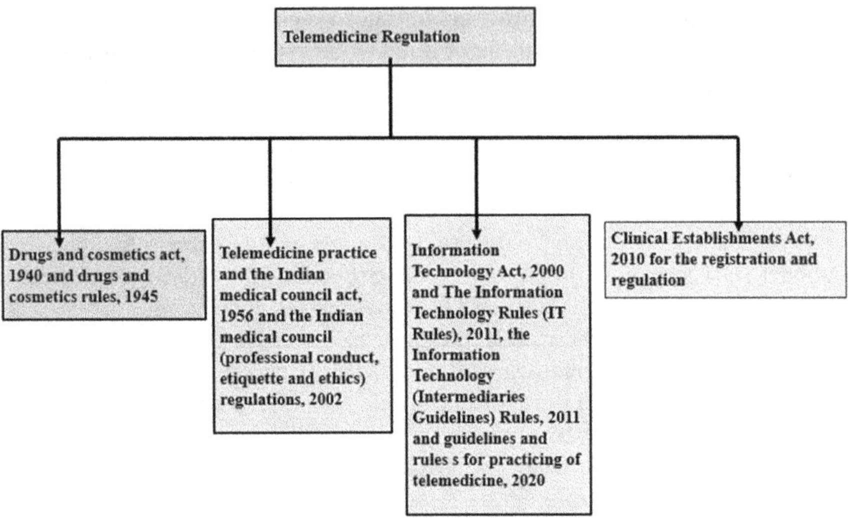

FIGURE 22.1 Telemedicine practicing regulated by different rules.

that no data leaks occur and that the individual's rights are protected. Understanding the legal aspects of telemedicine has briefly highlighted the relevant legislation with which a doctor must comply.

There is no current provision in health insurance policies regarding the effectiveness of telemedicine. If a refund claim is made for the use of telemedicine, it will raise a question about the debt of the equipment manufacturer, equipment dealer, equipment operator, repair service provider, and telecommunications company. It will be even harder if you are a health care provider at both ends or in a supportive hospital. The question of inadequate training or misuse and the decision to use or not to use or misinterpret the findings will be a major problem. Questions will also arise whether the whole process was necessary or not, whether it was simply to obtain financial benefits. Therefore, the practice of telemedicine has many of the challenges listed in Figure 22.1.

22.2 TYPES OF TELEPHONE CONSULTATIONS

22.2.1 Provision of Health and Hygiene Education

Any health promotion or hygiene practices, as well as disease prevention messages by doctors, e.g., advice on diet, prevention of infectious diseases, vaccination, exercise, exercise, mosquito control, etc., are included in this section.

22.2.2 Counselling or Advice

This is patient-centred counselling and treatment related to reducing the underlying condition, including dietary restrictions, home physiotherapy, use of a hearing aid, hygiene, etc. Suggestions for new research to be done before the next consultation are also considered at this stage.

22.2.3 Prescribing Medication

The doctor may prescribe medication via telemedicine after the completion of any diagnosis, and medication may be prescribed as a single rule for the benefit of the patient.

22.3 THE USE OF TELEMEDICINE IS SUBJECT TO THE CONSUMER PROTECTION ACT, 1986

Adapting to telemedicine is a legal consideration and there are many technical challenges. "Neglect" in a medical profession is conditionally challenging, and telemedicine cannot escape. The process of telemedicine is complex, and the chances continue that malfunction of software or computer systems can leads to death, where blame cannot be denied. The failure of the complex telemedicine process, resulting in death, could not be attributed to "*force majeure*," rather than to "ignorance."

The Supreme Court decision against Criminal Appeal Number 144–145 of 2004 (Jacob Mathew v. State of Punjab and others) that a physician should also be prosecuted as the case cannot be denied as it resulted in the death of a patient. But establishment of the facts is necessary because of the perceived negligence or incompetence of a physician. This is the basis for compensation on the basis of social responsibility.

Neglect is a simple word that is often associated with failure and lack of proper care and attention. This is in defiance of a breach of obligation directly related to breach of liability. When the question of a person's health or damage arises, an action will be rational and logical. The Indian Penal Code (IPC) under Section 304A imposed a penalty under a clause of negligence which attracts imprisonment for a period of up to two years, or a fine, or both. The discussion arises as to whether the doctor can be convicted of a crime by his passing. The Supreme Court recognised the right of citizens, and many cases were dismissed as civil cases against physicians and under the clause of "lack of service" under the Consumer Protection Act, 1986 arising out of negligence. IPC 336 is primarily designed for "rushed or reckless action that endangers human life." Also, the prosecution is provided under Section 337 of the IPC, where the provision is made for any negligence or reckless act that involves harming or endangering human life, whereas Section 338 is for instances where the content causes any serious harm to a person's life by negligence.

Establishment of criminal evidence is up to the complainant. The accused is innocent until the evidence is heard and presented by the prosecutor. Sometimes, evidence and the establishment of negligence in a civil court do not mean that the defendant is guilty of negligence or that it is established in a criminal court. Therefore, information in the medical field is needed to establish "negligence" and accept compensation. Sometimes, acquitted cases cause embarrassment and abuse as well as loss of dignity. The Supreme Court ruled in favour of the banning of such cases.

But telemedicine is a system in which everything is presented electronically and the maxim *res ipsa loquitur* (Let the event speak for itself; no other evidence needs to be emphasised): the principle that the mere occurrence of some types of accident is sufficient to imply negligence. Although there is a case for public prosecution and the establishment of negligence, it is not difficult to prove for telemedicine if someone has not understood a patient's right as described earlier. In telemedicine, "Major Violations" is the most common term used because the evidence is recorded in the system.

22.4 TELEMEDICINE AND THE DRUGS AND COSMETICS ACT, 1940 AND THE DRUGS AND COSMETICS RULES, 1945

The Drugs and Cosmetics Act and Rules need to be understood in the context of telemedicine implementation. Indian law is stringent in that, without the prescription of the doctor and the registered pharmacy, the drug cannot be sold. There is some relaxation on the selling of drugs which come under Schedules H, H1, C, C (1) and X of the Drugs and Cosmetics Rule,1945, so-called over-the-counter (OTC) drugs, but other scheduled drugs could not be sold without the involvement of a registered pharmacist and the prescription of the registered doctor. The schedule–k-listed drugs are not used for disease treatment but for prevention of diseases and can be sold without prescription. The boundary between the OTC drugs and schedule–k is broken and both category drugs are readily available. Psychotropic, anaesthetic, and neuroleptic drugs, etc., are strictly controlled and the selling or distribution of such a drug via telemedicine is difficult when we look at the regulations. Another important point is that every prescription requires the patient's name, doctor's name, doctor's signature on the prescription, so that the drug can be dispensed. Telemedicine is a challenge to honouring the Indian law and the correct way to dispense or prescribe drugs to the patient. Telemedicine involves the web-interface format and it is essential that the prescriptions, issued by the registered medical doctor, have the valid doctor's signature according to the Drugs and Cosmetic Rules 1945; any violation may treat the prescription as invalid according to the law.

22.5 TELEMEDICINE PRACTICE AND THE INDIAN MEDICAL COUNCIL ACT, 1956, AND THE INDIAN MEDICAL COUNCIL (PROFESSIONAL CONDUCT, ETIQUETTE, AND ETHICS) REGULATIONS, 2002

The Medical Council of India Act, 1956 (MCI Act) is important for practising under telemedicine. Section 27 of the MCI Act states that all doctors/medical practitioners should be registered with the Medical Council through the State Medical Registration Council. The MCI Act also directs that an individual having the recognised degree in medicine and with a valid MCI registration number has the right to practise medicine in India. Consultation or treatments via telemedicine must take place with a registered doctor/medical practitioner, according to the MCI Act.

Indian Medical Council (Professional Conduct, Etiquette and Ethics) Regulations, 2002 also covers important aspects of the telemedicine practice. Among the ethics elements, this regulation describes the interaction and relationship between the doctors and patients. The law enforced to doctor to obey, and declaration is commenced by the doctor. Understanding the more critically of telemedicine with the ethics parameter the patient consent forms is required with mentioning the benefits, consequences with the risks. Every patient has right to withdraw the telemedicine treatment without any reason. It is an important and without the consent the telemedicine treatment is treated as violation in the aspect of right to freedom of the Indian constitution and sometimes known as disharmony and complicated as professional negligence, duties liabilities and penalties. Under the telemedicine umbrella may be as called the tele-consultation, tele-health, military tele-medicine, tele-monitoring, prison tele-medicine, tele-treatment tele-care, tele-pathology, tele-radiology, tele-consultation, tele-diagnosis, tele-psychiatry, tele-cardiology, tele-dermatology, tele-emergency, tele-pharmacy, tele-endoscopy, tele-surveillance, robotic surgery or robotic follow-up etc and all comes in the regulation and there is no relaxation of informed consent. In the emergency or the treatment of minor required consent from the legal guardian. Any *sue* may be arises with the professional negligence and same liability are endorsed by local provider and distant provider or any involvement of caregiver. Sometimes all share the responsibilities if not clarified or documented of the patient party injury. The license to the doctor is required to practice the telemedicine and the same licensure is valid to across all states of India.

22.6 THE INFORMATION TECHNOLOGY ACT, 2000, INFORMATION TECHNOLOGY 2011, THE INFORMATION TECHNOLOGY (INTERMEDIARIES GUIDELINES AND DIGITAL MEDIA ETHICS CODE) RULES, 2021, AND GUIDELINES FOR PRACTICING OF TELEMEDICINE, 2020

The basic guidelines and standards practice guideline for practicing the telemedicine in India is acted from 25th March 2020 under the advocacy of Medical Council of India. 2003. The Department of Information Technology, Ministry of Communications and Information Technology guided two laws also required to understand which the Information Technology Act, 2000 is and Rules 2011 to practice the tale medicine.

The guideline issued to follow and honour of the two mentioned rules as mentioned and advisable to the medical professional and service provider. Service providers are also under the preview of legal framework of India including standards for using hardware, software, data storage system, data security and clinical devices. The most important to understand about the liabilities and legal window of practicing of the telemedicine without any conflict. The medical practitioner required to accord approval with the digital signature according to the Section 5 of the IT Act which should treated as the substitutes for written signatures of the individual.

The telemedicine based on the exchange of the information between the patient and the service provider. Thus, the process is involved with procedures where the sensitive personal information including the personal information, medical history and as per the rule 3 of the IT rule or more clearly data protection rule endorsed the personal information which the basic right to article 19 (1) of every Indian citizen. Telemedicine is under the deep scanner with the medico-legal parameters and required to compliance clearly because the treatment with telemedicine is involved the transfer of whole medical information of individuals through the telecommunications in the aim to better diagnosis and disease management of patients by the expertise may be another part of the world or country. The transmitting the data is required to taken care with the great caution and legal implication to be understood including the patient registration, insurance, licensing and confidentiality issues. The all information regarding the diagnosis, treatment and other procedure should be rational and actual because of all the communication are in the scanner and documented electronically. The most important to data preservation when the transmitting the radiological reports, live or real time video of the individual, hito-pathological report or the any confidential medical report like HIV, congenital infection etc. Most of the telemedicine are consulted with intranets, local area networks, World wide web, internet, E-mail in the forms of MMS, individual photographs and CT scans through mobile phones to get expert opinion. The consultation is both the user group, and the medical practitioner are benefited directly or indirectly and understanding the Section 43A of IT rule, 2011 involvement of "body corporate" clarify the anyone including firms, company or corporate sector involved the collect personal data, transform, transmit the data for the exploration of the commercial exploration are certainly preview the IT act or data protection act.

Rule 3 of the IT rule,2011 also conferred the individual data protection and the categorically mentioned that individual mental, physical, physiological condition, gender orientation and the medical records are classified as individual property as well as sensitive personal data information. Individual or legal consent mandatory for the dataprotection and the practitioners and the data operator both are required the recipient's consent or consent from the legal guardian in the case of emergency or minor in writing accordingly the rule 5(1) of the IT rule. In the consent have to affirmed by the patients without any objection that data collected could be transferred to the third party which accordingly with the rule 5(3) of IT rule, 2011. The Section 4(1) of the IT rule also conferred that the consent is mandatory to publish the data with privacy policy ensuring the data security. Also, Section 7 of the IT rule, 2011 confers that adequate security of the data transmitting of the third party. The IT rule 2011, mandate that when issues are in the personal data or the sensitive personal data information as per the rules have to conforms the international standard as per IS/ISO/IEC 27001 of information security management or the standard notified the Central Government for prevention of un-authorised interception. Rule 5(9) of IT rule, 2011 also directed for the designated the 'Grievance Officer' and the individual details are to disclose in the web as well as the follows the Rule 5(7) of user opt-out and provision of the modification related individual sensitive data protection should be conferred.

22.7 LEGAL AND ATTRIBUTIONS OF SECTION 79 OF THE INTERMEDIARY GUIDELINE BY MINISTRY OF COMMUNICATIONS AND INFORMATION TECHNOLOGY

Under Section 79 of the Ministry of Communications and Information Technology Intermediary Guidelines) Rules, 2011 accorded the delegate authority to the another for receive, store and transmitting data and the delegate power is often observed to the service providers including internet, network, hosting services, cyber cafes, online payments, e-portal etc. In rule 3 of the intermediary IT rule, the certain relaxation was given with the declaration of responsibility of third part communication. Enforcing the Rule 3 (2), any objectionable or unlawful shall be remove within 36 hours of a request and the involvement of the IT grievance officer. In March 2013 provided the clarification of the section 79 of IT rules, 2011 to understanding that the any third party are involved transaction of the sensitive personal data information mandatory to the get consent from the owner of the sensitive personal information data.

Some e-Health services mostly operated as the third party and have the limited facilities to interact the patients and the service provider. The section 79 awarded such e- health services as intermediary and not liable or exempted the liabilities. Such provision was challenged in the honourable Supreme Court in the case of Shreya Singhal v. Union of India in Writ Petition (Criminal) No.167 Of 2012) disclosed that this provision is the violation of Article 19 of the Constitution of India, which is the fundamental right to every Indian citizen guaranteed to the freedom of speech and expression. Moreover, this provisions not clearly drafted and having the ambiguities. The matter was great concerned that publications of the unlawful matter and the restriction is overlooked the restriction of the article 19 (2). It is hard to accept the logically the removing of such unlawful items required notification from the court, or any government agency and honourable Supreme Court taken the cognizance and stated that any such court order or notification for withdrawing the unlawful matter shall be under the ambit of reasonable restrictions under Article 19(2). More clearly honourable Supreme Court directed that the information removal for the interest of the sovereignty and integrity of the country, conferred the security of the State, maintains the foreign relation, morality, decency with the public relation, relation related the consumption of the court, dishonour of the any public or government order, defamation or incitement.

Unsolicited Commercial Communications Regulations, 2007 ("UCC Regulations") and Telecom Commercial Communication Customer Preference Regulations, 2010 ("TCCP Regulations").

The IT Act regulates and ensures the electronic documents as similar to the written documents. Every company and organisation have to registered with the IT for the doing business with the transmitting the electronic information. The IT act stipulates that ensure of the data protection, prevention of the leakage of any personal data, un-authorised access data, maximum security to the electronics user interface. The regular basis audit for ensuring the practice of telemedicine is in confidential and follows the rules and regulation. Understanding the UCC and TCCP regulations is very clear that Government of India prohibited the sending unsolicited commercial promotional communications by SMS or voice mail. But it is true the no legal bar is established or enforced for sending transaction messages. Therefore, the promotional information of the tele-medicine is not permissible. Understanding more about the statutory laws and the practice of telemedicine that every telemedicine consultation centre has own unique identifiable number or known as TCC code. The each of the telemedicine specialty centers (TSC) are also added to each telemedicine centre with the unique identity. Also, patient encouraged to register the universal identified number to relocate through the multiple providers without any data losing and build to comprehensive medical data of the individual patients. The specification of hardware and software, vendor responsibilities for legislation of governing of telemedicine should be clarified in the future concurrence if any requirement. The captive model of the practice with telemedicine is more comprehensive and controlled by only involvement of the telemedicine specialty centers and telemedicine control centers with the own operating entity and network. While the second model based on the multi-tier structure where the service or network provider is third party and incentive-based service provider. Most of service provider in India is follows the multit-ier based because of less investment with minimum risk involvement.

22.8 OTHER SERVICE PROVIDER'S REGULATIONS ("OSP REGULATIONS") IN TELECOM POLICY 1999

Telemedicine is categorised as the other "Application Services" where the medical or professional are practiced by using telecom resources and telecom service is the service providers. Therefore, any telemedicine is practicing within the India shall be registered with the department of the telecommunication as the 'Other Service Provider' ("OSP").

22.9 THE CLINICAL ESTABLISHMENTS ACT, 2010 FOR THE REGISTRATION AND REGULATION

Since the medical practice in under the roof or establishments by using the telecommunication and according to the law of Clinical Establishments Act such establishment is under the categorised definition of a 'clinical establishment'. The uniform Clinical Establishments Act are enforced to the many states like Uttar Pradesh, Uttarakhand, Arunachal Pradesh, Bihar, Jharkhand, Rajasthan, Himachal Pradesh, Mizoram, Meghalaya, Sikkim and all Union Territories except the NCT of Delhi. A few states such as Maharashtra, Assam, West Bengal and Karnataka regulated by their own established state clinical legislations. Therefore, telemedicine service centre and telemedicine service expert both have to register the Clinical Establishments Act 2010, for service providing or practicing with the telemedicine.

22.9.1 Liability and Dispute

The liabilities could not be denied for the violation of laws with practicing with telemedicine in India. Conventions may be with the various angle of defaulting the telemedicine practice which may be civil or criminal proceedings against the providing service by the establishment, service provider, institutions or individual doctor.

22.10 CIVIL CONTEMPT IN NEGLIGENCE OF TELEMEDICINE PRACTICE

Any breach of obligations of contractual in between the e-Health service provider and the patient/user leads to the civil contempt. The negligence of the duty from the service provider or the employees may be convicted toward to Trout law. Lack of negligence of the duty or the breach of trust may dispute to the liquidated damage or un-liquidated damaged to be decided by the court and to lead to payment damages.

A Contempt of negligence case of Jacob Mathew v. State of Punjab & Anr (2005), according to the honourable Supreme Court, a breach of duty results from doing something that a cautious and reasonable man would not do, or from failing to take a reasonable action that a reasonable man would do, guided by the reasons that typically govern the conduct of human affairs. It is matter of the negligence to establish to understand the failure of execute the legal duty with required care, secondly the breach of the duty and finally the eventual or consequential damage because of negligence of duty or the breach. The breach of negligence in the telemedicine consultation can be effectively established by drawing a correlation with a similar case, particularly Laxman Balkrishna Joshi v. Trimbak Bapu Godbole and Anr. 1969 SCR (1) 206, in this case, the respected Supreme Court made an observation that an individual who presents themselves as capable of providing medical advice and treatment implicitly assumes the responsibility of possessing the necessary expertise and knowledge in the relevant field. When a healthcare professional is approached by a patient seeking consultation, they are obligated to fulfill certain responsibilities. These responsibilities include the duty of care, which include making a careful assessment of whether to accept the case, determining the appropriate course of treatment, and ensuring the proper administration of the treatment. A violation of any of these duties grants the patient the ability to pursue a legal claim for negligence. Therefore, the relationship between the patients and the doctor is well understood with the assigned duty of the profession where the minimum of laxity to overrule the responsibility. Irresponsibility with the patients must be contempt in the angle of negligence of duty, thus claimed compensation has no limit of injury to the patient.

22.11 DISCIPLINARY ACTION BY THE MCI IN NEGLIGENCE OF TELEMEDICINE PRACTICE

Regulation 7.2 of the MCI is specified about the professional misconduct example of the operation without consent, unable to produce of medical records etc. Patients is treated as consumer whereas the doctor is service provider, and the doctor gets the financial gain because of the professionalism. A consumer has the right to raise the complaint in consumer forum or to the directly to the state medical council against doctor for the professional misconduct. State medicals have to take conclusive or refer to the ethical committee of the MCI for expeditious disposal as per Regulation

8.7 of the MCI act. As per the regulation of 8.8 of MCI act, in the event that consumers are dissatisfied with a decision, they possess the entitlement to lodge an appeal to the MCI within a certain timeframe of 60 days from the issuance of the order. If the complaint is established may led to suspension of medical license.

22.12 CRIMINAL LIABILITY IN NEGLIGENCE OF TELEMEDICINE PRACTICE

A criminal prosecution is brought before a criminal court for a variety of reasons, including the conduct of offences under any criminal legislation, which includes the Indian Penal Code, 1860 ("IPC"), which is the focus of the prosecution.

In the context of e-health services, should an individual exhibit recklessness or negligence while providing a service, resulting in physical harm or fatality to the patient or user, they may be subject to criminal prosecution. Doctors and other healthcare providers commonly face charges related to acts of negligence resulting in death (Section 304-A of the Indian Penal Code). Additionally, they may be charged with endangering the life or private safety of others (Section 336 of the IPC), causing harm by acts that endanger life or personal safety (Section 337 of the IPC), and causing severe harm by acts that endanger life or personal safety (Section 338 of the IPC). If an individual is found guilty of the aforementioned criminal offence, they may be subject to both incarceration and monetary penalties.

In contrast to criminal prosecution in typical circumstances, criminal prosecution in instances of medical negligence exclusively occurs when the negligence is characterised by a significant degree of severity. Indeed, the honourable Supreme Court has exhibited a disposition of empathy towards the criminal prosecution of medical practitioners. According to the Supreme Court, individuals who are burdened with the constant fear of criminal prosecution, regardless of whether it is their own fault or not, are unable to effectively carry out critical tasks such as performing surgery with a scalpel or administering life-saving drugs. This statement was made in the case of Jacob Mathew v. State of Punjab and Anr. (2005), 6 SCC 1. The honourable Supreme Court has established a distinct provision for the commencement of legal proceedings in cases involving medical malpractice. The initiation of a criminal prosecution necessitates the presence of a credible opinion from another medical professional, which serves to substantiate the allegations of recklessness or negligence against the accused doctor.

When it comes to questions concerning the detention of medical professionals, the honourable Supreme Court has created yet another unique and important exemption. The Court has established that a doctor who is accused of recklessness or negligence should not be subjected to routine arrest solely based on the accusation. Instead, the doctor's arrest should only occur if it is deemed necessary for the progress of the investigation, the collection of evidence, or if the investigating officer is convinced that the doctor will not cooperate with the prosecution unless arrested.

The legal doctrine of vicarious liability is not applicable in the context of criminal.

proceedings. This would imply that the institutions or online platforms offering e-health services would not bear legal responsibility for the actions committed by their workers.

22.13 VICARIOUS LIABILITY IN NEGLIGENCE OF TELEMEDICINE PRACTICE

In situations where there is a relationship between an employer and an employee, such as in the provision of e-Health services, the employer may also be subject to legal action due to the notion of vicarious liability. Under this principle, an employer is considered to be vicariously liable for the acts and omissions of an employee that occur in the course of the employee's employment. In the context of an employer-independent contractor relationship, it is typically uncommon for the service provider to possess significant control or supervision over the actions of the independent contractor.

22.13.1 The Consumer Protection Act (CPA)

The Consumer Protection Act (CPA) was implemented with the objective of providing customers with an alternative avenue to resolve their complaints, thereby avoiding the costly and time-consuming process of pursuing legal action in civil courts. CPA grants consumers the right to seek redress from service providers in the event of a service fault. In addition to the insufficiency of services, consumers also have the ability to initiate legal actions about defective items and unfair trade practises. Consumer forums have been established at several administrative levels, including district, state, and national, with the purpose of adjudicating such issues.

Previously, there was a degree of uncertainty regarding the inclusion of medical services rendered by physicians, hospitals, or other establishments under the scope of the CPA. The matter was clarified by the Supreme Court in the case of Indian Medical Association v. V. P. Shantha and Ors (AIR 1996 SC 550), which found that medical services would fall under the jurisdiction of the CPA given that the patient is being charged for the service. This decision was made in response to an appeal brought by the Indian Medical Association.

22.14 CATEGORY OF TELEMEDICINE AND REGULATION

According to the practice of the telemedicine divided in seven categories and have different mandatory relations which are as follows:

1	Category 1. The practice of telemedicine is delivered to a patient that is located in a hospital or clinic.	• It is imperative for the practitioner to adhere to both central and state legislation when engaging in their professional practice. • In order to prescribe a control scheduled drugs through telemedicine, it is imperative for the practitioner to possess registration in the state where the patient is situated. • In order to prescribe or conduct research on control scheduled drugs, it is imperative for the practitioner to possess a valid registration with the Drug Enforcement Administration (DEA). • In order to dispense or perform research on control scheduled drugs, the hospital and clinic are required to possess a DEA registration.

2	Category 2. The practice of telemedicine is conducted during an in-person examination with another practitioner.	• The practitioner is required to adhere to both central and state laws when engaging in their professional practice. • In order to prescribe a control scheduled drug, via telemedicine, it is vital for the practitioner to possess the necessary registration in the state where the patient is situated. • In order to prescribe control scheduled drugs, or carry out research on them, the practitioner needs to be registered with the DEA.
3	Category 3. The practice of telemedicine is conducted through the Indian Health Service (IHS).	• In order to engage in professional practise within this particular category, the practitioner must satisfy two specific prerequisites. In order to qualify as a practitioner, one must satisfy either of the following criteria: (1) being an employee or contractor of the Indian Health Service (IHS), or (2) being a member of an Indian tribe or a tribal worker engaged in a contract or agreement under the Indian Self-Determination and Education Assistance Act (P.L. 93-638). Furthermore, it is imperative that the practitioner is officially recognised as meeting the criteria for Internet eligibility.
4	Category 4. The practice of telemedicine is conducted during a public health emergency.	• The practitioner is required to make themselves available to deliver telemedicine services during a state of public health emergency. • The practitioner is obligated to offer telemedicine services to patients located in the area that has been deemed to be experiencing a public health emergency. • The Department of Health Services (DHS) secretary must declare a public health emergency.
5	Category 5. The practice of telemedicine is conducted by a health care practitioner that has obtained a special registration for telemedicine.	• A valid reason for the special registration must be shown by the practitioner. • The physician has to be registered in the state in which the patient resides in order to supply, distribute, dispense, or prescribe controlled scheduled drugs via telemedicine. • In order to ensure adherence to both central and state regulations, it is imperative for the practitioner to uphold compliance when engaging in the delivery, distribution, dispensation, and prescription of controlled scheduled drugs.
6	Category 6. The practice of telemedicine is conducted during a medical emergency situation.	In order to engage in professional practice within this particular category, the practitioner must satisfy three specific prerequisites. Initially, it is essential for the individual providing healthcare services to be a practitioner affiliated with the Department of Veterans Affairs (VA) or a practitioner contracted by the VA, and to ensure that their practise aligns with the parameters defined by their employment or contractual agreement within the VA. In addition, it is required that the practitioner have either a minimum of one state registration for the purpose of prescribing or conducting research on controlled scheduled drugs or engages in the prescription or research of controlled scheduled drugs within a VA health care facility, utilising the registration of said facility. In accordance with regulations, the prescribing practitioner is restricted from issuing a prescription for refillable and extendable controlled scheduled drugs to a single patient that exceeds duration of five days.

		There exist four conditions that classify a scenario as a medical emergency within this particular category. Initially, it is imperative that the circumstances exclude the patient from undergoing an in-person assessment conducted by a practitioner affiliated with the VA or a practitioner contracted by the VA. Furthermore, it is important that the circumstances effectively preclude the patient from receiving care within a VA health care facility. In addition, it is essential that the circumstances preclude the patient's primary care provider and other telemedicine practitioners within the VA system from conducting a comprehensive examination of the patient. Furthermore, it is imperative that the circumstances necessitate the prompt issuance of a prescription for a regulated medication to the patient.
7	Category 7. The implementation of telemedicine is subject to the discretion of the Drug Enforcement Administration (DEA).	The provision of tele-health services by the practitioner is subject to the discretion of the Drug Enforcement Administration (DEA).

22.15 TYPES OF THE TELEMEDICINE PRACTICE PLATFORM

22.15.1 Consultation by Using Telemedicine Platform

Much telemedicine mainly based on iOS and android mobile platform are using in India. These platforms are works through the website or mobile applications and connected both the patients and medical practitioner. The application is providing to the patents, a list of medical practitioners with the specialisation and the medical advice is provided to the patient in the printable format for medication. The medical practitioner to patient may advise to get certain tests underlying medical condition for concluding any medicine.

22.15.2 Consultation by Using Messaging Platform

These platforms are works through the messaging applications and connected both the patients and medical practitioner. This platform is different from telemedicine platforms, in this platform patient generated the medical consultation by a patient through the text messaging. The medical practitioner is provided to the patient in the printable format for medication and patient may advise to get certain tests underlying medical condition for concluding any medicine.

22.15.3 Consultation of Medical Practitioner to Medical Practitioner by Telemedicine

The consultations occur between two medical practitioners and such cases the treating physician or referring physician is involved to provide the consults a specialist regarding a patient under the care of the treating medical practitioner and expert medical practitioner.

This type consultants are takes placed between two medical practitioners informally where the discloses patient information to the specialist for the diagnosis or the course of treatment, thus the legality of the data confidentiality are to be maintained by two medical practitioners. The specialist medical practitioner conveyed the medical treatment to the treating medical practitioner to convey the patient.

22.15.4 Consultation by Cross-Border Opinion by the Medical Practitioner

Cross-border consultations are required the licence to Indian medical practitioner for practicing in foreign while the foreign medical practitioner is intended to practice in India is also required the licence. When Indian medical practitioner is considered as an advisor or referring to foreign medical practitioner is designated as specialist while the foreign medical practitioner an advisor or referring to Indian medical practitioner is designated as specialist. The Indian medical practitioner is executed the treatment through the prescription.

22.16 TELEMEDICINE PRACTICES SOME STANDPOINT, CONDITION AND GUIDELINES

The type of telemedicine practice is divided according to the type of consultation, type of consultation transmitted, purposes of consultation and involvement of the medical practitioner and patents.

22.16.1 The Condition where the Physical Verification Is Required

The telemedicine practice is based on the legal requirement as well the ethics and humanity. Thus, telemedicine practice is based on the professional judgment of medical practitioner and implemented methods.

The diseases where the visual observation is more logical like any diagnosis of skin diseases like psoriasis, lesions etc and medical practitioner should not conclusive or not prescribed by telemedicine.

22.16.2 Patient and Medical Practitioner Identity Disclosure before Consultation

Any anonymous consultation in both the patient and the medical practitioner is not permissible. The patient shall disclose the name, age, address, email ID, phone number while the medical practitioner shall disclose name, address, email, telephone number, registration number as per the National Medical Commission Act, 2019 previously Indian Medical Council Act, 1956, qualification etc.

22.16.3 Emergency Situation and Telemedicine Practice

The telemedicine us not practice in emergency situation and telemedicine practice is only limited to timely care. The telemedicine practice is allowed as first aid measures for life savings, counselling or the further referral. The impersonal care to the patient care is more advisable and the limitation of the telemedicine practice shall be kept in mind.

22.17 CONSENT FROM THE PATIENT

The consent is two types. First, any tele-consultation is initiated by the patient, no more consent is required, and it is self-implied. Furthermore, it is important that the initiation of any telemedicine service is carried out by a qualified health professional or medical practitioner, and that explicit agreement from the patient is properly documented. The record can be electronically retained through many forms such as texts, emails, recordings, or video messages.

22.18 CONSULTATION TO MINORS

The identifying of the age of the patient at the time of tele- consultation is very important. The tele-consultation of minor is legally could be done in the presence of legal guardian or in availability an adult is required, and their address shall be disclosed. Usually before the consultation, the medical practitioner is investigated of the pre-history or past reports or related information. Further, any additional test report is required, is to be tested and report to be submitted to the medical practitioner for further consultation.

Tele-consultation has the own limitation and emergency in life saving measure used as first aid, counseling and advice on referral. Such cases, the patient should be immediately to in-person consultation as soon as possible. The standard of care is the in-person care and the intrinsic limits of telemedicine. Therefore, medical practitioner shall maintain the MCI Code at the time of telemedicine practicing.

22.19 FORMAT OF PRESCRIPTION

The prescription issued according to the format as described by section 1.4.2 of MCI regulation, 2002 and Drug and Cosmetics rules. The practicing of tele medicine implemented the e-prescription and required the registration number. Further, the any form of scan, digital copy of this prescription is deemed to be valid considering the e- signature of the medical practitioner a per the IT rules. Therefore, according to the drug and cosmetics rule, IT rules and MCI code this prescription is endorsed as per the prescription.

22.20 PRESCRIBING MEDICINES THROUGH THE TELEMEDICINE

The government periodically determines the categories of drugs that may be prescribed using telemedicine. The all medicine could not prescribe through the telemedicine and only certain medicines can be prescribed depending upon the conditions of the patients, broadly classified in three list a s follows: -

22.20.1 List O: This list most of the drugs are the over the counter (OTC) medicines which are considered safest medicine. Such as antipyretics and analgesic category like Paracetamol, sodium diclofinac etc and antitussive or anti-common-cold agents like Lozenges or combinations of Guaifensen, Ambroxol, Acetylcysteine, Bromhexene, Ammonium Chloride, Dextromethorphan etc. The list also included the miscellaneous drugs like ORS, supplements of Iron, Zinc, Folic Acid tablets, Vitamin D, Calcium. List O also extended to the use of emergency medicine by the Government ordered like Chloroquine in endemic zone of malaria.

22.20.2 List A: This medicine is limited to practice only those conditions where the diagnosis could be done through the video conferences example diseases like skin, eye ear or any chronic diseases like diabetics. The first consult is over video, or follow-up consultations are to be deemed as required. The drugs like Clotrimazole, Mupirocin, Calamine Lotion, Benzyl Benzoate lotion, Ciprofloxacillin drop for Conjunctivitis etc, or local ear drops such as Clotrimazole ear drops, drops for ear wax etc. The follow up treatment like the management of hypertension like Enalapril, Atenolol management of diabetes like Metformin, Glibenclamide, management of disease like Asthma, Salmetrol inhaler etc are categorised to the list of A drugs.

22.20.3 List B: This medicine is limited to practice only those conditions where the drugs are prescribed by rewrite or new medicine added for follow-up consultations provided in the same medical conditions.

22.20.4 Prohibited List: The drugs are coming under the schedule X which are under the narcotic drugs and psychotropic substances, Act, 1985 (India's anti-drug legislation).

22.21 LIMITATION OF TELEMEDICINE

22.21.1 Applicability

The telemedicine has the limited applicability of the treatment and practices are done according to the MCI Act through the medical practitioner, patients and telemedicine platform or telemedicine service providers. In the telemedicine practice dental doctors and health worker are not included. Hence, tele-nursing, tele-ICU and tele-radiology are not included in the telemedicine. Another important issue that telemedicine practiced according to the MCI Code which bindis the medical practitioner but could not control over the platform are using during the telemedcibene practice. The MCI code also has lack of clarity about the procedure of implementation and how the penalised about any violation.

22.21.2 Security and Data Protection

The implementation of the information technology act for the data security, still the many issues are existed because information technology act and data privacy regulation does not provide guarantee of the manner/level of protection because if the privacy policy/terms of use regulating this data. The validation and standard of the software checking, no regulatory authority is available. Thus, the liability of the any damage to the patient by the data privacy could not establish.

Another challenge is development of many app developments and using without government approval and control where the privacy data are stored. India's data protection regulation is not providing any guarantee to the individuals and also virtually unprotected. In the context of patients seeking medical advice from individual healthcare providers using informal messaging applications, it is incumbent upon the healthcare provider to uphold patient data protection in accordance with India's or country's data protection regulations. Artificial intelligence (AI) and machine learning (ML) platforms aren't used by medical professionals in telemedicine practices. In telemedicine practice, medical practitioner shall be informed to the patients about the data privacy and mandatory of the informed consent. Any unsolicited health information is provided by the patient shall be kept with the privacy.

22.21.3 Protection to Minors

In telemedicine practice, medical practitioner shall be keeping the interest of minor patients and such case the consent is required from the legal guardian. The advice or the treatment shall be rendered without the parents of the sensitive subjects e.g., mental health/reproductive health consultations of the minor.

22.21.4 Prescribing Medicines

There is limitation of the prescribing of the medicine and only the medicine listed in the list B admitted in –person consultation and the in- person consultation limitation is only six months. Thus, the changing with the RMP and how the medicine of list –B is admitted is not clarified.

22.21.5 Telemedicine Practice within and Outside of the Jurisdiction of India

The ambit of the telemedicine practice is nor regularised within jurisdiction or outside of India and not enforced any laws. The NITI Aayog and the Board of Governors give the significant efforts to regulating telemedicine and excelled COVID-19 pandemic. The guidelines are only primarily guidance for consulting remotely rather than the regulation. How the regulatory guideline, penalised procedures of the violator and the hardware or software specifications to be used in the telemedicine practice are not mentioned. There is required to regulate and enforced the tele-health technologies. According to the MCI Act the doctors name is a part of the Indian Medical Register, which is considered central register are eligible to practice as a medical practitioner in any part of India. However, certain state medical council legislations enforced to medical practitioner to register under the state register for medical practice. In such conditions, the regulatory of the telemedicine shall be ensured that medical practitioner registered in any part of the country is unrestricted to practice nation-wide.

22.22 TELEMEDICINE PRACTICING IN USA

The using of information or information technology-based health care system including the medical apps are regulated in USA. Initially, the Food and Drug Administration Safety under the Food and Drug Administration (FDA) with the necessary directives of National Coordinator for Health Information Technology (ONC) first the drafted the regulatory framework for health information technology. Furthermore, in 2014, there was a further strengthening of regulations aimed at governing the field of m-Health (mobile health) and its utilisation. The parties involved have established a memorandum of understanding, outlining their commitment to collaborate within their respective areas of jurisdiction. This collaboration will focus on existing technologies and upcoming advances in the field of mHealth, with the intention of regulating their utilisation. On October 16, 2018, USA enforced the regulation for telemedicine under sections 822 and 831(h)(1) of Title 21 for the minimum requirement practitioners and required to special registration to practice including the prescription, dispensing of the controlled substances using telehealth from false or misleading claims. Federal Trade Commission (FTC) is the authority for the data protects and prevents data breaches associated with IT and convert the medico-legal cases.

FDA executed and promoted innovation concerning patient safety while FTC is acting against the unfair or deceptive acts or misleading claims and protects the patient interest. Also, FTC's controlling the effectiveness of the mHealth implementation and have the jurisdiction for the insurance cover and telemedicine in the enforcement of Health Insurance Portability and Accountability Act. The practicing of telemedicine is a challenging because of the logistic, insurance, reimbursement, standard of treatment and confidentiality. In US, individual practitioners have to registered or having licensed for practicing with telemedicine. The American Medical Association's encourages the physician–patient relationship and further encourages "face-to-face relationship" before telemedicine practicing.

22.23 TELEMEDICINE PRACTICING IN EUROPEAN UNION

European law regulated by 2011/24/EU about all health-related services, and the telemedicine regulated under the directives of 95/46/EU, 2000/31/EC and 2002/58/EC respectively. The practicing of telemedicine and practicing of medicine are very similar – understanding of the patient problems. Diagnosis and finally prescription or information about the treatment and EU provided to uniform laws including the medical liability and of medical *leges artis*. The mall practicing of telemedicine and accusation of criminal liability or trout law is not specific Probably such standardisation will never take place, since the European Union does not have, until now, a common set of norms regarding tort and criminal liability, much less specific which is one of the reasons jeopardise the practicing of EU telemedicine.

22.24 LEGAL PROVISION OF PRACTICING TELEMEDICINE IN EU

Article 3(1)(a) of Directive 2005/36/EC directed about the practicing of the medicine and health care by involvement of the health care professionals while Articles 56 and 57 provisioned the telemedicine practicing. The laws enacted the both the health care and information system as similar US and India. The main directive of telemedicine in EU as follows: -

	Directive	Summary
1	Directive 95/46/EU	Regulation on protection of individuals and personal data
2	Directive 98/34/EC	Regulation on information in the field of technical standards
3	Directive 2002/58/EC	Regulation on the electronic transformation of personal data and the protection of privacy
4	Directive 2011/24/EU	Regulation on patients' rights in cross-border healthcare
5	Directive 2011/890/EU	Implementation of National e-Health

Similar to the other countries like US and India, EU is also enforcement the telemedicine in the direction of patient's right, data protection, registration of the medical professionals and implementation of e-health care system. The EU ensures the telemedicine service as the standard health care services and accessible to every European patient. Addressing of Global health issues, EU enforced the e prescription system through the European Patients Smart Open Services project (epSOS). Further, EU recommended the cross-border health records system and exchanges among the EU. Directive 2011/24/EU is important for the e- medicine practicing and directive for the patients right and cross border medical claim and the European Communities Court of Justice (Court of Justice) has taken attention for the justice with the patients right according to Articles 3/d, 7/7 and 14 including the reimbursement of cross-border treatments.

22.24.1 Directive of Data Privacy (Article 8/1 and Article 9/1)

The similar to the other country regulation of the issue of data privacy, EU also enforced the provision of the data privacy as the telemedicine practice involved many sensitive data. The information is exchanged in telemedicine are defiantly in the category of the personal data protection. Categorically when the personal data are defined as the person can be identified by identity or many other identified factors like economic, cultural, physiological or societal identification and such it is challenge to the procedure of data privacy at the time of telemedicine practice. Some data are considered as legal related the health and gender or the diseases and regulated according to the Data Protection Directive of Article 8/1 and General Data Protection Regulation (GDPR) article 9/2.

According to the data protection directive article of 8/3 and GDPR article 9/2 confers that individual consent is mandatory when the data are related to diagnosis, preventive medicine and third-party data sharing, cross border data sharing. The controlling authority is liable for the data access, limit of collection of data as per medical act, the data preservation and consent of the patients.

One important consideration is to ensure that the data acquired is utilised exclusively for its intended purpose and not for any future purposes. One important consideration is to ensure that the data acquired is utilised exclusively for its intended purpose and not for any future purposes. Specifically, the commercialisation of data, such as selling it to insurance or marketing businesses, is strictly prohibited in order to generate financial gains from individuals' personal information. In the entire process mainly two authorities are involved among them first is healthcare professional. Health care professionals have to ensure that all the procedure adopted according to the laws and professional ethics. Second authority is data controller of the system and in the entire process is involved of handling of the medical, personal data. The obligation is vested to legal commitment of professional secrecy because handling the individual electronic health record rather paper or records. The subcontractor like the internet service provider also required to maintain secrecy and in the breach of trust prima facie the controller are counted as responsible person as the chairperson the selection process of the vendor where the grantee, security and reliability are required. The controller excises the power to allocate responsibility during the process. The guaranteed data safety is the right of the patient, and the data handler is worked between doctor-patients, server and data storage system. The data handler has to pay attention data collection, storage, unlawful or/and unauthorised disclosure or loss or any breach of trust. Therefore, the terms or agreement with the third party is very important to understand the legality where the action measure can be taken for more conservative in the data protection issue. The security measure is taken consideration like data encryption, electronic signatures and closed networks and maintained the data integrity, confidentiality, authenticity of all transmitted data.

22.25 APPS-BASED AND WEBSITE-BASED TELEMEDICINE AND E-COMMERCE BUSINESS IN INDIA AND EUROPEAN UNION

The real challenges area rising when mobile health applications (apps) and medical electronic devices. Multiple regulatory and security agency adhered with the laws of the country including GPS Location. The producer has the liability and complies with the regulation. In India, Telecom Regulatory Authority of India (TRAI) is authority for regulating the Over-the-top (OTT) apps and which are mostly TV stream Hotstar, Airtel, Sony TV etc. Now a day's smart phone user with internet user increased and TRAI bringing rules to regulate the TV, broadcasting and apps-based industry in India. Apps based telemedicine practice and other services are regulated by TRAI in India. OTT based service including WhatsApp, Netflix, Skype, Hotstar Voot, Zee5, Arre, SonyLIV, ALT Balaji, Jio Digital Life and many more has been signed under the self-regulated aegis of industry body Internet and Mobile Association of India (IAMAI) and it is mandated that content producers should refrain from exhibiting any form of disrespect towards the national emblem or flag, endorsing acts of terrorism, or inciting religious emotions that may cause offence within the nation. It is imperative to consistently uphold the dignity and reverence of the country.

The Supreme Court has issued a notice to Central Government on May 10, 2019, to regulate the content featured on OTT platforms after the petition has been filed by an NGO-Justice for Rights Foundation (JRF). TRAI also regulated the through the licensing mode offer voice, messaging and video call services through applications and whether the revenue losing by over-the-top growth network.

The app application is not limited to the telemedicine and using the buying vegetable to doctor appointment and ensures that the penetration of e- commerce have to follow the basic of regulatory requirement to Indian regulation like Companies Act, Income Tax Act, Service Tax Act, Copyright Act, Patents Act. Also requires complying with Founder's agreement, Vendor agreements, Business registration, App Platform, App charges and data security Disclaimer, Terms of Use and Privacy etc.

22.25.1 Platform for App Application for Telemedicine App

The legal question is arrived when the app shared the platform or where it is functioning or distribution of the app. Most popular platform of the app user is App store, Google play, The Microsoft Window Phone and has their own license agreement like Apple's iOS Developer Program License Agreement or Google's Google Play Developer Program Policies for Android devices. The user license or agreement required to establish for app service.

22.25.2 Legality of Third-Party App for Telemedicine App

It is nothing but the app developed by another other than mobile manufacturing or operating system. The apps Apple used own iOS operating system while Google used for Android devices. Most of third parties are developed apps used by these two platforms. The security is a big concern third-party app stores and chances to infect the mobile device with malicious codes like ransomware and adware. The using of third-party sensitive information may be passed on like Phone numbers, Device information or email addresses and usually to understand celerity the app privacy statement or risk.

22.25.3 Agreements of Legality of Third-Party App for Telemedicine App

An app development required developers, designers, and copywriters and NDA (Non-Disclosure Agreement) is very important legal document while founder Agreement is important to understand equity distribution, obligations, fixed roles and responsibilities and vesting provisions. Development agreement is an important when the joint development with IPR related issue and absence of any agreement of third-party app development is contrary. Noncommercial exploitation if any or future commercial use shall be mentioned in joint ownership.

22.25.4 Disclaimer, Terms of Use and Privacy Agreements for Telemedicine App

Indian Telecommunication rules 2011 enforced to all mobiles apps operating in India declare about the intermediary terms of use and privacy policy available to their users. The whole app has to disclose the grievance officer's name and contact number which is legal binding of the mobile app-based businesses or use and government also extended the huge punitive implications. The Term of app discloses the conditions where the service is provided while the privacy policy explains the use of information collected from them and disclaimer establishes the rights and liabilities of a particular product or service.

The right to privacy is important issue and protected by Indian constituents under Article 21 as an intrinsic part of the right to life and personal liberty. The personal data or sensitive personal information (SPI) collection like name, phone number, email etc and this data could not share with third party. Therefore, fundamental and legal consideration of any mobile app how to maximum provide security to end user. When the app intended to use multi-country required data protection agreement and adhered to the individual country data protection law. Any app attracts below 13 years and mostly online games, or cartoon app comply the Digital Personal Data Protection Bill, 2022 in India or Children Online Privacy Protection Act (COPPA) in USA.

Specially designed the mapping apps where the location can be identified by app server and easily calculate directions, desired destination or location. This app should be third-disclosed third party libraries. Most libraries collect sensitive data and deposit the online servers. Such app makes the digital profiles of users. Such thing can be illustrated a person may give permission to an app to know the location and may another app access to the contacts. But this two individual app used the same third-party library and shared different pieces of information together which is legally not correct. It is important to disclose the software libraries and a few apps declared the policies on user privacy. Thus, every app should be clear, accessible, and comprehensive and adhered to strict privacy policy. Any app shared private data with third parties, required permission from user.

Under Section 43A of the IT rules enforced the Security Practices and Procedures and Sensitive Personal Data or Information (SPDI) Rules (2011) and empowerment for protection of the personal data or sensitive personal information and personal information. Further, the Digital Personal Data Protection Bill, 2022, empowered the data protection and strengthen the legal position on privacy and data protection. The piracy data and beach of personal data protection is liable severe punishment. The confirmatory guideline for standard quality management BS 7799 and ISO 17799 standards are implemented to the employee. The data security, confidentiality and privacy of client information are maintained by the Reserve Bank of India. Also, Indian banks maintains the banking codes and issues guidelines time to time and enforced internal grievance redressal mechanisms within each bank with the designated officer "Code Compliance Officer" and an Ombudsman. The medical practice also kept the confidentiality by the act of Professional conduct, Etiquette and Ethics Regulations, 2002 or Code of Ethics Regulations, 2002. Thus, confidentiality shall be guaranteed to the client according to the Constitutional right and commendation upto INR 50,000,000 is payable according to merits of defaults.

22.25.5 Designs and Trade Secrets of Telemedicine App

The App developed via outsources and the vendor agreement according the "work for hire" clause where the IPR claiming, and rights vested to the developed company. IPRs is important – it is not only protection also equally gives free from infringing on someone IPR. Alternative, intellectual rights can be protected by trade secret agreements where the unauthorised public disclosures are prohibited exceptional for promotional activities. The app code also required to register for prevention of duplicity of the app designs/features.

22.25.6 Telemedicine App Charges and Data Security

Distribution and mostly uses the platforms of the Android, IOS or Windows the app charges required to mention. The offence is counted by IT Act, 2000 under Section 43 (h), when charge the services availed by one person to the account of another person. The collection, storage and protection of the data particularly in the sensitive area addressed with caution. Intermediary data to preserve and retain information as per the Section 67C of the IT Act and the "Intermediary" definition included all telecom, web hosting, internet and network service providers.

BIBLIOGRAPHY

AMD Global Telemedicine. I want to "do telemedicine": What is involved and how much does it cost. July 9, 2015. Available from: http://www.amdtelemedicine.com/blog/article/i-want-do-telemedicine-what-involved-and-how-much-does-it-cost.

Case C-372/04. Judgment of the Court (Grand Chamber) of 16 May 2006. The Queen, on the application of Yvonne Watts v Bedford Primary Care Trust and Secretary of State for Health. European Court Reports. 2006 Available from: http://eur-lex.europa.eu/legal-content/EN/TXT/?uri=CELEX:62004CJ0372.

Cavoukian V. Privacy by design [cited 2015 September 15]. Available from: https://www.ipc.on.ca/images/Resources/privacybydesign.pdf.

Commission implementing decision of 22 December 2011 providing the rules for the establishment, the management and the functioning of the network of national responsible authorities on eHealth. *Official Journal*. 2001; L 344:48–50. Available from: http://data.europa.eu/eli/dec_impl/2011/890/oj.

Council Directive 85/374/EEC of 25 July 1985 on the approximation of the laws, regulations and administrative provisions of the member states concerning liability for defective products. *Official Journal*. 1985; L 210:29–33. Available from: http://data.europa.eu/eli/dir/1985/374/oj.

Council Directive 93/42/EEC of 14 June 1993 concerning medical devices. *Official Journal*. 1993; L 169:1–43. Available from: http://data.europa.eu/eli/dir/1993/42/oj.

Dinakaran D, Manjunatha N, Kumar CN, Math SB. Telemedicine practice guidelines of India, 2020: Implications and challenges. *Indian J Psychiatry*. 2021 January–February;63(1):97–101. doi: 10.4103/psychiatry.IndianJPsychiatry_476_20. Epub 2021 Feb 15. PMID: 34083829; PMCID: PMC8106416.

Directive 95/46/EC of the European Parliament and of the Council of 24 October 1995 on the protection of individuals with regard to the processing of personal data and on the free movement of such data. *Official Journal.* 1995; L 281:31–50. Available from: http://data.europa.eu/eli/dir/1995/46/oj.

Directive 98/34/EC of the European Parliament and of the Council of 22 June 1998 laying down a procedure for the provision of information in the field of technical standards and regulations. *Official Journal.* 1998; L 204:37–48. Available from: http://data.europa.eu/eli/dir/1998/34/oj.

Directive 2002/58/EC of the European Parliament and of the Council of 12 July 2002 concerning the processing of personal data and the protection of privacy in the electronic communications sector (Directive on privacy and electronic communications). *Official Journal.* 2002; L 201:37–47. Available from: http://data.europa.eu/eli/dir/2002/58/oj.

Frequently Asked Questions [FAQs] on telemedicine practice guidelines, Medical Council of India, Ministry of Health and Family Welfare, Guidelines. Available from: https://www.nmc.org.in/MCIRest/open/getDocument?path=/Documents/Public/Portal/LatestNews/Final_FAQ-TELEMEDICINE%20%206-4-2020..pdf (Accessed on 6 October 2023).

Hari Subramaniam Subramaniam & Associates (SNA) Aditi Subramaniam Subramaniam & Associates (SNA) Idia Data Protection 2019: Laws and regulations | India | ICLG. Available from: https://iclg.com/practice-areas/data-protection-laws-and-regulations/india 4/39.

Available from: https://www.shoneekapoor.com/legal-requirements-for-mobile-app-ecommerce-business-in-india

Information technology (intermediary guidelines and digital media ethics code) rules, ministry of electronics and information technology 2021. Available at: www.meity.gov.in/writereaddata/files/IT%20Intermediary%20Rules%2C%202021%20updated%20on%2028.10.2022.pdf) (Accessed on 6 October 2023).

Kadzielski MA, Kim JY. Telemedicine: Many opportunities, many legal issues, many risks. AHLA Connections. 2014 July. Available from: http://www.pepperlaw.com/resource/178/2412.

Kelly B. E-Health: Ethical and data privacy challenges in the EU [cited 2015 February 4]; Informa. 2011 Available from: https://www.cov.com/~/media/files/corporate/publications/2011/04/e-health---ethical-and-data-privacy-challenges-in-the-eu.pdf.

Krupinski EA, Bernard J. Standards and guidelines in telemedicine and telehealth. *Healthcare (Basel).* 2014 February 12;2(1):74–93. doi: 10.3390/healthcare2010074. PMID: 27429261; PMCID: PMC4934495.

McLaughlin P. The proliferation of mobile devices and apps for health care: Promises and risks. Privacy & Security Law Report. 2011 June 27; Available from: https://www.foley.com/files/Publication/384118ed-894a-48e0-9594-6b4b1cf13d1c/Presentation/PublicationAttachment/197c3d9f-5c8e-4762-8284-7102074d86e3/PVLR.pdf

Nair MH. Nair Supreme Court judgement on criminal medical negligence: A challenge to the profession. *Indian J Med Ethics.* 2005;II(4) October–December 110–111.

Order dated July 25, 2018, in Criminal Anticipatory Bail Application No. 513 of 2018 passed by Justice Sadhana S. Jadhav of the Bombay High Court.

Proposal for a Regulation of the European Parliament and of the Council on the protection of individuals with regard to the processing of personal data and on the free movement of such data (General Data Protection Regulation) /COM/2012/011 final - 2012/0011 (COD)/. Available from: http://eur-lex.europa.eu/legal-content/en/ALL/?uri=CELEX:52012PC0011.

Raposo VL. O fim da "letra de médico": Problemas suscitados pelo processo clínico electrónico em sede de responsabilidade médica. *Lex Medicinae.* 2013;10(19):51–77.

Sánchez-Caro J, Abellán F. *Telemedicina y protección de datos sanitarios.* Granada: Editorial Comares; 2002.

Silverman RD. Current legal and ethical concerns in telemedicine and e-medicine. *J Telemed Telecare*. 2003;9(1_suppl):67–69. doi:10.1258/135763303322196402.

Telemedicine in India. Nitin Desai Associate, 2020 October. Available from: https://nishith-desai.com/fileadmin/user_upload/pdfs/Research_Papers/Telemedicine-in-India.pdf (Accessed on 4 January 2021).

Telemedicine Practice, Medical Council of India, Ministry of Health and Family Welfare, Guidelines. Available from: https://www.mohfw.gov.in/pdf/Telemedicine.pdf) (Accessed on 6 October 2023).

The digital data protection bill 2018. Ministry of Electronics and Information Technology, 2023. Available from: https://www.meity.gov.in/writereaddata/files/The%20Digital %20Personal%20Data%20Potection%20Bill%2C%202022_0.pdf (Accessed on 6 October 2023).

The special registration for telemedicine: In brief. Available from: https://fas.org/sgp/crs/misc /R45240.pdf (Accessed on 3June 2019).

Venkatesh U, Aravind GP, Velmurugan AA. Telemedicine practice guidelines in India: Global implications in the wake of the COVID-19 pandemic. *World Med Health Policy*. 2022 September;14(3):589–599. doi: 10.1002/wmh3.497. Epub 2022 Feb 21. PMID: 35601469; PMCID: PMC9111269.

WHO. A health telematics policy in support of WHO's Health-For-All strategy for global health development: Report of the WHO group consultation on health telematics, 11–16 December 1997. Geneva, World Health Organization, 1998.

23 Compressed Medical Gases
Regulations and Quality Control

23.1 INTRODUCTION

Medical and pharmaceutical gases are compressed liquids that are only used for therapeutic and pharmaceutical purposes. Medical gases are classified as therapeutic (pharmaceutical) when used to treat disease, provide life support, and protect individuals from breathing emergencies. The COVID-19 pandemic has brought to light a persistent issue in the world's medical oxygen supply. This crisis was already causing problems prior to the rise in COVID-19 cases that occurred around the world. Oxygen is absolutely necessary for the treatment of a wide variety of otherwise fatal illnesses, including pneumonia and acute respiratory failure.

Many accidents have occurred as a result of the improper use of medical gases, and medical gases are strictly regulated by the Government. A 20-year-old patient who suffered brain damage during a dental procedure (2009) claims that two gas lines, oxygen and nitrous oxide, were crossed at the time of design. A patient went into a coma after being given nitrous oxide incorrectly during surgery at Nagercoil Government Hospital (India) (Madras High Court W.P. (MD) No.4301 of 2013), and the petitioner was compensated. Another example is the death of over 60 children at the BRD Medical College in Gorakhpur (India) from August 7 to 12, 2018 due to a lack of oxygen. Every country has established its own regulatory system to ensure patient safety. Medical gas is strictly regulated in terms of quality, standard, and handling.

Many accidents occur around the world as a result of inappropriate medical gas administration. In Castellaneta (Italy), eight heart patients died after inhaling nitrous oxide instead of oxygen. Contaminated gas is another major concern. As a result, medical gas regulations are strictly enforced in the United States, India, the United Kingdom, and throughout the world. A medical gas is a compressed liquid before being packaged and administered to a patient for treatment. Medical gas is used as an anaesthetic in surgery and as a drug delivery agent. Because medical gases fall under the drug category in Indian regulation, every manufacturer is required to obtain a licence and adhere to the regulating agency's quality controls. The purity of medical gases should be extremely high (99.5%). Medical gases are stored in containers made of materials such as aluminium, stainless steel, or non-corrosive, non-reactive metals. Gas pipelines in hospitals are designed to provide medical gases, vacuum,

 DOI: 10.1201/9781003397854-7

and manage waste anaesthesia exhaust systems. Safety is crucial in the installation and maintenance of gas lines.

Various safety features such as alarm systems, gauges, and testing facilities are integrated to ensure safe operations. The maintenance of gas lines involves the collaboration of various professionals, including anaesthesiologists, engineers, maintenance personnel, pharmacists, nurses, and gas suppliers.

- Oxygen (O_2): Used for treating hypoxaemia or hypoxia.
- Nitrogen (N_2): Utilized for hypoxic challenge.
- Nitrous Oxide (N_2O): Mixed with diluents for anaesthesia and analgesia treatments.
- Carbon Dioxide (CO_2): Employed for extracorporeal oxygenation or respiratory stimulation.
- Medical Air: Used to reduce the risk of hyperoxia.

Medical gases serve diverse medical applications, addressing conditions such as oxygen deficiency, hypoxia, anaesthesia, analgesia, and respiratory support.

23.2 CATEGORIES OF MEDICAL GAS PRODUCTION

Medical gas production can be classified into three categories.

23.2.1 Air Separation Units (ASUs)

Standardised processes such as pre-cleaning, compression, and chilling, followed by fractional distillation of liquefied air are used to separate according to the liquefaction temperature the three gases, namely oxygen, nitrogen, and argon, that are found in atmospheric air. These gases are then collected and stored in separate containers. This method results in the production of oxygen and nitrogen of a quality suitable for medical and industrial use. The operation of ASUs is a continuous process that occurs seven days a week, twenty-four hours a day; as a result, some level of technical personal engagement is required. Because of the presence of individuals at the production site, vital steps in medical gas production, such as the validation of the batch record, are stringently regulated or inspected by the authority. This is the rationale behind the implementation of Good Manufacturing Practice (GMP) standards for the testing, validation, and in-process control of automated processes and equipment functionality. In the manufacturing process, the mixing of medical gases is a greater risk, and, at times, it can be dangerous; mishaps like those described previously can be caused as a result.

23.2.2 Transfers

Low-temperature liquefaction of air results in the production of oxygen, nitrogen, argon, and other mixes of rare gases, and this liquefaction is achieved according to the individual gas liquefaction temperatures. This common process is used to manufacture medical gases. The entirety of the process is carried out in accordance with the requirements of the ASTM F2773—13 standards (2017). The technique of fitting larger tanks with smaller containers and then appropriately separating the various gases into their respective compartments is known as cascading.

23.2.3 Chemical Synthesisers

Chemical synthesisers are instruments that are utilised in the bulk production of compounds such as nitrous oxide or carbon dioxide. Nitrous oxide can be generated through either the thermal decomposition of ammonium nitrate or the reprocessing of waste streams resulting from the production of adipic acid; carbon dioxide that is produced as a waste stream in various types of industrial production operations can also be treated. Additionally, compliance with GMP requirements is obligatory for the documentation, handling, quality control, and testing of the gas produced gas.

23.3 MEDICAL GASES ARE IN THE REGULATION

Medical gases are treated as "drugs" in most of the country because they are used to treat pneumonia, acute respiratory failure, anaesthesia, and medical support. There are many standards for medical gases, but most countries follow National Fire Protection Association-99 (NFPA 99) in the United States and the Health Technical Memorandum 02-01 (HTM 02-01) in the United Kingdom. Every country adheres to its own rules, and each manufacturer should have the highest level of training to pass the basic examination for Medical Gas Installer Certification. In the US, medical gases can't be sold until they are approved under Section 505 or 512 of the Food, Drug, and Cosmetic Act. In India, medical gases can't be sold, stored, or used until approved by the DCGI, a part of the government. Other governing bodies in the US, such as the Department of Transportation (DOT), the Compressed Gas Association (CGA), and the NFPA, also put the standards in place for compressed gases.

Medical gases are considered drugs and can only be used with a doctor's prescription. Because of this, they are governed by the Drugs and Cosmetics Act or the Rules for the drug for which they are used. Gas Cylinders Rules, 2016 are used across India to carry out the powers given by Section 18 of the Explosives Act, 1884 (4 of 1884), and to get rid of the Gas Cylinders Rules, 2004. The Gas Cylinders Rules, 2016 regulate the transport, possession, and storage of gas cylinders. The Drug and Cosmetics Act, 1940, which is enforced by the CDSCO, regulates the manufacturing of medical gas.

23.4 CHALLENGES IN ENFORCEMENT OF THE ACT

Medical gases are classified as "drugs" due to the important role they play in the treatment of pneumonia, acute respiratory failure, induction, or recovery anaesthesia, and other medical support health care systems. As a result, medical gases are categorised as a "drug" under Section 3(b)(i) of the Drugs and Cosmetics Act

1940. Oxygen is frequently utilised as an emergency medicine as well as for a wide range of medical purposes. Nitrous oxide is used as an anaesthetic in surgery and dentistry. Using the common parlance test, there is no dispute that the products in question are used to treat diseases and disorders and thus fall under the purview of Entry 88 as drugs as defined in Section 3(b)(i) of the Drugs and Cosmetics Act, 1940. The Indian Pharmacopoeia, which prescribes drug standards, includes medical oxygen and nitrous oxide. Section 16 of the Drugs and Cosmetics Act, 1940 grants legal standing to the Indian Pharmacopoeia. Furthermore, the Supreme Court stated unambiguously that Medical Oxygen IP (Indian Pharmacopoeia) and Nitrous Oxide IP represent drugs. They were widely employed in human diseases and disorders for diagnosis, treatment, mitigation, and prevention. As a result, they obviously fell under the purview of Section 3(b)(i) of the 1940 Act. As a consequence of this, medical gases have been given the status of regulated products, which means that they must be produced and transported in compliance with specific regulations. Many different restrictions pertaining to medical gases have been put into place by various regulatory authorities in order to guarantee the highest possible degree of compliance in terms of the quality of the product for the patient. These rules ensured that the Good Manufacturing Practices (GMP) were followed, which contributed to the sector being regulated. The provisions of Subsection 501(a)(2)(B) of the Food Drugs and Cosmetics Act in the US, which controls the manufacture, processing, and packaging of medical gases, apply to all three of these activities. In addition, the European Union (EU) is responsible for regulating the actions taken by the European Directorate for the Quality of Medicines (EDQM), as well as the monographs of medical gases that are included in the European Pharmacopeia (Ph. Eur.) In a similar vein, medical gases have defined specifications in the United States Pharmacopeia (USP40, NF35 (2017)), the Japanese Pharmacopeia (17 (2016)), and the Indian Pharmacopeia (2007) for the United States, Japan, and India, respectively.

In India, the Central Drugs Standard Control Organization (CDSCO) is the regulatory organisation responsible for controlling the manufacturing, storage, and distribution of medical gases. Accidental mixing of gases is still being recorded, despite the fact that the CDSCO established the necessary labelling, colour coding, and warning to avoid mixing of gases. In order to manufacture medical gases and then administer them to patients, one needs to be a trained and experienced specialist in the relevant profession.

23.5 ENFORCEMENT OF THE VIOLATION OF THE REGULATIONS

23.5.1 Dangerous Practices

As a direct consequence of the above, medical gases have been given the status of regulated products, which means that they must be manufactured and transported in compliance with specific regulations. Many different restrictions pertaining to medical gases have been put into place by various regulatory authorities in order to guarantee the highest possible degree of compliance in terms of the quality of the product for the patient. These rules ensured that the GMP are to be followed for manufacturing the medical gases and that GMP regulated most of the drugs and pharmaceuticals being manufactured or those considered a "drug" under Section 3(b)(i) of the Drugs and Cosmetics Act 1940. Precautions with regard to hazards to public safety or the physical safety for the storage conditions of medical gases, with or without violation of the licensing agreement, are audited by the DCGI and noted to the manufacturer; rectification must be made within the defined period, if any are found not to be in accordance with the regulations.

It would appear that a violation of this rule has occurred if the DCGI does not consider the licence anymore, the fails to appeal it, or does neither within the allotted amount of time for doing so. The options to search, seize, detain, remove, and prosecute are all included in the first paragraph of the Seventh Section of the Drugs and Cosmetics Act, 1940. The laws are enforced by the deputed officer assigned to do so by the laws, which include the DCGI of India, the deputy commissioner of each respective district, each magistrate of the relevant jurisdiction, and the commissioner of police or police officer of each presidency town.

23.5.2 Protection of Action Taken in Good Faith

With the intention of implementing the pursuance of rules, no legal proceedings could be taken against the Central Government or Chief Controller or Controller who acted in good faith since they did not deliberately break the rules. In addition, there will be no legal action taken against the Central Government, the Chief Controller, or any Controller for anything that was done in good faith for the purpose of enforcing the regulations (Table 23.1).

TABLE 23.1
Regulation and Enforcement of Rules for Compressed Medical Gas

S. No.	Title	India	US	UK
1	The authority	Ministry of Commerce and Industry and Drugs Control Authority of State.	Center for Drug Evaluation and Research (CDER) under the riles of US Food and Drug Administration (FDA)	Medicines and Healthcare products Regulatory Agency (MHRA)
2	The Act	Gas Cylinders Rules, 2015 Drugs and Cosmetics Act, 1940	Federal Food and Drug Cosmetics Act/ Compressed Medical Gas Guideline 1989	Medicines Act 1968.
3	Official listing of the country	Indian Pharmacopeia	US Pharmacopeia (USP), USP-National Formulary	British Pharmacopoeia, European Pharmacopoeia

23.6 REGULATIONS FOR MEDICAL GASES IN THE USA

The United States Pharmacopoeia (USP) and the National Formulary (NF) both include medical gases in their lists of drugs because they are regarded to be pharmaceuticals. It is necessary to have a prescription in order to use medical gases, and the administration of medical gases should only be done under the supervision of a qualified medical professional. In the United States of America, the guidelines included in the USP and NF regarding medical gases, such as oxygen, helium, nitrogen, nitrous oxide, carbon dioxide, medical air, and combinations of these gases, are legally enforced by the FDA. In contrast, the admixture of gases such helium, carbon dioxide, oxygen, nitrogen, nitrous oxide, nitrogen, medical air, and admixing or combinations come under drugs and pharmaceuticals, which are governed by Section 201(g) of the Act of FDA. As stated earlier, medical gas is the most utilised pharmaceuticals and is endorsed by a special category, including all hardware piping, tubing, regulators, which come under the purview of biomedical equipment.

USP provides a description of medical gases and requires that information regarding the quality, including the strength, purity, and traces of impurity along with the identification by colour coding, be disclosed prior to marketing the products. In the US, the FDA is linked to the Joint Commission on Accreditation of Healthcare Organizations (JCAHO) and USP for the purpose of research and adverse reporting related to medical gas accidents. As a result of the fact that medical gases are classified as oxidants, in the context of the US, the fabrication and installation of gas lines must comply with stringent fire safety regulations in addition to meeting the prerequisites for regulatory clearance. Therefore, the guideline NFPA 99 must be followed when dealing with medical gases.

The FDA is in charge of enforcing Title 21 of CFR, which governs the manufacturing and quality control of medicinal gases. The Act includes provisions for controlling the production of medical gases in Sections 201(g)(1), 321(g)(1), 503(b)(1)(A), and 353(b)(1)(A). Both Section 501(a)(2)(B) and Section 351(a)(2)(B) are accountable for the enforcement of the regulation that was designed to prevent the adulteration of medical gases. Both Part 501(a)(2)(B) and Section 351(a)(2)(B) specified safety standards during the manufacturing process, and this section also describes compliance of the prescribed strength and purity levels. Section 211.165(a) describes the test of the finished products of medical gases. Briefly, the regulation can be summarised as follows:

23.6.1 Equipment Design, Size, and Locations

This would be a specific section within the regulations outlining requirements related to the manufacturing process for finished pharmaceuticals. The section likely provides details on the manufacturing process, including the location (facility), equipment used, and operational procedures. The mention of GMP indicates that the section is related to ensuring compliance with Good Manufacturing Practices, which are regulations and guidelines that ensure the quality and safety of pharmaceutical products. The clause ensuring appropriate gases are contained in the appropriate enclosures emphasizes the importance of controlling the manufacturing environment, which is a key aspect of GMP.

The quality assurance of the finished product is discussed in Section 211.84(a), which details procedures such as sampling from the minimal lot, undergoing testing, and reporting the results.

23.7 QUALITY CONTROL OF MEDICAL GASES AS PER FDA REGULATION

1. Section 211.84(b) explains the minimum number of samples that must be taken from the test
2. Section 211.84(d)(1) The provision may be emphasizing the necessity for a minimum testing requirement to identify or verify the quality of packed gases used in the manufacturing process.
3. Section 211.84(d)(2) describes the requirements for testing and ensuring that the strength, purity, and quality meet all specifications. The test report should include information about the component, a specific identity test, and an analysis of the supplier's reliability. It is hard to know when the gas is supplied in bulk, and sometimes it may not be possible.
4. Section 211.160(b) describes the requirements for scientific credentials for testing laboratories, including the right specifications, sampling, qualitative and quantitative requirements for tests of identity, strength, quality, and purity.
5. Section 211.84(d)(3) specifies requirements for the containers and lids, along with written instructions.
6. Section 211.94(c) describes the requirements for specifications, testing methods, and the cleanliness of the container.

Impurities or gas residues are seen as important factors that should be eliminated. In an ideal situation, 25 inches of Hg pressure is used to apply the vacuum for free. Cryogenic vessels don't need any extra vacuuming before being filled.

23.8 LABELLING AND PACKAGING, AND LABELLING AS PER FDA REGULATION

1. Section 211.125(c) describes the requirements and details of the standard procedure for issued, used, and returned labels of gas cylinders.
2. Section 211.130 describes the requirements for the design and placement of correct labels, including the primary packaging and secondary packaging materials. Most compressed gas cylinders don't need to have their labels changed every time. Once it's labelled, it doesn't need to be replaced until the label is no longer legible or is damaged. This is because a compressed medical gas cylinder is known as a "multiple use" item. The FDA said that

each compressed medical gas cylinder should have a batch number and an expiration date so that it can be found again in the future. Also, for best practice, there should be a record of how many levels are issued and how many labels are destroyed.

23.9 TESTING AND RELEASE FOR DISTRIBUTION OF MEDICAL GAS AS PER FDA REGULATION

1. Section 211.165(a) describes the overall GMP requirements for making compressed medical gases. The requirements for specifications, identity, and strength should match the official monograph requirements. Also, this section describes the testing procedure and quality control requirements that must be adhered to before putting the product on the market.
2. Section 211.165(c) describes the overall requirements, the testing procedure, and the sample taken from the manufactured bulk. The minimum number of samples is taken, and the testing details should be written in the inventory, which can be checked.

23.10 COMPONENT AND RECORDS OF MEDICAL GAS AS PER FDA REGULATION

Section 211.184(c): This appears to be a specific subsection within the broader regulations that pertains to the requirements for records or inventory related to individual components and their use in the manufacturing lot or batch process. The section may outline the specific information that should be documented or maintained for bulk manufacture, particularly in the context of compressed medical gases. It seems that a practical difficulty is acknowledged in measuring bulk compressed medical gas that goes through a vaporisation process and experiences losses. Mention of FDA relaxation suggests that there may be some flexibility or relaxation granted by the FDA for accountability in certain situations. This may emphasize the importance of rationalizing or reconciling the operating losses and the actual use of components, even in situations where some relaxation is provided.

23.11 BATCH PRODUCTION AND CONTROL RECORDS OF MEDICAL GAS AS PER FDA REGULATION

In Section 211.188, the requirements for production and control records of batch processes are outlined, and it is imperative that the records be correctly described.

(a) A control record for the master production, which must include the date, an indication of its accuracy, and the signature of the person responsible for monitoring the entire procedure.

(b) Records of each significant implemented procedure, including the manufacturing process, finishing, packaging, distribution, batch sampling, and other procedures, as appropriate.

23.12 LABORATORY RECORDS OF MEDICAL GAS AS PER FDA REGULATION

In Section 211.194(a)(2), the standards for the laboratory records technique of the testing of crude medical gas and the final product after purification and concentration are outlined in the regulation. In addition to this, the appropriate standards of accuracy should be indicated, and the limit should be contained within the USP or the NF and according to testing prior to the release of each batch. The compliance with pharmacopoeias or any other non-official procedures for quality check should be of an exceptionally high standard, and the details should be documented with precision.

23.13 MISLABELLING AND MISCELLANEOUS PROVISIONS OF MEDICAL GAS AS PER FDA REGULATION

FDA regulates and controls the GMP rule and ensures that it is enforced correctly. It should be notable that any infringement of FDA regulation is subject to prosecution, civil contempt actions, procedural injunctions, and inspectional warrants to enforce the GMP requirements as they pertain to medical gases. For any violations of laws, the FDA enforcement is subject to possible legal action under the following conditions

- Gas filling and delivery staff have insufficient training
- Failure to do quality control on completed goods—medical gas
- Failure of quality control tools, such as stainless-steel joints, hoses, and cryogenic tanks
- Failure of process control, Standard Operating Procedure (SOP) production process, and written manufacturing, processing, and testing procedures

23.14 REGULATIONS OF MEDICAL GAS IN EUROPE

It is possible to implement a framework for a therapeutic or medical gas pipeline if it is deemed acceptable as a risk-free, user-friendly, and cost-effective option. In addition, the system must be user-friendly in order for the nursing staff to accumulated filth.

23.15 BRITISH COMPRESSED GAS ASSOCIATION (BCGA)

The rule that was put in place by the BCGA was followed by the majority of European countries, including the UK. This legislation governed the distribution of medical gases (Table 23.2).

23.16 REGULATIONS OF MEDICAL GAS IN INDIA

Over the previous few decades, the desire for better human health care has grown dramatically in India. Medical gases are crucial components for any health care facility,

TABLE 23.2
Brief Regulation of BCGA (British Compressed Gases Association)

Sl no	Regulation No.	Subject
1	BCGA CP 44	Describes the criteria for medical gas storage as well as the methods involved in use
2	BCGA GN 26	Guarantees the maintenance and identification of the high-pressure gas
3	BCGA GN 32	Defining the distribution scope of medicinal gases
4	BCGA L 7	The misuse of industrial gases is defined here
5	BCGA L 13	Specifies the features of the vehicle that transported medical gases
6	BCGA L 16	The prohibition of electronic cigarettes and other tobacco products-cigarettes in close proximity to medical oxygen installations is defined here
7	BCGA TIS 6	Specifies the colours associated with the various medical gas cylinders
8	BCGA TIS 20	Outlines the policy statement about the use of colour coding for several types of medical gases.
9	BCGA TIS 36	Outlines the procedure for handling and using gas cylinders with integrated pressure regulators and valves.
10	BCGA TIS 37	The required level of cleanliness for medical gas cylinders is specified.
11	BCGA TIS 39	The quality control and batch certification standards for liquefied medical grade oxygen in bulk are specified here.

and their demand is always increasing. Conditions need to comply with the IS/ISO 13485 for the uniform Medical Devices Quality Management Systems (MDMS) Certification Scheme including medical gases. Furthermore, India also recognised the directive of EU along with CE (Conformity European)/European Certificate (EC) as per Directive 93/42/EEC. In addition, the ISO 13485: 2016 is considered to comply for the design of medical systems while EN ISO 7396-1/ EN 737-3 is also considered, in accordance with medical device Directive 93/42/EEC.

23.17 MEDICAL GAS RULE ENFORCED IN INDIA

In India, the Drugs and Cosmetics Act of 1940 governs the manufacture, marketing, and distribution of compressed medical gases. The state authorities are the enforcing agencies, whereas the central authorities are responsible for approving medical gases in India. The Drug Controller General of India is the authority responsible for approving licences for the manufacture, distribution, storage, and sale of medical gases in India. The Central Government delegated authority under Sections 5 and 7 of the Drugs and Cosmetics Act of 1940 and established the Gas Cylinder Regulations, 2016, which defined the manufacturing, filling, ownership, and distribution of medical gases. These guidelines assure the general population's safety and the quality of health care delivery.

23.18 MANUFACTURING OF MEDICAL GASES AS PER REGULATIONS OF INDIA

The company must have a valid manufacturing licence issued by the state Drug Controller in accordance with the Drugs and Cosmetic Act 1940 and the requirements for manufacturing the medical gases, namely medical oxygen IP, medical carbon dioxide IP, and nitrous oxide IP.

23.19 GENERAL REQUIREMENTS OF MEDICAL GAS MANUFACTURING AS PER REGULATIONS OF INDIA

The location, building, and premises should be free of any pollution risks.

23.19.1 Personnel

An accountable individual who possesses sufficient knowledge and qualifications in the relevant fields should be in charge of supervising each and every step of the production process for medical gases. Such personnel are responsible for any violation according to the said Act.

23.19.2 Buildings and Premises

The premises, facility, and operating area are designed, constructed, adapted, and maintained in accordance with the GMP guideline. This ensured that all manufacturing processes are carried out under hygienic conditions. The Factories Act of 1948 must be complied with in order to produce medical gases. In addition, all other regulatory clearances, including those pertaining to fire safety and environmental pollution, must also be obtained.

23.19.3 Production Area

The production area must have inflows of direction of air in order to eliminate the risk of cross contamination and should be developed in accordance with GMP requirements. The entire operational facility should be composed of logical sequences of operations of the process and should be constructed accordingly in a logical manner. While planning the construction of a facility for the production of medical gases, it is critical to give careful consideration to the placement of instruments and the flow of workers in order to reduce the risk of cross contamination to an absolute minimum. As a result, every aspect of the installation, including the piping, ventilation apertures, gas lines, and electrical fittings, is planned, developed, and put in place. It is important to clearly designate both the flow direction and the colours used for the service lines.

23.19.4 Quality Control Area

The quality control area that is used for quality control is required to have a layout that is suitable for the operations that will be performed inside of them. In order to avoid error and cross-contamination through mixing of different gases, an adequate space must be made available. It is imperative that sufficient and appropriate storage space be made available for test samples, stored samples, reference standards, chemicals, and records.

23.20 MANUFACTURE OPERATIONS AND CONTROLS OF MEDICAL GASES AS PER REGULATIONS OF INDIA

The Drugs and Cosmetics Act of 1940 says that the licensing authority should approve the technical staff that will be in charge of supervising the production of medical gases. On each label of a finished product, the name of the product, the number of the batch, the size, and the stage of production should be written, and the label should be signed by a member of the technical staff with the date.

23.20.1 Equipment

In order to perform the operation successfully, it is necessary to install equipment that is inert, non-reactive, accurate, precise, and calibrated. The instrument is expected to undergo routine inspection and testing on a regular basis. In addition, the standard operating procedures (SOP), and any and all relevant records that are required to be kept need to be maintained, and any potential hazards need to be assessed.

- Compressed Air
- ISO 8573-1 :2010: Contaminants and purity classes as per specification
- ISO 8573-2:2018: Comply with the contaminant measurement like oil and aerosol mixtures
- ISO 8573-4: 2019: Comply with the contaminant measurement particle content
- ISO 5011:2020: Comply with performance testing of inlet air cleaning equipment for internal combustion engines and compressors
- ISO 13485: 2016: Comply with the design of medical systems

23.20.2 Records

As an important component of the medical gas manufacturing process, maintaining the GMP is a vital requirement for quality assurance, and accurate documentation of this is required.

Its purpose is to establish the requirements for all of the materials, the manufacturing process, and the process control, as well as the validation and individual participation in the manufacturing process. The records may all be audited, while retaining the documents guarantees that the correct batch was produced, as well as identifying any substandard batches, which are often withdrawn or not released.

In order for any of the documents to be legitimate, they need to be signed and dated by an authorised person, and they also need to have a header that specifies the document's purpose, type, page numbers, and title. Every document may be audited and is organised in such a way that it is simple to get it when needed. In order to make use of the reproducibility, the documents in question need to be legible and clearly written. It is mandatory that each and every document be evaluated on a consistent basis. The documents have to be kept up to date at all times, and any changes to the formula have to be signed off on by an authorised individual. The entire process of the production must be carried out in accordance with the master records, including the batch size that is ultimately produced.

23.20.3 Processing Records

In order to reduce the risk of transcription errors occurring throughout the manufacturing process, processing records are maintained according to batch number, as specified by the master formula. Each stage, including the receiving of material, sampling from the lots, batch number, methods of testing, and keeping records, was outlined in the Standard Operating Procedures (SOPs), which were included in this document.

23.20.4 Labels

Labels are necessary for both the identification of the gases and their application. Labels must be written in a legible and clear manner, and each label must use a different colour code to indicate the state of the product, such as "under test," "passed," "rejected," or "approved." At the time of the containers' release, the quality control check needs to be successfully completed.

23.20.5 Quality Check

This is a mandatory procedure for guaranteeing that the manufactured products are of the requisite quality to meet the safety, efficacy, and regulatory criteria for their intended use. The quality check is applicable for single unit, a whole batch, or the entire manufacturing process. The GMPs should be adhered to throughout the entire process, and all of the procedures, including testing and validation, should be carried out in accordance with the Good Laboratory Practices (GLP). The quality check must be strictly adhered to by all of the materials, including the raw materials, the products used in the intermediate steps, and the products used in bulk. Validated quality control checks and established processes need to be followed in order to ensure that in-process controls, end-product controls, batch sampling, lot sampling, and effluent discharge are carried out correctly. Before a product can be released onto the market, it must first pass a quality inspection and bear the signature of an authorised person in order to comply with all applicable regulatory standards.

23.21 QUALITY AUDIT OF MEDICAL GASES

The quality assurance procedure is applicable to various levels, including a single unit, an entire batch, or the entire manufacturing process. This flexibility allows for a comprehensive approach to ensuring product quality. The primary goal of quality assurance is to verify that the manufactured products meet predefined standards and criteria, ensuring their safety and effectiveness for their intended use. Adherence to regulatory criteria is crucial in industries like pharmaceuticals and medical devices. This includes compliance with guidelines and standards set by regulatory bodies to guarantee the quality and safety of products.

ISO 9001:2008 is a quality management standard that provides a general framework for quality management systems. While ISO 9001:2008 is not specific to medical gases, it is a widely recognized standard that can be applied to various industries, including those involved in manufacturing and production. ISO 13485:2012 is a specific standard for quality management systems in the design, production, installation, and servicing of medical devices. It is particularly relevant for ensuring the quality of medical devices throughout their lifecycle.

The quality assurance process typically involves quality control measures during production and post-production, as well as a commitment to continuous improvement to enhance processes and product quality. Industries dealing with medical gases and devices often need to comply with regulations from health authorities, such as the Food and Drug Administration (FDA) in the United States or the European Medicines Agency (EMA) in Europe.

GMPs are crucial for maintaining the quality and safety of pharmaceutical and medical products. Adhering to GMP guidelines ensures that manufacturing processes are controlled, documented, and validated to meet quality standards. All procedures, including testing and validation, should align with GLPs. This ensures that laboratory activities, such as testing and data recording, are conducted with accuracy, consistency, and reliability.

Strict adherence to quality checks is essential for all materials involved in the manufacturing process. This includes raw materials, intermediate products, and bulk products. Ensuring the quality of materials contributes to the overall quality of the final product. Validated quality control checks and established processes are necessary to verify that in-process controls, end-product controls, batch sampling, lot sampling, and effluent discharge are carried out correctly. Validation ensures that these processes are reliable and effective.

Before a product can be released onto the market, it must undergo a rigorous quality inspection. The release process typically involves the signature of an authorized person, indicating that the product meets all applicable regulatory standards. Compliance with regulatory standards is a fundamental aspect of the entire manufacturing and quality control process. Meeting regulatory requirements ensures that products are safe, effective, and meet the standards set by health authorities..

Periodic inspection and testing of compressed gas cylinders should follow in accordance with Rules 35 and 36 of the Gas Cylinder Rules of 2004. The minimum frequency of inspections and tests should be performed on the cylinders as mentioned. In accordance with the prescribed regulation, it is imperative that no cylinder be filled with compressed gas unless it has undergone a thorough examination and has been subjected to either the hydrostatic test or the hydrostatic stretch test, as specified in Schedule IV. This must be done within the specified time period as mandated by ISO:15975, which is issued by the BIS. Furthermore, any testing facility accredited for the periodic testing and inspection of cylinders is required to offer the facilities listed in Schedule IV and is required to submit to the Chief Controller of Explosive (CCOE) of the Government of India the particulars of the facilities provided in addition to a scrutiny charge as indicated in Schedule V.

23.21.1 Product Containers and Closures

It is recommended that all pharmacopoeia requirements be made mandatory for the product labels, product containers, and stoppers. In order to guarantee that no materials are reactive, absorptive, or leachable, end-product test techniques, sample size, and specifications, as well as cleaning and sterilisation processes, should be described. This will ensure that the quality of the products is not compromised in any way.

23.21.2 Distribution Records

Before being distributed or dispatched, each and every product needs to have its safety verified and be examined on a randomised basis according to the Standard Operating Procedure. Before the products are made available for sale, the quality control shall pass audit and be approved by the authorised quality control officer.

23.21.2.1 Distribution through Gas Line

- ISO10083/ENISO7396-1/EN737-3: Comply with the gas line system.
- ISO 10083/ EN ISO 7396-1/ EN 737-3: Comply with the medical gas distribution networks.
- *ISO 7396-1:2026: Comply with the* specific safety requirements for pipeline systems used in health care facilities.

23.21.3 Validation and Process Validation

Procedure and process validation are essential parameters of GMP for ensuring that the process that is adopted is correct and as per the norms. The validation of all procedures, including those pertaining to processing, testing, and cleaning of the empty cylinder must be carried out in accordance with the Standards Operating Procedures. It is required that the processes be revalidated on a regular basis, and important processes must either be prospectively or retrospectively validated in the time gap.

23.21.4 Product Recalls

Standard operating procedure should be in written format, including the distribution procedure, so that, in the event of an emergency, a defective product can be recalled promptly before it reaches a large number of customers.

23.21.5 Complaints and Adverse Reactions

The quality of the compressed medical gases is an essential factor in ensuring the safety of their use and the proper functioning of the product. Each complaint or adverse reaction that is recorded should be carefully monitored, and appropriate action should be taken to remedy the situation. The significant action is going to be documented and kept up to date by the designated personnel of the business.

23.21.6 Site Master File

The site master file is one of the most important documents and is required to be maintained during the operation of medical gas production. It contains the specific and factual information that was adopted in order to comply with GMP during the stage of production and/or control of medical gas manufacturing in licenced premises. Each medical gas producing unit is required to comply with the test facilities to control in-process and final medical gases to detect trace impurities in ppm/ppb concentrations for all noxious impurity gases such as CO, phosphines, NO, SO_2, polymers, argon, etc., and the facilities themselves should be verified and inspected by the authorities for the issuing of the licensing. The minimum storage space and conditions of compressed medical gases are specified in accordance with the Explosives Act of 1884 or the Gas Cylinders Rules of 2004.

Regulation of Filling Gas Cylinders while filling the gas into CCOE-approved cylinders in CCOE-licenced premises, the company should perform the dragger test in accordance. Additionally, the company should fill out Forms E and F (Rules 50, 51, and 54) to obtain a licence to fill compressed gas in cylinders and a licence to store compressed gas in cylinders, respectively. The different offices of the Department of Explosives are the ones who are authorised to issue the licence in Form F. However, if there is a storage shed for cylinders that are attached to the gas filling plant, then the Chief Controller of Explosives in Nagpur will issue a licence for storage of cylinders at the filling plant, in addition to a licence for filling the cylinders.

23.21.7 Transport of Medical Gases

The Gas Cylinder Rules, 2004 include a provision in Schedule VI Rule 20 that governs the transport of cylinders. Cylinders that have been filled with any type of compressed gas must be transported, including loading, unloading, and transportation of cylinders, in accordance with the provisions that have been laid down as stated and while adhering to the relevant provisions of any other statutes that are applicable.

23.22 REGULATION ON QUALITY CONTROL OF COMPRESSED GAS CYLINDERS AS PER SCHEDULE I OF RULE 3(1) OF GAS REGULATION, 2004, GOVERNMENT OF INDIA

When transporting any compressed gas cylinders, an authorised individual is required to accompany them and ensure that all applicable regulations, which are outlined in

Schedule VI, are followed. The Gas Regulation, 2004 requires that occasional examinations of compressed gas cylinders be carried out in accordance with Rules 35 and 36.

Before being filled with compressed gas, each cylinder must undergo several tests, including a hydrostatic test, a hydrostatic stretch test, and any other tests deemed necessary. These testing requirements are outlined in Schedule IV of IS 15975. IS 15975 is the relevant standard published by the Bureau of Indian Standards. It serves as the reference document for establishing the testing procedures and requirements for compressed gas cylinders.

The testing facility conducting these tests must be recognized or accepted in accordance with the requirements specified in Schedule IV of IS 15975. Recognition ensures that the facility meets the necessary standards and qualifications for conducting these critical tests. The testing facility is required to appoint a Chief Controller in accordance with Schedule V of the Gas Regulation, 2004. The Chief Controller plays a crucial role in overseeing the testing processes and ensuring compliance with regulatory standards.

The appointment of a Chief Controller is also referred to as Scrutiny Charge for Quality Control. This position is responsible for scrutinizing and overseeing the quality control aspects of the testing procedures. The testing and quality control processes are governed by the Gas Regulation, 2004, which provides the regulatory framework for the industry.

The institution or business is supplying medical gases in cylinders to hospitals, and does so only after conducting appropriate testing and keeping appropriate documentation. In accordance with Rule 3(1) of Schedule I of the Gas Regulation, 2004, the quality management of compressed medical gas is subject to regulation in India. Section 201(g) (1) of the Federal Food, Drug, and Cosmetic Act (FD&C Act) (21 U.S.C. 321(g)(1)) regulates the product in the US. Additionally, section 503(b)(1)(A) of the FD&C Act (21 U.S.C. 353(b)(1)(A)) regulates the product. Both of these sections can be found in 21 US Code. These additional equipment, calibration, and codes, as well as certification from the Medical Gas Professional Healthcare Organization (MGPHO), are required for the re-validation in order to achieve a higher level of proficiency. The NFPA 99 Regulation, which serves as validation for the American Society of Sanitary Engineering (ASSE) 6030 standards, is the one that is followed in Europe. In addition, both the NFPA and the ASEE 6030 standard impose a restriction on the gas line attachment.

The guidelines established by the International Organization for Standardization (ISO) are followed in order to ensure the quality of composite compressed gas containers. This standard is applicable to the worldwide federation and is enforced by national standards agencies (ISO member bodies). All technical committees at ISO were brought into conformity with the ISO 11623 standard. After the technical meeting that was held in accordance with the specification ISO/TC 58 (Subcommittee SC 4), the operation of compressed gas was carried out. In addition, an agreement on technical collaboration between ISO and Comité Européen de Normalisation (CEN) was reached (Vienna Agreement). The same was decided upon for "Transportable gas cylinders" according to the specification described in EN ISO 11623:2002 and the specification drafted by technical committees CEN/TC 23 and ISO/TC 58. The regulations of the European Committee for Electrotechnical Standardization (CEN/CENELEC) countries now adhere to the EN ISO 11623:2002 guideline. These countries include Austria, Belgium, Denmark, the Czech Republic, Finland, France, Greece, Germany, Iceland, Ireland, Luxembourg, Italy, the Netherlands, Norway, Malta, Spain, Portugal, Sweden, Switzerland, and the United Kingdom. In the United States of America, the power to implement the standard ISO 11623:2002(E) was placed in Part 5 of the United States Code 552(a) and in Part 1 of the Code of Regulations 51, respectively. This gave the government the authority to carry out the standard's implementation throughout the entire country (Table 23.3).

TABLE 23.3
Specification of the Compressed Gas Cylinder (Excluding LPG (Liquefied Petroleum Gas) Quality Control

Sl no	Contents	Specifications
1	Gas cylinders (Transportable) Part 2: Checking the gauge: 25E taper thread for connecting valves to gas cylinders.	EN 629-2: 1996
2	Gas cylinders (Transportable)—identification of gas cylinder—Part: Marking of Stamp	EN 1089-1:1996
3	Gas cylinders (Transportable)—identification (excluding LPG)—Precautionary labels (Part 2)	EN 1089-2:2002
4	Identifying gas cylinders (Transportable) by their colour coding (Part 3)	EN 1089-3:2011
5	Procedures for change of gas service	EN 1795:1997
6	Gas cylinders (Transportable)—Testing and inspection of seamless aluminium alloy gas cylinders	BS EN 1802:2002
7	Gas cylinders (Transportable)—Inspecting and testing seamless stainless steel gas cylinders	BS EN 1968:2002
8	Gas cylinders (Transportable)—Conditions of filling for single gases, including medical grade	BS EN 13096:2003
9	Gas cylinders (transportable) for medical use—Identification of contents and marking	ISO 32:1977
10	Precautionary conditions and labels	ISO 6406: 1992
11	Checking and testing gas cylinders made of seamless aluminium alloy on a regular basis	ISO 10461: 1993
12	Gas cylinders (Transportable)—Compatibility between the materials used to make the cylinder and valve and the gas inside—Part 1: Metallic materials	ISO 11114-1: 1997
13	Gas cylinders (Transportable) Part 2: Non-metal materials—Compatibility between the materials used to make the cylinder and valve and the gas inside	ISO 11114-2:2021
14	Gas cylinders (Transportable)—25E taper thread to connect gas cylinder valves—Inspection gauges	ISO 11191 :1997
15	Procedures for changing gas service	I SO 11621: 1997
16	Gas cylinders (Transportable): valves and fittings for gas cylinders	ISO 13341: 2010
17	Toxicity testing of a gas or gas mixture	ISO 10298:2018
18	Stamping on gas cylinders	ISO 13769:2018

23.23 INTERVALS BETWEEN PERIODIC INSPECTION AND TESTING OF COMPRESSED GAS CYLINDER

The container containing the compressed gas needs to be inspected and tested at regular intervals. After the gas canister has reached the expiry periods, it is typically thrown away, and the inspection is only valid for a re-test. Consequently, the requirement that the test be performed on each and every filing is not implemented by regulations, despite the fact that the test interval time may have already lapsed. In the event of an emergency, used cylinders, most commonly containing compressed medical gases, are required to be periodically tested and inspection reports submitted.

23.24 INSPECTION INTERVALS FOR ALUMINIUM ALLOY LINERS OF GAS CYLINDERS

In accordance with ISO 11114-1:1997, the compatibility of gases and aluminium alloys is checked. The suitability of a non-reactive gas that is going to be loaded into an aluminium alloy cylinder needs to be checked. The gases are categorised based on the requirements of the specification BS EN 13096 (Table 23.4).

23.25 INSPECTION INTERVALS FOR STEEL LINERS OF GAS CYLINDERS

In compliance with ISO 11114-1:1997, tests are conducted to determine whether or not steel is compatible with the gas in order to guarantee that the polymerisation and decomposition reactions take place at dew points. It is recommended that the expiration date on the cylinders used with self-contained breathing apparatus in the marine dive or combat fighter aircraft re-inspection/test not exceed five years. If there is no water in the cylinder and it is dry, the time it takes to re-inspect and re-test the cylinder may be increased. In this particular instance, the supportive evidence with regard to the quality of the filter unit will warrant the additional testing time. Every two to five years, the gas cylinder that is used for medical purposes or in an emergency situation that requires artificial respiration must undergo a visual inspection both internally and externally, and it must be completely retested every five years. In a cylinder

TABLE 23.4
Periodicity of Inspection of Container Having the Aluminium Alloy Liners with Compatibility of the Gases

Sl no	Gas Type with Aluminium Alloy Liners	Periodicity in Years
1	Compressed gases, e.g., air, Ar, He, H_2, Ne, N_2, O_2, etc.	5 or 10
2	Liquefied gases, e.g., CO_2, N_2O and liquefied gas mixtures	5 or 10
3	Very toxic gases LC_{50}: less than 200 ppm, e.g., AsH_3, PH_3	3

like this, the tensile strength as well as the surface condition are both very significant factors. It is important that the hydrogen canister conforms to the specifications laid out in ISO 11114-1:1997. When switching filling from one type of compressed gas to another in the same cylinder, the service changing each cylinder should correspond to either EN 1795:1997 or ISO 11621:1997 (Table 23.5).

23.26 INSPECTION INTERVALS FOR NON-METALLIC LINERS OF GAS CYLINDER

It has been determined that the gas's compatibility satisfies the requirements of ISO 11114-2. During the polymerisation and decomposition processes, it is necessary to ascertain whether or not mercury was present, as well as the role of stress hydrogen and the end products. The cylinders that are used for underwater operations, space, aircraft, and self-contained breathing apparatus, in addition to this form of cylinder, are required to undergo re-testing every five years. It is also recommended that if the finished product's toxicity LC_{50} is greater than 200 ppm, then the period of time between 5 and 10 years should be re-tested (Table 23.6).

TABLE 23.5
Periodicity of Inspection of Container Having the Steel Liners with Compatibility with the Gases

S. No,	Gas Type	Periodicity in Years
1	Underwater breathing apparatus, e.g., air, O_2	2,5 (visual) and 5 (full)
2	Gas mixtures	5 or 10
3	Very toxic gases LC_{50}: less than 200 ppm, e.g., AsH_3, PH_3	Shortest period of any component

TABLE 23.6
Periodicity of Inspection of Container Having the Non-metallic Liners with Compatibility with the Gases

S. No.	Gas Type	Periodicity in Years
1	Underwater breathing apparatus containing compressed gas, e.g., air, Ar, He, H_2, Ne, N_2, O_2	5 or 10

23.27 INSPECTION INTERVALS FOR CGAS CYLINDERS WITHOUT LINERS

The test is carried out in accordance with ISO 11114-2, and the determination of any decomposed products must be recorded. The cylinder that is used for underwater operations, space, aircraft, and self-contained breathing equipment must undergo re-testing within the five-year time frame. Once a cylinder of this type has been utilised for highly toxic gases, it is no longer permissible to use it (Table 23.7).

23.28 PROCEDURES FOR PERIODIC INSPECTION AND TESTING OF GAS CYLINDERS

Identifying the cylinder, inspection, and testing is a system, with well-written procedures to be followed as described in the guideline.

- Conforms to ISO 11623:2002 for external visual inspection (E).
- Internal visual inspection conforms accordingly for steel or aluminium alloy liners; the inspection shall be in accordance with prEN 1968 or ISO 6406, or prEN 1802 or ISO 10461 respectively.
- Supplementary tests as per ISO 11623:2002(E).
- Pressure test as per ISO 11623:2002(E).
- Valve check according to ISO 11623:2002 (E).
- Cylinders were rejected and deemed unusable after testing according to ISO 11623:2002 (E).

Before the pressure test, all of the internal visual inspections should have been done. If the inspection or testing fails, the item will be rejected. The extra tests are recommended to make sure that the cylinder is fit for use.

23.29 HEAT EXPOSURE OF GAS CYLINDERS

Refurbished cylinders are subject to periodic examination for their ability to withstand heat exposure. This is done to ensure that there is no damage caused during

TABLE 23.7
Periodicity of Inspection of Containers without Liners with Compatibility with the Gases

S. No.	Gas Type	Periodicity in Years
1	Underwater breathing apparatus containing compressed gas, e.g., air, Ar, He, H_2, Ne, N_2, O_2	5 or 10

the initial cleaning, operation, or powder or paint coating processes. After the heat shocking has been completed, the mechanical properties of the liners and/or composite cylinder are to be established. The temperature of the cylinder was maintained at not more than 70 °C for a duration of twenty-four hours, or in accordance with any guideline that is recommended. The terms and conditions of storage for the gas cylinder are to be written down on the container.

23.30 IDENTIFICATION OF CYLINDER

The cylinder is identified in accordance with the specified specification of EN 1089-1:1996 or ISO 13769:2018 and the gas content are identified in accordance with the aforementioned specification of EN 1089-2:2002 or ISO 7225:2005. The gas canister is handled carefully before being depressurised, drained, and finally having its valves removed.

23.31 PERMEABILITY TESTING OF CYLINDER

The permeability test is carried out with soapy water, and any leaks to the valve and the connections of the liner (if present) with the metallic bosses or rings are observed. After the leak has been fixed, an additional test called a weight variation test will be performed with corresponding weight variations after 23 hours. If the cylinder's weight loss is less than 0.25 ml/h (per litre of cylinder water capacity), the test will be considered successful; otherwise, the cylinder will be rejected (Table 23.8).

23.32 BIS ACT OF COMPRESSED MEDICAL GAS (1986)

The specification of the BIS has been streamlined to make it easier to comprehend regulation for use by country, and the Government of India has committed to enforcing both BIS and another accepted standard. BIS takes a significant role to educate the people, their rights, and the public safety. The standard well characterised the seamless steel, transportable gas cylinder of compressed and liquefied gases under pressure, from the smallest (0.5 litre) up to 150 litres. For the periodic inspection and testing for the integrity of such gas cylinders, BIS specifications are to be observed. However, this standard does not correspond to the periodic inspection and testing of acetylene cylinders or any composite cylinders. Those cylinders are not covered by this standard (Tables 23.9 and 23.10).

The categorical statement needs to be mentioned on the cylinder with the word “WARNING” written in bold. Only a registered practitioner or someone working under the practitioner's supervision should administer the medicinal gases. The medical gas is handled by a classified practitioner who is sufficiently familiar with the administration of medical gases, including the indications, methods, effects, and dosages, as well as having knowledge of the risks, contraindications, side effects, and precautions associated with medical gases.

TABLE 23.8
International Standard with the Test Conditions

Sl No	Test	Origin	Specification
1.	Cylinders	Indian	Specification must comply with IS: 3196 Part 1(2006), Part 2 (2012), and Part 4 (2001), IS: 7142 (1995), and Dissolved Acetylene Cylinders (DA) must comply with IS: 7312:1993, both of which must be validated by the BIS. Only cylinders made of low-carbon steel that have been welded together and filled with low-pressure liquefiable gases are authorised.
		USA	Gases that are permanent and liquefiable are compliant with DOT:3A/3AA, and canisters made of aluminium alloy are compliant with DOT:3AL.
		UK	Aluminium alloy cylinders conform to BS:5045: Pt. 3 (1984) or EN Specification according to BS:5045: Part I (1982), which conforms the seamless steel cylinders for use with liquefiable gases and also conforms the specification to DOT:3, whereas seamless steel cylinders shall be according to the FM-200 gas service regulation, which corresponds to DOT:4BA:500.
		China origin	Cylinders made of seamless steel for use with high-pressure gas that correspond to the IS:7285 standard
2	Cylinders	Austrian origin	The BS 5045: Part I: 1982 specification is appropriate for both non-liquefiable and liquefiable gases.
			The NZS:5454-1989 specification is applicable for seamless steel cylinders that are used to store compressed natural gas (CNG) gas, with a workable pressure permitted up to 200 Bar and a test pressure of 335 Bar.
3	Containers	Indian	In accordance with the requirements outlined in BS:1500 (1958) or those specified in ASME Section VIII Division 1, IS:2825 (1969).
4	Valves	Indian	According to the requirements of the specification IS: 3745:2006, while respiratory equipment must comply with the requirements of the specification IS: 7302:1974, it must be certified by the BIS and given approval by the CCOE.
		Europe/Italy	With the pressure set at 2.2 MPa and in accordance with the specification of ECER-67-01
5	Hydrostatic test		In accordance with the IS: 5844:1970 for pressurised gas. Measure the sensitivity of the volumetric equipment using 1/20,000 of its overall capacity.

(Continued)

TABLE 23.8 (CONTINUED)
International Standard with the Test Conditions

Sl No	Test	Origin	Specification
6	Another test		Non-destructive methods are also recommended like ultrasonic flaw techniques, auditory emission techniques, etc. These tests are helpful for detecting stress corrosion cracks that have developed throughout the course of operation. In addition to its measurement and testing functions, a dead-weight pressure gauge can be used to ensure that an appropriate pressure range is covered. Boroscopes or extra-low voltage lamps can be used to measure the internal view of the cylinder, while lights can be utilised for investigation of the cylinder's external surfaces.
7	Inspection and periodicity		In accordance with the requirements of ISO 11114-1:2020 (Amendment 2023).
8	Identification label		Satisfies the requirements of either the EN 1089-1:1996 or the ISO 13769:2002 specification and includes a label bearing permanent inscriptions as well as the pertinent design document.
9	LC_{50}		Complies with the requirements of ISO 10298:2018 or the 50% lethal concentration
10	Toxic gases		When the LC_{50} value is greater than 200 ppm, the gas is classified as hazardous and complies with ISO 10298:2018.
11	Very toxic gases		According to ISO 10298:2018, substances with an LC_{50} of less than 200 ppm are considered to be extremely hazardous.
12	Identification of cylinder and preparation for inspection and test		Both the data of the cylinder and the gas content are compliant with EN 1089-1:1996 or ISO 13769:2018, and EN 1089-2:2002 or ISO 7225:2005 (amendment 2012), respectively.
13	Internal visual inspection		The aluminium liner meets the requirements of specification prEN 1968 or ISO 6406:2005, and the stainless-steel liner meets the requirements of specification prEN 1802 or ISO 10461:2005. Neck and shoulder cracks correspond to specification prEN 1802 or ISO 10461:2005 for aluminium liner, and prEN 1968 or ISO 6406:2005 for stainless steel, respectively, for neck and shoulder cracks. The EN 629-2 standard for 25E threads is met by this specification.
14	Pressure test		Specified in accordance with either prEN 1968 or ISO 6406, prEN 1802 or ISO 10461, or ISO 10461.

(*Continued*)

TABLE 23.8 (CONTINUED)
International Standard with the Test Conditions

Sl No	Test	Origin	Specification
15	Cylinder re-valving		Complies with the requirements of specification ISO 13341:2010. It is important that the lubricants and sealing substance be compatible with the gas service. The international standards ISO 11114-2:2021 and ISO 13341:2010 are met by medical oxygen.
16	Check on cylinder tare		Meets the requirements of EN 1089-1:1996 or ISO 13769: 2018.
17	Marking		Maintains compatibility with either EN 1089-1:1996 or ISO 13769:2018.
18	Identification of contents		The content consistency is defined according to the specifications ISO 7225:2005 and EN 1089-3:2011, which this product satisfies. Any change to the gas utility should comply with EN 1795:1997 or ISO 11621:1997. Specification
19	Transportable gas cylinders		Compatibility of cylinder and valve materials with gas components according to EN ISO 11114-1 1997—Part 1: Metallic materials or ISO 11114-1:2020. Compatibility of cylinder and valve materials with gas components according to ISO 11114-2:2021.
20	Taper thread (25E) for connection of valves to gas cylinders		Complies with either the EN 629-2: 1996 or the ISO 11191:1997 standard.
21	Provisions of changing of gas service		Meets the requirements of EN 1795: 1997 or ISO 11621:1997.
22	Stamp marking on gas cylinders		Complies with either the EN 1089-1:1996 or the ISO 13769:2018 standard
23	Labels of precaution		Meets the requirements of either EN 1089-2:2002 or ISO 7225:2005.

23.33 MEDICAL GASES AS PER BIS SPECIFICATION

In India and throughout the rest of the world, medical gases are utilised for a variety of applications, including use as drugs (*in vivo*) and along with medical devices (*in vitro*). Air, carbon dioxide, helium, nitrous oxide, oxygen, blood gas calibration mixtures, lung diffusion mixtures, anaerobic and aerobic growth mixtures, and other gases are included in the category of medicinal gases.

As per Section 3(b) I of the Drugs and Cosmetics Act, 1940, the definition of "Drugs" encompasses medicinal substances intended for both internal and external

TABLE 23.9
BIS Specification for the Test Conditions of Compressed Gas

Sl. no.	Test	Specification
1	Yoke-style connections on the valves of the smaller medical gas canisters (Second Revision)	Conforms to IS3745: 2006
2	Identification of gas cylinders for medical use and the associated apparatus via coloration	Conforms to IS3933: 1966
3	Identifying commercial and industrial gas canisters	Conforms to IS 4379: 1981
4	Inspections of gas canisters at regular intervals	Conforms to IS8868: 1988
5	Gas canisters made of seamless steel that are refillable in 2004. Quenched and hardened steel cylinders with a tensile strength of less than 1 100 MPa (112 kgf/mm^2) are required for this part of the specification (Third Revision)	Conforms to IS 7285 (Part 2): 2004
6	Code of practice for steel containers containing compressed gases such as atmospheric gases, hydrogen, high-pressure liquefiable gases, and dissolved acetylene gases.	Conforms to 8198: 2004
7	Procedures for inspection of instruments with type 2 taper threads on gas cylinder valves, with taper 3 in 25	Conforms to 9122: 2008
8	Refrigerants. Identifiers by number and name	Conforms to 10609:1983.
9	identifying markings on the canister of medical-grade compressed gas	Conforms to IS 7285(Part2):2004 and duly approved from CCOE.
10	Fire safety	Conforms to IS 7285(Part- 2):2004.

TABLE 23.10
Colour-coded Cylinder are Used for Easy Identification and to Avoid Accidental Mix-ups

	Name	INDIA (Official Monograph I.P 2007)	USA (USP 31) (Official Monograph United State Pharmacopoeia USP 31)	UK (British Pharmacopoeia 2008)
1	Medical Air	-	Yellow	White
2	Medical Oxygen	Shoulder white and remainder in Black	Green	Shoulder white and remainder in black
3	Medical Nitrogen	-	Blue	Shoulder black and remainder in grey
4	Medical Helium	-	Black	Brown
5	Medical Carbon Dioxide	-	Grey	Grey
6	Medical Nitrous Oxide	Blue	Blue	Blue

administration to humans or animals. It also includes any substances intended for use in the prevention, treatment, mitigation, or diagnosis of diseases or disorders in humans or animals. This definition further encompasses preparations applied to the human body with the purpose of repelling insects, such as mosquitoes. This definition of "Drugs" applies to "all medicines for internal or external use of human beings in the case of the State of Andhra Pradesh vs. Linde India Ltd (AIR 2020SC2148), the Supreme Court of India ruled that medical oxygen is considered a "medicine" because it can be used for or in the diagnosis, treatment, mitigation, or prevention of any disease or disorder in human beings. This ruling means that medical oxygen falls under the purview of Section 3(b)(i) of The Drugs and Cosmetics Act, 1940. Hence, the manufacturing, distribution and import of medical oxygen in India is regulated by The Drugs and Cosmetics Act, 1940, and guidelines framed thereunder. Any individual or organisation that produces medical gases, such as medical oxygen IP, medical nitrous oxide IP, or medical carbon dioxide IP, is required to possess a valid manufacturing licence that has been granted by the respective state Drug Controller in accordance with the provisions of The Drugs and Cosmetics Act of 1940 and the rules that are enacted under that Act. This is not limited to medical oxygen but extended to other gases used for medical purposes.

The Indian Pharmacopoeia Commission (IPC) is an autonomous organisation operating under the Ministry of Health and Family Welfare, Government of India. Its primary function is to create and enforce standards pertaining to the identification, purity, and potency of pharmaceutical products made, distributed, and utilised within India. The compendium of standards referred to as the Indian Pharmacopoeia is published. The Indian Pharmacopoeia holds a legally recognised status as stipulated in Section 16 of The Drugs and Cosmetics Act 1940. The drugs that are listed in the Second Schedule of The Drugs and Cosmetics Act 1940 are mandated to adhere to predetermined requirements. The purity necessary for medical oxygen is very high, due to the fact that it is utilised in healthcare facilities, primarily hospitals and clinics, for the treatment of patients, in particular for ventilation for patients who are unable to breathe on their own. The purity recommended under the Indian Pharmacopeia for medical oxygen is 99.9%.

In spite of this, the World Health Organization (WHO) came out with a set of interim guidance technical specifications for pressure swing adsorption (PSA) plants in June, 2020. These specifications state that "pressure swing adsorption technology to generate medical oxygen 93% from ambient air" must be used. In addition, WHO made it perfectly clear that the manner in which medical oxygen is administered depends on the clinical medicinal necessity as well as the clinical guidelines. Medical oxygen may be administered either in its undiluted form, or as mixtures of oxygen concentrations of 93% or 99.5% or other oxygen products, or in its undiluted form or as mixtures in conjunction with ambient or compressed air of an appropriate quality or other medications. At the 56th meeting of the WHO Expert Committee on Specifications for Pharmaceutical Preparations, the monograph on medicinal oxygen was approved for publication in the International Pharmacopoeia, 11th Version. In accordance with the specification, Oxygen 93% must contain at least 90.0% and no more than 96.0% (v/v) of O_2; the remaining volume must primarily be composed of

TABLE 23.11
Monograph of Medical Gas and the Specification as per Regulatory Requirement

Nitrous oxide	Nitrous oxide is used as a solvent for a variety of gas anaesthetics, including halothane, enflurane, desflurane, isoflurane, and ethane, amongst others. For the purpose of relieving pain during a short surgical treatment, for instance the dressing of wounds and burns, the suturing or debridement of wounds, or the extraction of teeth, 50% oxygen is used. Additionally, it is frequently utilised as an insufflating substance in laparoscopy and cryosurgery by being administered via inhalation at concentrations of up to 80% with oxygen. Below the threshold of 70%, neonatal operation is performed.	DOT Classification: 2.2. (Non-Inflammatory) Specified Volume: 8.7 ft 2/lb The specific gravity is 1.53 at 68 °C Specification in accordance with United States Patent 31, European Patent, Chinese, Japanese, and Vietnamese law. Includes not less than 98% Volume/Volume of Nitrogen in Gaseous Phase (Eur P), 99% Volume/Volume of Nitrogen in Gaseous Phase (USP), 99-100% Volume/Volume of Nitrogen in Gaseous Phase (Eur P) (IP). Maximum for Impurities: CO: ≤ 5 ppm (Eur P), ≤ 0.001% V/V (USP). CO_2: ≤ 300 ppm (Eur P), ≤ 0.03% V/V(USP). ≤ 300 ppm (IP). NO/NO_2: less than 2 ppm V/V combined in the gaseous and liquid phases (Eur P), NO less than 1 ppm (in the gas phase), and NO_2 less than 1 ppm (in the liquid phase) (USP). NH_3: < 0.0025 % V/V (USP and IP) (USP and IP) H_2O: ≤ 67 ppm V/V (Eur P), ≤ 150 mg/m3 (USP). Halogen Gas: < 1 ppm (USP).

argon and nitrogen. Pressure swing adsorption (PSA) and vacuum swing adsorption (VSA) are two methods that can be used to extract oxygen from atmospheric air. Throughout the manufacturing process, the oxygen concentration is constantly checked. The production process has been validated to demonstrate that oxygen 93% complies with the following limits, which can be found below: carbon dioxide: maximum 300 ppm (v/v); carbon monoxide: maximum 5 ppm (v/v); total nitrogen monoxide and nitrogen dioxide: maximum 2 ppm (v/v); sulphur dioxide: maximum 1 ppm (v/v); oil: maximum 0.1 mg/m^3; water: maximum 67 ppm (v/v); and that viable and non-viable particulates are eliminated or minimised and appropriately controlled in the product (Table 23.11).

23.34 INSTILLATION OF THE LIQUID MEDICAL OXYGEN (LMO) PLANT *IN INDIA*

As a source of medical oxygen, liquid medical oxygen (also known as LMO) is considered to be superior for a number of factors, including the following: (a) According to IP 2018, the oxygen coming from this source has a purity of 99% volume percent oxygen. In addition, there is no variation in the purity, not even when considering factors such as movement or temperature and it is also an excellent choice for use in conjunction with ventilators and at critical ICU units; (b) LMO does not have any restrictions on the flow rate, and it can accommodate or adjust any flow rate as per hospital requirements, and other systems have limitations, which could not exhibited at the high rate of flow; (c) LMO has a significant potential for the storage capacity because of liquefaction of oxygen. One litre of medically graded liquid oxygen is comparable to approximately 870 litres of oxygen in its gaseous state. Large bulk cryogenic liquid oxygen tanks can be installed in healthcare facilities, and these tanks are occasionally refilled by a truck that comes from the supplier. Independent of the power source, the liquid oxygen tank provides a centrally piped system known as the Medical Gas Pipeline System (MGPS) that is located throughout the medical facility. Distribution of LMO requires an MGPS; (d) In order for any source of medical oxygen, including LMO, to be delivered up to an individual's bedside in the hospital, it is necessary for there to be a network of medical gas pipelines that are part of the Medical Gas Pipeline System (MGPS). The high-pressure oxygen cylinders (Type D) that are connected to the gas manifold continue to serve as the backup or secondary source of oxygen, which is necessary according to the norms and standards established by MGPS; (e) The administration of LMO does not incur any expenditure related to operational expenses. As soon as it is introduced into the canister within the walls of the hospital, it automatically enters the MGPS of the facility and begins to circulate. There is no requirement for additional personnel, additional electrical power, or additional maintenance.

23.34.1 Regulatory Requirement for Installing of LMO

All statutory requirements are to be followed precisely as prescribed under the rules of the Explosives Act of 1884, The Static and Mobile Pressure Vessels (Unfired) Rules, 2016, The Gas Cylinders Rules, 2016, and the necessary licence is to be obtained from them. The manufacturing of LMO is licensed through the Central Drugs Standard Control Organisation (CDSCO), under The Drugs and Cosmetics Act 1940 and Rules. An authorisation from the Petroleum and Explosives Safety Organization (PESO) is necessary in order to operate the LMO installation and to have the LMO filled. In accordance with the PESO guideline, information was provided regarding the fencing, gate, provision of the fire extinguisher, water connection, illumination, concerns regarding safety, earthing pit, and lightning arrestor.

23.34.2 Quality Controls

The LMO tank is an essential component and, in order to design it correctly, there are a few parameters that need to be taken into consideration. Cryogenic liquids are vapours that have been liquefied and have a boiling point that is between –150 and –270 °C. Liquid oxygen is in a cryogenic state at –183 °C. A cryogenic storage tank, vaporisers, and a pressure control system are the three main components that make up a standard liquid oxygen storage system. The LMO reservoir should be designed as a double-walled vacuum-insulated container, capable of withstanding a maximum operating pressure of 16 to 18 kg/cm^2. It should meet the certified guidelines outlined by ASME/EN or their equivalents, specifically ASME Sec. VIII/

EN-13458-2 or equivalent specifications. The tank's capacity should be adjustable within the range of 2 kilolitres to 20 kilolitres. The LMO tank's capacity should be able to meet ASME Sec. VIII In order to insulate the contents from the surrounding air temperature; the walls are made of stainless steel and are intended for a positive pressure at a cryogenic temperature. In addition, there is a vacuum in between the walls for insulation.

There are a few different kinds of containers that can be used to store, transport, and handle liquid oxygen. The type of container used is determined by the quantity of oxygen that is needed by the user. The dewar, the cryogenic liquid cylinder, and the cryogenic storage tanks are the different kinds of containers that can be found in use. Each tank is equipped with insulation from vacuum and incorporates numerous circuits to control various aspects such as product filling, pressure accumulation, pressure release, product extraction, and tank vacuum. Tanks are also insulated against vacuum. Insulated liquid transfer or withdrawal lines are utilised for the secure removal of liquid product from either cryogenic liquid cylinders or dewars. This helps to reduce the amount of liquid product that is converted to gas during the process.

The LMO storage tank is equipped with many safety features and control mechanisms. These include a pressure valve, safety devices, two separate liquid withdrawal valves with a dual parallel regulator system to ensure a continuous supply, and a three-way gauge valve that allows for the isolation of line pressure with operator intervention. Additionally, the tank has a dual parallel regulator system. The tank ought to have a PESO certification, and the substance used for the outer shell ought to be in compliance with EIGA IGC 73/08/E/IS2062/SA36.

The double-walled Vacuum Insulated Evaporator (VIE) is constructed with an interior vessel made of stainless steel that is contained within an outer vessel made of carbon steel. The non-combustible insulation substance known as perlite was packed into the annular space that was left between the vessels after the vacuum was applied. The VIE is of the self-pressurising variety and achieves this through the partial evaporation of liquid oxygen that occurs within a pressure building coil that is controlled by a non-ferrous imported pressure regulator. The container was provided as a fully functional unit, including all of the construction components and the cleaning protocol that were appropriate for medical-grade liquid oxygen. The materials that are utilised, which also include lubricants, comply with the requirements of EIGA IGC 73/17/E (the revised version of Doc 73/08).

When oxygen comes into contact with the temperature of the surrounding environment, it undergoes a phase transition from the liquid to the gaseous state as it undergoes an expansion of approximately 860 times. The tank comes equipped with its own evaporator, which ensures that the liquid oxygen continues to transform into oxygen gas at a rate that is less than 1% of the total volume per day (the natural evaporation rate).

Liquid oxygen requires special vessels that can withstand the high pressure and temperature that is present. The construction of piping must also adhere to the same design principles and comply with all applicable national standards and codes.

23.35 PRESSURE SWING ABSORPTION (PSA) *OXYGEN PLANT INSTILLATION IN INDIA*

The setting up of a medical oxygen facility requires approval from Government bodies. First, permission is needed from the local pollution control board for installation. Secondly, the applicant and operator of the medical oxygen facility must have an "Establishment Registration Licence" from the Labour Department of the respective state government. Third, approval from the Petroleum and Safety Organisation (PESO) is required, including the chemical facility, engineering drawings such as plant layouts and area classification. Other requirements may include No Objection Certificate (NOC) from collector or district authority and a licence as per The Drugs and Cosmetics Act, 1940 is required, since medical oxygen is under the purview of drugs.

BIBLIOGRAPHY

BOC Products 2011. Available from: http://www.bochealthcare.co.uk/en/products/index.shtml. Accessed 12 March 2021.

British Pharmacopeia Commission. *British Pharmacopeia*. London: T.S.O; 2008.

CGMP-Guidelines 2006. Available from: http://frwebgate.access.gpo.gov/cgibin/getdoc.cgi?dbname=2006_register&docid=fr10ap06-17. Accessed 12 March 2021.

CGMP-Guidelines [Internet]. 2006 [cited 9 March 2018]. Available from: http://frwebgate.access.gpo.gov/cgibin/getdoc.cgi?db name=2006_register&docid=fr10ap06-17. Accessed 12 March 2021.

Churchill-Davidson A. *Practice of Anesthesia*. 7th ed. London: Arnold; 2003.

Civil Appeal No 2230 of 2020 The Hon'ble Supreme Court on April 14, 2020, in the matter of State of Andhra Pradesh v. M/s Linde India Ltd.1 Has Held That 'Medical Oxygen IP' and 'Nitrous Oxide IP' Are Classified as 'Drug' and Fall Within the Meaning of Section 3(b)(i) of the Drugs and Cosmetics Act 1940.

Compressed Medical Gases 1992 [Revised 31 August 1992]. Available from: http://www.fda.gov/ICECI/ComplianceManuals/CompliancePolicyGuidanceManual/ucm074381.htm. Accessed 12 March 2021.

Draft Guidance Note on Liquid Medical Oxygen (LMO) Storage Tanks. Available from: https://nhm.gov.in/New_Update-2021-22/PIP/ECRP-II/Guidance_Note_on_LMO_Storage_Tanks.pdf. Accessed 12 March 2021.

European Directorate for the Quality of Medicines. *European Pharmacopeia*. 7th ed. France: EDQM; 2006.

Fatal Mix Up Doctor Can Work 2001. Available from: http://news.bbc.co.uk/2/hi/health/1235745.stm. Accessed 12 March 2021.

Gas Cylinder Rule 2015, Ministry of Commerce and Industry, Department of Industrial Policy and Promotion, Government of India [Internet]. 2015 [Cited 11 March 2018]. Available from: http://peso.gov.in/PDF/GCR_Draft_Notification_201 5_English.pdf. Accessed 12 March 2021.

Gas Cylinder Rule, 2016, Ministry of Commerce and Industry, Department of Industrial Policy and Promotion, Government of India [Internet]. 2016 [Cited 12 March 2018]. Available from: http://peso.gov.in/Work_Mannual/Gas_cylinder_Rule _WM.pdf. Accessed 12 March 2021.

Government of India. Ministry of Health and Family Welfare. *Indian Pharmacopoeia Vol. I & II*. New Delhi: The Controller of Publication; 1996, 762–10.

G.S.R. 907(E). —Whereas the Draft of Explosives Rules, 2006 Were Published, as Required by Sub-Section (1) of Section 18 of Explosive Act, 1884 (4 of 1884) vide.

http://www.gawdawiki.org/headlines/index.php/Medical-Gas-Mix-up-at-Dentist-1448.

Lawrence L, Keith L, editors. *Goodman and Gilman Manual of Pharmacology and Therapeutics.* McGraw Hill; 2008, San Diego La Jolla, California.

Medical Gas Containers and Closures; Current Good Manufacturing Practice Requirements 2006. Available from: http://federalregister.gov/a/06-3370. Accessed 12 March 2021.

Medical GAS Mix-Up At a Dentist 2011. Available from: Accessed 14 March 2021.

Medical Gas Solutions 2011. Available from: http://www.medicalgassolutions.co.uk/fill.html. Accessed 12 March 2021.

Medical Uses of Helium 2011. Available from: http://www.suite101.com/content/medical-uses-of-helium-a188726. Accessed 12 March 2021.

Ministry of Commerce and Industry 2006. Available from: http://peso.gov.in/Roles_Respons.aspx. Accessed 12 March 2021.

Proposal for USP Standards Based on Medical Gas Mix-Ups 2011. Available from: http://www.gmptrainingsystems.com/files/u1/pdf/Medical_gas_Q&A.pdf. Accessed 12 March 2021.

Rahul V. Regulation Applicable in the Manufacturing and Supply of Medical Oxygen in India- A Legal Overview Tanks 2021. Available from https://www.linkedin.com/pulse/regulations-applicable-manufacture-supply-medical-oxygen-rahul-varma. Linked in Accessed 12 March 2021.

Rebecca J. Medical Grade Compressed Air. *Update in Anaesthesia.* 2001;13:1–2.

Soni NN, Maheshwari DG. Current Regulation of Medical Gases in India and Future Aspects. *Int J Drug Regulatory Affairs.* 2018;6: 35–40.

Stoeling RK. *Pharmacology and Physiology in Anesthetic Practic*e. 4th ed. Philadelphia: Lippincott Williams; 2006.

Sweetman SC, editor. *Martindale the Complete Drug Reference.* 36th ed. London: Pharmaceutical Press; 2009.

The Gas Cylinders Rules, 2016 Published vide Notification No. GSR. 1081(E), dated 22 November 2016. Accessed 12 March 2021.

The Static and Mobile Pressure Vessels (Unfired) Rules, 2016 Published Vide Notification No. G.S.R. 1109(E), dated 1 December 2016.

Trail Begins in a Medical Gas Mix-Up. 2010. Available from: http://www.gawdawiki.org/headlines/Trial-Begins-In-Medical-Gas-Mix-up-893/128. Accessed 12 March 2021.

Twigg SJ. Helium-Oxygen Mixtures in Adult Critical Care Medicine. 2011 Available from: http://www.avon.nhs.uk/bristolitutrainees/dissertations/Helium%20Dissertation%20-%20Twigg.pdf. Accessed 12 March 2021.

United States Pharmacopeial Convention. *United States Pharmacopeia.* 31th ed. National Formulary. 26thed; 2008.

Working Document QAS/20.867/Rev6 May 2022 for Publication in the 11th Edition of Ph.Int. Available from: https://cdn.who.int/media/docs/default-source/essential-medicines/norms-and-standards/qas20-867-medicinal-oxygen.pdf?sfvrsn=ab60e2fe_5. Accessed 12 March 2021.

24 Regulation of Radiopharmaceuticals in the Preview of the Drugs and Cosmetics Act, 1940

24.1 INTRODUCTION

The use of radioactive compounds is common in present times for exploration into their applications in fields such as medicine, industry, agriculture, and research, etc. Radiopharmaceuticals are included under "drugs" and fall into a unique subset of the drug classification system and are put to use in clinical practice as diagnostic and therapeutic agents. Depending on the drug definition, the manufacture, use, and storage of this product are subject to the special requirements of the regulatory authorities, such as the production falling under the purview of the Drug Control Government of India (DCGI), and the regulation of the Atomic Energy Regulatory Board (AERB) in India. The implementation of Good Manufacturing Practices (GMP), which are national requirements for the manufacture of radiopharmaceuticals, must be a prerequisite for any preparation.

Any establishments in India that manufacture radiopharmaceuticals must follow primarily two regulations for India, i.e., The Drugs and Cosmetics Act, 1940 for the manufacturing process, and the Atomic Energy Act of 1962 for the transportation and installation of the facilities. In the United States, the Code of Federal Regulations (CFR) Title 21 and the Nuclear Regulatory Commission (NRC) are in charge of regulating the radiopharmaceuticals, whereas, in Europe, radiopharmaceuticals are subject to regulation under Directive 89/343/EC and are subject to supervision in that region. Before using any radiation or radioactive substances, to ensure their safety, operation, possession, and disposal, they are strongly regulated by government. The United States Food and Drug Administration (FDA) enforces the regulation of radiopharmaceuticals in the US, The Drugs and Cosmetics Act, 1940 enforces the regulation for India, whereas EU Directive regulates them in Europe. The regulations govern manufacturing, standardisation, and marketing of the radiopharmaceuticals.

24.2 CLASSIFICATION OF RADIOPHARMACEUTICALS

Radiopharmaceuticals are divided into four main types:

1. Preparation of a Radiopharmaceutical

   A radiopharmaceutical preparation with radionuclide can be used on humans directly for diagnosing or treating medical conditions.

DOI: 10.1201/9781003397854-8

2. Radionuclide Generator
   The daughter radionuclide, having a short half-life, fused and separated from the parent radionuclide which has a longer half-life and is used for production of a radiopharmaceutical. Example: Technetium-99m (Tc-99m) generator. In this system, Molybdenum-98 (Mo-98) serves as the parent radionuclide with a relatively longer half-life, and it decays to produce the daughter radionuclide Technetium-99m (Tc-99m), which has a shorter half-life. Tc-99m is widely used in nuclear medicine for the production of radiopharmaceuticals.
3. Radiopharmaceutical Precursor: In the radio-labelling process, a specific radionuclide is formed, which is known as a radiopharmaceutical.
4. Kit for Radiopharmaceutical Preparation

The components mentioned are used in the preparation of radiopharmaceuticals. These components likely include sterilized and validated precursors or radionuclide products. The prepared radiopharmaceuticals are diluted before medical use. This dilution may be part of the final steps in the preparation process to achieve the desired concentration for medical applications

24.3 THE MANUFACTURE OF RADIOPHARMACEUTICAL PREPARATIONS IN ACCORDANCE WITH GMP

Radiopharmaceuticals are used as drugs, and their quality is maintained throughout the preparation and dosage form formulation processes. In order to complete the preparation of the radiopharmaceuticals, an excipient is added to them. This step is necessary for quality control and manufacturing in a GMP facility.

24.3.1 The Incorporation of Antibacterial Preservatives

The vast majority of radiopharmaceuticals come in the form of injections intended for multiple patients and packaged in containers designed to hold multiple doses. Because of this, prolonged preservation at the optimum concentration is necessary in order to withstand the contamination caused by the withdrawal of multiple doses.

On the packaging, there needs to be an endorsement of the antimicrobial agent that was used. Injectable drugs that have a half-life of less than one day are typically packaged in single-dose containers, even when only a single dosage is required. Where the half-life is greater than one day, and consequently, antimicrobial agents are typically not used after the initial dosage has been withdrawn in an aseptic manner. The container is stored at a temperature between 2° and 8°C for 7 days.

24.3.2 Sterilisation

The validation of sterilization procedures is linked to the half-life of the isotopes used in radiopharmaceuticals. The validation process demonstrates the effectiveness of sterilization methods, ensuring the safety and integrity of the final product. A validated production method is applied specifically when working with ultra-short half-life isotopes, defined here as less than 20 minutes. Validation ensures that the production process meets predetermined criteria for quality, safety, and efficacy. Radiopharmaceutical preparations with ultra-short half-lives are designed for parenteral administration, indicating that they are intended for injection or infusion into the body.

Final sterilization is identified as the preferred method for sterilizing radiopharmaceuticals. This step is crucial for eliminating or reducing microbial contamination, contributing to product safety. Ultrafiltration is recommended as a technology for use with short-lived radiopharmaceuticals. Ultrafiltration involves the use of a semipermeable membrane to separate particles based on size, allowing for the removal of impurities.

Good Manufacturing Practice (GMP) protocols for radiopharmaceuticals have been successfully validated through the use of sterilization techniques. GMP compliance is essential for ensuring that radiopharmaceuticals meet quality standards throughout the manufacturing process.

24.3.3 Identity Tests

The radiopharmaceuticals are identified in accordance with the half-life and energy of their radiation as described in the corresponding monograph.

24.3.4 Determination of the Half-life

It is possible to determine the half-life with a Geiger-Muller counter, a scintillation counter, an ionisation chamber, or a semiconductor detector. This is done while avoiding dead time losses by diluting the sample appropriately. The calculated half-life is within a range of 5% from the calculated half-life that is given in the particular monograph.

24.3.5 Radionuclide Purity

Before the expiration date, the gamma-ray spectrum of the radionuclide should be comparable to that in the particular monograph for that radionuclide. The impurity also slowed down the half-life; for instance, thallium-202 had a $t_{1/2}$ value of 12.23 days according to the monograph, but, in practice, the manufacture of thallium-201 could have resulted in a $t_{1/2}$ value of 72 hours. In conclusion, the contaminant is the driving force behind the shifts in the half-life.

24.3.6 Radiochemical Purity

There are a variety of sensitive analytical techniques available, such as paper chromatography, liquid chromatography, electrophoresis, and thin-layer chromatography, for determination of radiochemical purity of radioactive pharmaceuticals. The alternations in radioactivity that occur in the chromatography techniques are indicative of the purity of radiopharmaceuticals. The interpretation of purity needs to exclude the artifacts of the diluents of chromatographic techniques or any interaction between the reaction impurity and radiochemical impurity. The evaluation of radiochemical purity frequently makes use of high-performance liquid chromatography (HPLC) techniques. Additionally, the biological distributions of the radiopharmaceutical are taken into account when determining the concentration.

24.3.7 Chemical Purity of Radiopharmaceuticals

The original chemical component that is present in the actual forms is what is known as chemical purity, and this is true independent of the radioactivity. The purity of radiochemical changes over time, so the time scale should be stated when the purity is mentioned. The radiochemical purity is the determining factor throughout for the shelf life.

If the radioactivity breaks down, extra isotopic radionuclides are made, which are then called impurities. For example, 99mTc-DTPA (diethylenetriamine-pentaacetic acid) is made from diethylenetriamine-pentaacetic acid, and 99% of the complex is present. But the free 99mTc-pertechnetate anion made by the radiochemical decay of 99mTc with reduced hydrolysis is not a contaminant.

The specific activity of radiopharmaceuticals is an essential factor to take into consideration, and it is denoted as the rate of disintegration with the unit mass. Specific radioactivity and radiochemical purity are two different things, and most pharmacopoeias address the activity of the radiation. Sometimes, a chemical impurity is an extra radionuclide that is made during storage by radiation-radiolysis. This is called a radiochemical impurity with a high specific activity. So, figuring out the chemical impurity predictor is an important part of making sure of quality. For example, ion exchange resins or reactions like *o*-iodohippuric acid, which is used to replace iodine-131 atoms, are used to figure out the amount of iodine in a sample. Sometimes, chemical impurities cause toxins and interfere with the human body's biological processes, like when an impurity in the aluminium present which caused 99mTc flocculated forms. Stereo-isomeric purity is also important for ligand bonds, whereas organ toxicity is caused by inorganic impurities like heavy metals.

24.3.8 Bacterial Endotoxins/Pyrogens

This describes the planning needed to pass the bacterial endotoxins test. Because of the characteristics of the radiopharmaceutical, it is necessary to conduct the required test, as well as the validation, in order to determine the test. Because the high level of radioactivity could mess up the test, it had to be validated.

24.3.9 pH

The pH of radiopharmaceutical preparations should be isotonic with blood adjusted to pH 6.5–7.5. pH is one of the key factors to take into account.

24.3.10 Labelling

Labelling the radiopharmaceuticals is conducted according to GMP rules. The label includes the following:

- A bold, easy-to-read statement that mentions radiation and has the international symbol for radioactivity.
- The name of the radiopharmaceutical, its symbol, and the amount of radioactivity in the whole mixture.
- The whole process of getting a test or treatment ready to use.
- Administration process details.
- The details of the radioactivity in the measure should be written with the date, such as MBq per ml.
- The expiration date and time must be mentioned.
- The batch process ID number.
- Conditions for storage, such as time, light, and temperature.
- Details should be given about the stabiliser, antimicrobial agents, or any other additives.

24.3.11 Storage

Storing radiopharmaceuticals is important. They should be kept in a covered container so that the operational person gets the least amount of radiation possible and so that the maximum radiation doses can be kept in the container. The necessary government regulations for protecting against harmful radiation must be followed. Radiopharmaceuticals for parenteral use should be kept in a clear or amber glass bottle, ampoule, or single-dose syringe, and they should be inspected so that they can be seen clearly.

24.3.12 Safety of Critical Organ Exposure

Any radiopharmaceuticals used to image a vital organ exposes it to radiation, and the maximum safe dose is used to figure out the safety level of radiation exposure.

24.3.13 Other Important Data Requirements for Approval of Radiopharmaceuticals in India

The Indian government put into place rules for using and disposing of radiopharmaceuticals properly. Radiopharmaceuticals are medicines or drugs that have radioactive materials in them and are used to treat or diagnose health conditions. These radiopharmaceuticals actively participate in the biological activities, and they have a variety of physicochemical characteristics, including the fact that they degrade over time. Radiopharmaceuticals can be classified as either simple radiochemicals or radiopharmaceuticals, and they were among the chemicals used for diagnosis and treatment purposes. In addition, radiopharmaceuticals have intricated molecular and supramolecular structures with active homing abilities, which allow them to specifically deliver the radioactive payload to the region of disease or dysfunction, which can then be used as a diagnostic or treatment tool. The homing characteristics and natural consequences of radiopharmaceuticals increased the sophistication of the requirements for nuclear medicine. This necessitated the adoption of targeted approaches that engaged at the level of cells and organelles. Radiopharmaceuticals have the same regulatory windows as other drugs, as was already stated.

24.3.14 *In vivo* Study

Therapeutic radiopharmaceuticals, like other medicines, need to go through pre-clinical testing, which includes both *in vitro* and animal studies. Animal pharmacology and animal toxicology studies will have to be done, and the details of these studies will be listed in Schedule Y of Appendix III and Appendix IV of the Drugs and Cosmetics Rules, respectively. Radiopharmaceuticals, on the other hand, are nothing like other types of chemical compounds like drugs. When testing radiopharmaceuticals is carried out in pre-clinical studies, there are a lot of aspects that need to be taken into account, such as dose preparation and the use of radioactive substances, evaluation, especially signal acquisition, and animal handling, particularly animal housekeeping, euthanasia, and organ or tissue withdrawal for future treatments. This makes it possible to collect sufficient data on the potential behaviour of the radiopharmaceuticals in animal models and extrapolate them to human patients, with respect to both their safety and their efficacy. Studies should be designed in the same way that diagnostic radiopharmaceuticals are studied to figure out their chemistry, toxicology, and dosimetry. When it comes to the preclinical assessment of therapeutic pharmaceuticals, the reality is that biodistribution and dosimetry play an even greater role. Because the findings of these tests can be used to evaluate radiation-induced toxicity, which is frequently the only type of toxicity caused by this class of agents, and because they can also provide data regarding efficacy when dose escalation studies are carried out, this is the case. Toxicology and dosimetry are two very important aspects that must be considered in the process of determining whether radiopharmaceuticals should be used for diagnostic or therapeutic purposes. Dosimetry prediction is a method for figuring out the absorbed dose, which is the amount of energy that is received per unit of mass in all irradiated tissues or organs. In diagnostic radiopharmaceuticals, they are mostly used to comprehend if any unintentional damage has been done to a living system. This damage may have been caused by a radiation dose that was too high or by a pharmacological effect of the carrier that was used to transport the radioactive label.

Radiopharmaceuticals are sorted by their possible diagnostic, theranostic, or therapeutic uses based on the type of radiation, the amount of energy, and the half-life of the radiopharmaceutical. The cytotoxic or modulatory effects of therapeutic radiopharmaceuticals are also taken into account. However, the preclinical assessment of these radiopharmaceuticals cannot be complete without a thorough study of these toxicological effects. The pharmacological profile of many radiopharmaceuticals is unknown, as are their affinity and selectivity for plasma binding. Because of this, biodistribution and dosimetry studies need to be carefully planned and done in order to correctly simulate how the substance is meant to be used in a clinical setting. This is essential in order to comprehend the radiometabolite analyses, which originate from different uptake in various tissues compared with the parent tracer.

It is best to use lead radiopharmaceuticals that do not get broken down in humans or whose breakdown products are excreted from the body quickly. The radionuclides' lipophilicity has a small effect on both its ability to bind to non-displacing plasma and its ability to be removed from the body. One of the significant parameters could be to identify the effect of radiopharmaceuticals on the target-to-background ratio of its metabolism. This ratio is affected by a number of significant parameters. Also, many post-translational interactions of radionuclides happen after metabolism. A high affinity and selectivity or a low selectivity or a low affinity toward the intended target of the radiopharmaceutical are common ways to classify it so that it can be quickly removed from the rest of the body. *In vivo* testing is the only way to figure out pharmacodynamic properties like target retention, which are needed to understand pharmacokinetic characteristics. Biodistribution studies need to be done before organ distribution and whole-body dosimetry can be calculated. Understanding the target binding and figuring out whether a radiopharmaceutical can bind in a way that is competitive, non-competitive, or allosteric is one of the most important steps in learning about radiopharmaceuticals. It is crucial to emphasise the fact that the specific activity has the potential to have an impact on the biodistribution of the radiopharmaceutical. Specific activity is the amount of radioactivity in a radiopharmaceutical that is measured per unit of mass and takes into account all of its isotopes. As a direct result of this, specific activity generally decreases with the passage of time as the decay continues and the radioactivity decreases. On the other hand, the molecular mass, which is mostly decided by derivatives that don't decay, will stay about the same.

24.3.15 *Ex-vivo* Testing of Radionuclides

Iodine-123, technetium-99m, xenon-133, thallium-201, and indium-111 are the radiopharmaceuticals that are most frequently utilised in the process of Photon Emission Computed Tomography (SPECT) imaging. After the radionuclides have been injected into the animals, the number of radionuclides that have been deposited in an animal is determined, and the animal is then euthanised. This is an illustration of the spatial distribution of radionuclides deposited in biological tissues. The distribution of these radionuclides in biological tissues depends on the affinity of the tissue. The amount of radioactivity can be determined based on the amount of substance that was present in the sample at the moment in time when it was collected.

24.3.16 Organ Biodistribution of Radionuclides

This study is important for a number of reasons, including the fact that it will help to understand whether or not radionuclides are safe to inject into experimental animals. According to the affinity of the metabolites, radionuclides are disseminated in a certain way; for example, fluorine compounds are deposited in bone, whereas copper compounds are deposited in the liver. The distribution of the radiopharmaceutical throughout the organs of the animal provides a picture or a general notion of how the radionuclides are distributed and retained within the animal. In practice, after a radiopharmaceutical is given, the affected organs and tissues are removed after a particular period of time so that the amount of radioactivity can be measured. In most cases, the organs serve as sink conditions, which are places where the majority of radiopharmaceuticals are transformed to metabolites and deposited.

24.3.17 Autoradiography of Tissue Sections for Radionuclides

Autoradiography is one of the most common techniques that is used to determine the distribution of radioactivity throughout the tissues of animals, which is an essential step in comprehending the toxicity of the substance. In *ex-vivo* autoradiography, the tracer is injected into a living animal, so the tracer–target interaction has already happened, and the tissue is already radioactive when it is cut. Therefore, *ex-vivo* autoradiography provides a significantly higher resolution (0.2 mm) than any other technique.

24.3.18 Radio Metabolite Analysis

After being administered, radiopharmaceuticals undergo metabolism and biotransformation, and the products of this transformation, which are known as radiometabolites, themselves become radioactive after their transformation. However, radio-metabolites can cause a radioactive signature to be produced, whereas active radio-metabolites typically do not interfere with the function of non-radioactive metabolites. Because of this, the pharmacokinetics and target affinity tracer of the offspring are substantially different from those of the parent. As a result, radiometabolites cause changes to the imagery, and these changes must be taken into account when quantifying the images because of the background radio-metabolites noise. In addition, tailored radiotherapy and radio metabolites can make the risks of radiation exposure to healthy tissue even greater. Therefore, in the safety research, this should be taken into consideration.

24.3.19 Plasma Protein Binding of Radionuclides

In the case of therapeutic radiopharmaceuticals, a plasma protein binding is an essential factor to take into consideration. Studies of a drug's effectiveness in living organisms, or *in vivo*, are necessary for determining whether or not it possesses the pharmacological activity that is desired. Additionally, plasma protein binding plays a significant part in determining whether or not the drug has increased toxic effects that compromise its effectiveness.

Dietary conditions, medical treatments (both invasive and non-invasive), radiation therapy, surgical procedures, prostheses, cardioversion, intubation, chemoperfusion, external massage, immunotherapy, blood transfusion, and haemodialysis are mentioned as factors that can significantly impact protein bindings. These factors can affect the degree to which a particular drug, including radiopharmaceuticals, binds to proteins in plasma. The nature of the drug and the patient's physiological state can influence the likelihood of protein binding.

Radiopharmaceuticals in the blood can exist in two forms: bound and unbound. The binding status is determined by the interaction between the drug and proteins in the plasma. The degree of protein binding establishes an equilibrium between the bound and unbound states of a drug. This equilibrium is affected by the specific characteristics of the drug and the conditions in the patient's body.

If protein binding is reversible, an equilibrium state is achieved between the bound and unbound states. This equilibrium ensures that the drug remains in a dynamic balance, with some portions bound to proteins and others remaining unbound. The equilibrium state results in the formation of complexes between radiopharmaceuticals and proteins. This complex composition may influence the behaviour, distribution, and pharmacokinetics of the radiopharmaceutical within the body.

A strong affinity of radiopharmaceuticals for a receptor can sometimes result in toxic effects, and the majority of radiopharmaceutical kinetics and plasma kinetics are based on a competitive reaction. The receptor is also a protein. Although the unbound radiopharmaceuticals component of the drug is metabolised in the liver and other tissues, both bound and unbound radiopharmaceuticals are ultimately excreted through the urine. Ideally, radiopharmaceuticals with high efficacy and low toxicity have enough "clinical promise" to be used on people.

24.3.20 Toxicology of Radionuclides

The *in-vivo* animal model is used to conduct an assessment of the risks and benefits associated with radiopharmaceuticals. Before beginning experimentation on humans, it is beneficial to conduct preclinical research using radiopharmaceuticals since it can provide helpful ideas. Diagnostic radiopharmaceuticals, in contrast with therapeutic radiopharmaceuticals, are often supplied at low doses as tracer levels (micrograms per kilogram of body weight). These tracer levels are at such a low dose that there is no detectable biological effect from the radiopharmaceutical. In conclusion, non-clinical toxicity studies should be carried out in a laboratory that is certified as adhering to good laboratory practice (GLP), should follow the guidelines established by the International Council for Harmonization of Technical Requirement for Pharmaceuticals for Human Use (ICH), and should implement the ICH M3 (R2) guideline, which is standardised for primarily optimising dosages and fulfilling regulatory requirements. According to the ICH guideline, Approach 1 is used when the total dose total dose administered is $\leq$100 µg and the NOAEL ("No observed adverse effect level") dose is $\leq$1/100. This is called the "accepted dose," and it is measured in mg/kg for intravenous administration and in mg/m^2 for oral administration. In addition, the ICH guideline specifies that when numerous administrations or more than one administration are required advocates the Approach 2 study and cumulative dose administered is $\leq$500 µg, whereas the NOAEL dose is $\leq$1/500.

A maximum limit of five administrations is mentioned for radiopharmaceuticals. This suggests that there are restrictions on the number of times a patient can receive this type of treatment or imaging agent. To ensure safety and allow for proper elimination of the radiopharmaceutical from the body, there is a specified elimination phase between each dose. This approach helps manage the potential accumulation of radioactive material. The statement suggests that in-actuality half-lifetimes of radiopharmaceuticals can be calculated based on the elimination time. This calculation provides insights into how long it takes for the radiopharmaceutical to be eliminated from the body and helps determine the appropriate timing for subsequent administrations. Limiting the number of administrations and incorporating elimination phases are considerations aimed at ensuring patient safety. Managing radiation exposure and allowing the body time to eliminate the radiopharmaceutical are important factors in clinical practice.

The approach of allowing a maximum number of administrations and incorporating elimination phases may be part of individualized treatment plans. Factors such as the specific radiopharmaceutical used, the medical condition being addressed, and patient characteristics may influence these decisions.

Approach 3 of the guideline can be used for any dose as long as it falls within the range of a single dose at a sub-therapeutic or expected dose. The initial dose should be on the order of the particular toxicity, and the maximum dose might be regarded up to half of the NOAEL dose for sensitive animals. However, such a dose should not have produced toxicity; otherwise, the dose should have been reversed.

24.3.21 Studies of Toxicity, Along with Dosage of Radionuclides

Studies of toxicity at Approach 1 dosages are conducted using an "extended single-dose toxicity study," and only one species (often rodents) is employed for the research. In each group, ten animals of each sex are used, and, on day 14, necropsy data, haematological, electrolyte, and bio-chemical chemistry results, as well as histopathology examinations, are performed, whereas using Approach 2, a repeated dosage toxicity study in one species of rodents over the course of seven days has to be carried out at the same dose level that was specified earlier. After a seven-day observation period, data from necropsy as well as hematological, electrolyte, and biochemical chemistry as well as histopathology are evaluated. The dose that was employed in the prospective microdose studies is $\leq$1/100 of the NOAEL of the NOAEL. This indicates that, in clinical practice, a dose that is one hundred times higher might be administered to humans without causing any adverse reactions. In order to properly evaluate toxicity studies, it is necessary to conduct plasma kinetics studies (also known as PK) and dosimetry for the purpose of determining the organ-specific toxicity caused by radiation exposure.

24.3.22 First Dose Calculation to be Given to a Human Being (Also Known as the FIH Dose)

First-in-Human (FIH) studies involve the initial administration of a therapeutic radiopharmaceutical to human subjects. These studies are crucial for assessing safety, dosage, and potential therapeutic effects. Dosage selection is a critical aspect of FIH studies. Determining the appropriate amount of radioactivity and the ligand (molecule) used is essential. This process involves balancing therapeutic efficacy with minimising the risk of adverse effects, particularly radiation exposure. The choice of ligand is mentioned as a factor that minimises the chance of patients being affected by radiation. Ligands play a crucial role in targeting the radiopharmaceutical to specific tissues or cells, contributing to both therapeutic efficacy and safety. Time-Activity Curves (TAC) are derived from pre-clinical experiments in relevant animal models. These curves provide information about the biodistribution of the radiopharmaceutical over time. Compartmental modelling is used to analyse and interpret TAC data. Compartmental modelling is a mathematical approach to characterize the distribution and kinetics of a radiopharmaceutical within the body. It involves dividing the body into compartments and describing the movement of the radiopharmaceutical between these compartments.

The statement refers to the FDA (U.S. Food and Drug Administration) as a regulatory authority that provides guidance on the development of therapeutic radiopharmaceuticals. Compliance with regulatory guidelines is essential for the approval and marketing of such products. Information from pre-clinical experiments in animal models is used to inform the design and dosing strategies for FIH studies. This data helps predict how the radiopharmaceutical will behave in humans.

These curves are then used to calculate the exposure to radiation that a patient obtains from a radiopharmaceutical, as well as the duration of residence and time-integrated activity in human organs.

The development of therapeutic radiopharmaceuticals occurs in conjunction with the development of a diagnostic analogue and the determination of the human dose that is to be administered by primary diagnostic agents. Therefore, the pharmacokinetics of the primary diagnostic agents is an essential factor in determining the effective therapeutic dose or the maximum dose that is indicated, the Maximum Recommended Starting Dose (MRSD). In addition, the total radioactivity of the therapeutic radiopharmaceutical being investigated in a FIH trial is an essential element, as is the mass dose of the pharmaceutical. Animal dosimetry studies can also provide useful information for determining the appropriate beginning radiation dose for a FIH investigation. The measurement of radiation from animal key organs, such as the thyroid, bone marrow, small and large intestine, brain, stomach, heart, liver, lungs, kidneys, muscles, ovaries, and pancreas, might be used to create an organ Time Activity Curve (TAC) graph. Other parameters that could be measured include radio intervals for five times the effective half-life of the radiopharmaceutical. As a result, MRSD selection is an important element that can be addressed in two different ways. In the first step, conversion factors for deriving a Human Equivalent Dose (HED) need to be established. In the second step, a method of dose selection based on animal studies needs to be developed in order to convert NOAELs to HED. According to FDA guidelines, the MRSD is nothing more than the NOAELs in the animal species that were tested and the conversion of the NOAELs to HED. However, other various elements may be taken into consideration such as the safety of the parent molecule, clinical modalities, and so on. The determination of scaling factors is in accordance with the NOAEL of each species and their subsequent conversion to the HED. A dosimetry study is a type of preclinical study that offers extrapolation information regarding the quantity of dosage that can be safely injected for initial clinical testing. The biodistribution of radiopharmaceuticals is an essential component in gaining an understanding of TACs in physiological organs, and the biodistribution of any radiopharmaceuticals can be ascertained through quantitative imaging through the dissection of an individual animal. The HED can be calculated by looking at the toxicity and the dose that is absorbed in animals.

24.3.23 Small-scale Dosimetry Models of Radionuclides

Short-ranged particle emitters, such as beta particles or low-energy electrons, could be used in autoradiography to diagnose relatively small organs like the kidney, spleen, etc. Calculating the absorbed dose values in organs or target locations are done with the help of a camera.

24.3.24 Dosimetry Phantoms and Models for Use with Smaller Animals

Phantoms that are standardised or used as references for dosimetry calculations can provide true anatomical images if they are used. The diagnosis of a tumour or other illness conditions or any abnormality off the organ reference dosimetry may be greater or lower than the reference of the particular organ. One of the most significant drawbacks of this approach is that the radiopharmaceutical exhibits non-uniform absorption when applied to organs that are carrying malignancies.

24.3.25 Extrapolation of Animal Dosimetry to Human Dosimetry

Clinical trials provide insights into potential dangers associated with the absorption of high doses, offering a hint about the risks posed to specific organs. Correlation studies are conducted to understand the relationship between dosage levels and potential hazards, especially at high doses that may be considered hazardous. Preclinical trials involve the establishment of dosage limits to assess toxicity. These limits are determined through experiments conducted on animals before moving on to human trials. Dosage limits are set in preclinical trials to determine the equivalence of toxicity, helping researchers understand the potential adverse effects of the substance being tested. The dosage limits identified in preclinical trials are translated to human doses, considering differences in morphology between animals used in preclinical studies and humans.

The translation process takes into account the morphological differences between animals and humans. This ensures a more accurate estimation of safe and effective dosages for human subjects. Preclinical trials play a crucial role in identifying potential risks and establishing safety limits before exposing humans to experimental substances. This risk mitigation approach is fundamental for ethical and regulatory reasons. Observations from preclinical trials serve as early indicators of potential toxicity, guiding researchers in making informed decisions about the safety profile of the substance. Adhering to ethical principles and regulatory guidelines is essential throughout preclinical trials to ensure the responsible and safe progression of experimental substances to human testing.

PK investigations are necessary in order to extrapolate the findings from research conducted on small animals to those conducted on humans. The organ time-activity curves (TACs) data were obtained from preclinical investigations conducted in relevant animal models in order to determine the residence duration and the time-integrated activity in human organs. According to what was stated before, the majority of therapeutic radiopharmaceuticals are developed from diagnostic radiopharmaceuticals since it is simpler to understand the absorption, distribution, metabolism, and excretion of diagnostic radiopharmaceuticals. The calculated dose is going to be put to use in order to arrive at a decision regarding the first application of the medication to human patients.

24.3.26 *In vivo* Pharmacokinetic Data to Formation of Time–Activity Curves of Radionuclides

The absorption of radionuclides with regard to the time–activity curves with time limit, i.e., TAC (A(t)), in each organ is derived from biodistribution data or from quantitative imaging investigations and then translated into pharmacokinetic models. Any research on biodistribution, the timing of animal euthanasia, and the scan times all need to be taken into mind. In addition, any PK investigations are appropriate when the characteristics of the radiopharmaceuticals, such as their absorption time, are examined, along with the association between elimination and physical decay. In a PK study, the radioactivity in plasma at different times, also known as the area under the curve, is measured, and two main constants, namely the plasma absorption constant (PKa) and the elimination rate constant (PKe), are derived. Accordingly, many conclusions, including plasma distribution, volume of distribution, and elimination rate of radiopharmaceuticals, can be drawn.

24.3.27 Stability Assay Radiopharmaceuticals

24.3.27.1 Plasma/Serum Stability Assay Radiopharmaceuticals

The stability of plasma and serum in the presence of radiopharmaceuticals is an important parameter that must be considered in order to comprehend the behaviour of plasma or serum. The *in vivo* stability is also important to examine the radiopharmaceutical in order to determine whether or not it is metabolized *in vivo* and distributed in the target organ. In the majority of instances, an HPLC system equipped with a particular type of column is used to carry out the analysis.

24.3.27.2 Ex-vivo *Autoradiography of Radiopharmaceuticals*

Autoradiography is an essential method for understanding the organ distribution in the target organ through comparison with that of a marker or reference radiopharmaceuticals having shorter half-lives that have completely decayed (six half-lives or more in a short amount of time) with standard radiopharmaceuticals in the same animal. In dual-label autoradiography, the radiopharmaceuticals are administered at various time intervals and the animals sacrificed in order to find the ideal kinetic behaviour of each radiopharmaceutical. During the process of converting from density light units to radioactivity units, the pixel values should also be corrected for radionuclide decay. This is done so that the resulting data are accurate.

An individual who is familiar with the legal provisions of the Atomic Energy (Radiation Protection) Rules, which were published in the Gazette Notification GSR 303, 2004, and the Atomic Energy (Safe Disposal of Radioactive Waste) Rules, which were published in the Gazette Notification GSR 124, 1987, is qualified to hold the position of a radio safety officer. This individual is in charge of managing radioactive chemicals that are afterwards utilised in medical applications. The manufacture of radiopharmaceuticals is said to follow the unique or own Standard Operating Procedure (SOP) throughout the entire manufacturing process of radiopharmaceutical products, as stated by the pharmaceutical business or institutes.

24.3.27.3 Clinical Trials of Radiopharmaceuticals

Clinical tests performed on radiopharmaceuticals were subject to the Drugs and Cosmetics Regulations, 1945. In particular, these regulations included rules 122A, 122B and 122D, 122 DA, 122DAA, and 122E of the Drugs and Cosmetics Rules, in addition to Appendices I, IA, and VI of Schedule Y. In addition, the National Ethical Guidelines for Biomedical and Health Research with Human Participants in 2017 have been recently updated by the Indian Council of Medical Research. These guidelines sheds light on radiopharmaceuticals as one of the elements that are required to carry out a clinical trial in any research or study. Radiopharmaceuticals are one of the features that are required to be carried out and to pay more attention to conduct clinical trials. These guidelines also promote the inclusion of human participants or patient groups in one or more health-related investigations so that the consequences of such investigations can be reviewed. This evaluation can take place so that the guidelines can be improved. The only types of radiopharmaceuticals that are specifically covered by the rule are diagnostic and therapeutic radiopharmaceuticals, and the maximum exposure dose that can be utilised in clinical research needs to be in accordance with the standards that have been established by Bhaba Atomic Research Centre (BARC), Mumbai. The fundamental facts of radiopharmaceuticals, such as the maximum tolerated dose, pharmacokinetics, and pharmacodynamics, as well as early measurement of the activities of pharmaceuticals, are required in order to provide the Institutional Ethical Committee with the information it needs to come to a decision about, regarding the modalities of clinical trials. Every Institutional Ethical Committee should be registered with the CDSCO. The dossier that must be submitted to CDSCO in order to receive clearance for clinical trials needs to be prepared in compliance with the following guidelines:

Introductory Comments

A concise explanation of the diagnostic or therapeutic radiopharmaceutical class to which it belongs.

Information on Chemicals and Radiopharmaceuticals

Information on chemically active parts of radiopharmaceuticals, such as generic name or chemical name

Physicochemical Data

The essential pieces of information consist of the molecular weight, as well as the chemical name, the structure, and the empirical formula of the radiopharmaceuticals. In addition, the information addressing the physical properties of radiopharmaceuticals must include not only a description of the radiopharmaceuticals, but also statistics regarding their solubility, partition coefficient, optical rotation, and dissociation constant.

Analytical Data

The purpose of this section is to ascertain whether or not other materials are integrated into radiopharmaceuticals. Infrared radiation (IR), nuclear magnetic resonance (NMR), and ultraviolet light (UV) spectra are required in order to determine the identity of radiopharmaceuticals and their polymorphic properties.

Reference Monograph Specification

These data comprise the identification and measurement of impurities, as well as enantiomeric purity, and the method of quantification, which includes the validation of the procedure.

Studies on Stability

This part covers stability in serum and plasma, binding assay, and final delivery specification, reference standard characterisation, and Material Safety Data Sheet (MSDS).

Formulation Data

These data includes the dose form and the master manufacturing formula's ingredients. In addition, the description needs to include information regarding the content's uniformity, pH, an accelerated degradation research, stability evaluation, storage circumstances, and packing criteria. A comparison evaluation with any applicable overseas brand(s) or any applicable Indian brand(s) that has been approved should also be included, if appropriate.

Animal Pharmacology

This part needs an overview of animal pharmacology, including the manner in which each major organ responds to radiopharmaceuticals. In addition, research is being conducted on the pharmacokinetics aspects of radiopharmaceuticals, including absorption, distribution, metabolism, and excretion, as well as follow-up further safety pharmacology investigations.

Regulatory Status in Other Countries

These data are essential to comprehend the state of the radiopharmaceuticals to the other countries and the information such as marketed, approved status as Investigational New Drug (IND), withdrawal (if applicable), and the reason for it. Other requirements include a limitation on the sale of radiopharmaceuticals in any other country, a Free Sales Certificate, prescription information, or anticipated full prescribing information.

Submission of Samples

The samples of the completed product or an equivalent of 50 clinical doses (under GMP manufacture), or a greater number of clinical doses, if necessary, with testing protocol/s, along with quality controls and specifications, are to be sent to the CDSCO. In addition to this, quality controls and specifications are to be included.

Approval of Clinical Trial

Once it had the application in its possession, the CDSCO proceeded to conduct an initial evaluation of the submission. If any missing data are identified, the applicant will be notified, and, if not, the applications will be forwarded to members of the IND committee in the case of Investigational New Drugs (INDs), or to members of the New Drug Advisory Committee (NDAC), in the case of radiopharmaceutical evaluation of new chemical entities. Form CT-10 is used to make applications for the grant of permission to manufacture new or investigational new radiopharmaceuticals in order to conduct clinical trials, whereas Form CT-04 is used to make applications for the grant of permission to conduct clinical trials of new or investigational new radiopharmaceuticals. On the other hand, according to Clause 1(3) of Schedule Y in The Drugs and Cosmetics Rules, there is provision for the reduction, postponement, or exclusion of toxicological and clinical data requirements for pharmaceuticals intended for the treatment of life-threatening or serious disorders, or diseases that hold particular significance in the context of the Indian health care environment. This is determined by what the CDSCO considers to be the most appropriate course of action in each individual case. In this scenario, applications for the authorisation to produce a formulation must be made using Form CT-12 in order to be considered. This form is only to be used for active pharmaceutical compounds that have not yet been licensed for use, and they must be used in clinical trials. On the other hand, the use of Form CT-13 is required for the submission of applications seeking approval to produce unapproved active pharmaceutical ingredients for the purpose of employing them in the development of formulations that are intended for use in clinical trials. After receiving the application, the CDSCO carried out an initial evaluation of the submission. In the case of Investigational New Drugs (INDs), the applications will be sent to the members of the IND committee. In the case of evaluations of new chemical entities or radiopharmaceuticals, the applications will be sent to the members of the NDAC.

In addition to this, the location that is carrying out the investigation needs to have a licence from the relevant government that enables them to keep, handle, and distribute the radioactive substance. Furthermore, they need to have the necessary permission from BARC that enables them to handle and dispose of the radioactive material. The possible radiation dosage to which participants are likely to be treated should be indicated in quantitative terms, either to the overall body or to each organ individually, in both the protocol and the informed consent document (ICD). These statements should be included in both documents. The Ethics Committee (EC) needs to have the appropriate qualifications to evaluate these types of procedures, and it needs to be registered with CDSCO. In clinical tests using radiopharmaceuticals, it is unethical to include any volunteers who satisfy any of the following criteria: women of childbearing age, children, radiation workers, or anyone who has received a dosage of radiation that is greater than the permissible limit in the preceding year.

Registration of Radiopharmaceuticals

The provisions for the award of registration certificate and import permission for the import radiopharmaceuticals are specified in Rule 23 to Rule 27(A) of The Drugs and Cosmetics Rules from 1945. After receiving CDSCO approval, Form 10 may be issued for *in vivo* radiopharmaceutical items without a registration certificate pursuant to Rule 24 for those radiopharmaceuticals that do not have an indigenous manufacturing facility. For import of such non-indigenous radiopharmaceuticals, Form 10 is mandatory, in accordance with the provisions of The Drugs and Cosmetics Rules 1945, and such radiopharmaceuticals are to be tested for quality at the time of import. The term "Registration Certificate" refers to a certificate issued by the licensing authority in Form 41 under Rule 27A of The Drugs and Cosmetics Rules, 1945, for the registration of the premises for manufacturing radiopharmaceuticals for import and use in India after examining the requisite data as filled in Form 40 by the applicant. In this context, the term "import licence" refers to either a licence in Form 10 to import radiopharmaceuticals, with the exception of those listed in Schedule X. Applications for the registration of radiopharmaceuticals are submitted using Form 44, and the following information is necessary:

- Specifications of the precursor of the radiopharmaceuticals.
- Stability of the radiopharmaceuticals.
- Information of the radiopharmaceuticals as well as analyses and quality control.

- Specifications of particular radionuclides of radiopharmaceuticals, and analytical data.
- Details about the finished product, excipient used, stability, quality assurance formulation development, storage conditions, analytical control validations, and impurity profiling.
- Clinical trial data.

24.4 ROLE OF CENTRAL DRUG STANDARD CONTROL ORGANIZATION (CDSCO) FOR LICENSING AND APPROVAL PROCESS OF RADIOPHARMACEUTICALS

The radiopharmaceuticals are governed by the Central Drug Standard Control Organization (CDSCO). The working and power of CDSCO is under the delegate to regulate the radiopharmaceuticals and other drugs under the Ministry of Health and Family Welfare, Govt. of India. The Indian government has established an effective regulatory framework for radiopharmaceuticals and has made it more efficient. There has been some modification of provisions of The Drugs and Cosmetics Act of 1940 and rules established thereunder in order to accommodate radiopharmaceuticals. According to Schedule Y of The Drugs and Cosmetics Act of 1940 and the Rules of 1945, radiopharmaceuticals are considered to be drugs for the purposes of the definition. Taking into account that the new radiopharmaceuticals are considered to be a drug, and that it is timely for it to be regulated under the new drug approval process, an application for approval was submitted to the licensing authority, i.e. the Drug Controller General of India (DCGI) with Form 44 to ascertain the submission of the requisite data to establish the efficacy and safety in the Indian population with the support of clinical trials, as mentioned in the regulation of Schedule Y. The requisite data for clinical trial are to be submitted to CDSCO through Form CT-04 whereas the clinical trial permission is granted by CDSCO by issuing Form CT-06.

In the provision of The Drugs and Cosmetics Act 1940 and Rules 1945 titled 122A schedule Y, the DCGI has been assigned the capacity to waive the clinical trial in the interest of public health and to provide approval for the importing of radiopharmaceuticals with validated trials into other nations. In such instances, the case may be referred to the BARC for the purpose of remark and transportation approval of the radiopharmaceutical in concern. Further, Schedule Y, Section 2.4 (a) advocates that all medical products or drugs must have been found in India and must have passed all phases of clinical testing for the rule to apply, with radiopharmaceuticals not being an exception. Therefore, in order to comply with the requirements of the aforementioned rule, new radiopharmaceuticals need to demonstrate that they have successfully completed the clinical trial. A further point of Section 2.4 (b) of Schedule Y and Rules described that any drug or medical component that falls under the definition of a drug and was invented in a country other than India is required to submit all clinical trial data to CDSCO and for the Phase III clinical trials to be repeated on the Indian population. Therefore, import radiopharmaceuticals are to undergo Phase III clinical trials. In accordance with Section 2.8 of the aforementioned Schedule and Act, the licensing authorities demanded that any experimental findings pertaining to the pharmacokinetic or bioequivalence studies be confirmed with the Indian population.

The current status indicates that Schedule K of the Drugs and Cosmetics Act has not been amended to relax regulations on radiopharmaceuticals, and any future changes in this regard would be contingent on decisions made by the Drug Controller General of India.

The radiopharmaceuticals have already been approved for use in other countries, so the approval process is made somewhat simpler by the fact that only a bioequivalence study needs to be performed on the Indian population. The radiopharmaceuticals don't receive the status of approval as new for use in India until after the data on their safety and efficacy have been established. In accordance with Section 3, Clause (b) and Sub-clause of The Drugs and Cosmetics Act of 1940, the CDSCO is responsible for evaluating radiopharmaceuticals, including their safety, efficacy, and quality.

24.5 THE RESPONSIBILITY OF THE ATOMIC ENERGY REGULATORY BOARD (AERB) IN THE PROCESS OF AUTHORIZING THE USE OF RADIOPHARMACEUTICALS

The Atomic Energy Regulatory Board (AERB) was founded in November 1983 by the President of India with powers provided by Section 27 of the Atomic Energy Act, which was passed in 1962. AERB falls under the purview of the Department of Atomic Energy, which is part of the Government of India. By enforcing the Atomic Energy Act of 1962 and the Environment (Protection) Act of 1986, the government was able to control and regulate the use radioactive instruments, their installation, safety, and functions, as well as the transportation of radiopharmaceuticals. The BARC, which is part of the Department of Atomic Energy, is the responsible authority for regulating the use of radioactive materials and advancing their medical applications, is also involved in these activities.

The order came from the Doctorate General of Health Services, DCGI, and was recorded in File DCGI(I)/MISC/2017(11), dated May 1, 2017, put into effect Rules 23–27(A) of The Drugs and Cosmetics Rules, 1945, which say that radiopharmaceuticals must be registered for any import. This order allows for a window of only forty-five days for the relaxation of certain constraints, one of which is the Tc-99m generator. According to the aforementioned rule, a radiopharmaceutical could not be imported or be transported if it did not have a registration number. In order to import radiopharmaceuticals, domestic manufacturing facilities are required to apply for and receive the licence under Form 10. This order superseded the earlier order 1/ RIA(NOC) /2003 –DC dated 6th February, 2006, where the BARC was authorised to grant a non-objection certificate of radioisotope or tracer for radioimmunoassay for import. Further, radio-active instruments are to be installed according to AERB Safety Guide for Consenting Process for Radiation Facilities (AERB/RF-SG/G-3) (Figure 24.1).

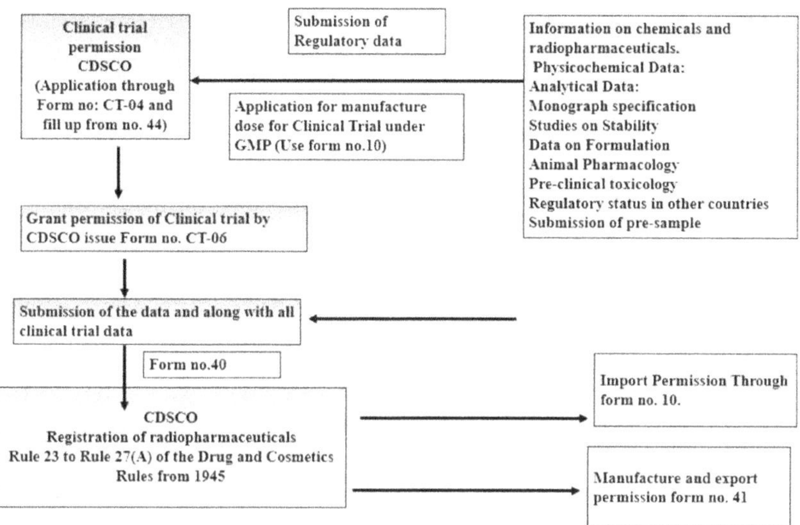

FIGURE 24.1 Procedure approval of radiopharmaceuticals from the regulatory authority in India.

24.6 THE INDIAN PHARMACOPOEIA AND THE OFFICIAL MONOGRAPH FOR MEDICINES AND RADIOPHARMACEUTICALS

As stated earlier, radiopharmaceuticals are considered to be drugs according to both the definition and the legislation. The Indian Pharmacopoeia (IP) included a number of radiopharmaceuticals, as well as the monograph, and they mentioned some examples of them as well. First, the 19 radiopharmaceutical monographs that were published in IP-2014 are included, together with the ten monographs that were published in 2015 (this is referred to as the 206/17 status).

In 2014, radioactive sodium fluoride (^{18}F) injection, fluorodeoxyglucose (^{18}F) injection, samarium (^{153}Sm) ethylene diamine tetramethylene phosphonate injection, sodium iodide (^{131}I) capsules for diagnostic use, and meta-iodobenzyl guanidine injection for diagnostic use, sodium iodide (^{131}I) capsules for therapeutic use, and sodium iodide. The following are the ten radiopharmaceutical monographs that were included in the Addendum-2015: gallium citrate (^{67}Ga) injection, strontium (^{89}Sr) chloride injection, technetium (99mTc) colloidal rhenium sulfide injection, technetium (99mTc) exametazime injection, technetium (99mTc) HYNIC-TOC injection, and technetium (99mTc) macrosalb injection.

In 2018, the IP Commission brought out the Eighth Edition of IP. Three new radiopharmaceuticals monographs were included in IP-2108 and those were gallium (^{68}Ga) chloride, sodium iodide (^{123}I) solution, and sodium iodide (^{123}I) injection. Subsequent to those, two more radiopharmaceuticals, gallium (^{68}Ga) and sodium chromate (^{51}Cr) injection were added in Addendum 2019.

24.7 THE REGULATORY FRAMEWORK FOR RADIOPHARMACEUTICALS IN THE UNITED STATES

The Center for Drug Evaluation and Research (CDER) of the United States governs the radiopharmaceutical industry within the sub-delegated United States regulatory authority for Food and Drugs Administration (FDA). These days, there has been a substantial amount of research conducted on radiopharmaceuticals, and robust regulatory guidelines have been implemented from the beginning of the process all the way through its development, uses, and the reporting of adverse drug reactions. The amendment to the constitution that initiated the process of regulating radiopharmaceuticals was not implemented until 1938. In 1944, the FDA took control of the radiopharmaceuticals and began the process of regulating them. The Atomic Energy Commission's (AEC) regulation stipulated that a licence needed to be obtained before materials could be used or transferred. Between the years 1944 and 1963, the majority of Investigational New Drugs (IND) was given the go-ahead for release, but, in 1971, this provision was overturned, and, from that point on, radiopharmaceuticals were considered to be New Drugs (NDA). After 1989, the FDA began mandating compliance with the GMP when it came to the production of radiopharmaceuticals. Manufacturing of GMP products is covered by the Federal Regulations Code (FRC), and GMP for radiopharmaceuticals is expressly implied by Title 21, Parts 210, 211, and 212. The radiopharmaceuticals are governed in FRC 21, Part 315, 601 of Subparts 601.30 to 601.35. The regulation of *in-vivo* radiopharmaceuticals was implemented later, in 1998.

In the United States of America, there are two regulatory agencies that work together. One of these agencies, the FDA, has the jurisdiction to approve radiopharmaceuticals and manufacture them, while the other, the Nuclear Regulatory Commission (NRC), regulates medical equipment and issues linked to radiation. Other regulatory authorities have specific limited roles, such as the Occupational Safety and Health Administration (OSHA) for the safety of individual operators, the Environmental Protection Agency (EPA) for the disposal of radiopharmaceuticals, and the Department of Transportation (DOT) for the safety of radiopharmaceuticals in transportation. These regulatory authorities are examples of those with limited roles.

24.8 RADIOPHARMACEUTICALS AND THE UNITED STATES' NATIONAL LEGISLATION

The national legislation of nuclear medicine exercises the power of control, subject to approval, over radiopharmaceuticals, including possession of radiopharmaceuticals and the precise facility in which they are stored. The licence is only used for patients and radioactive equipment, as well as radioactive substances.

The licence issued on radiopharmaceuticals is utilised by the federated state government of the particular area. These states are known as "Agreement States," and they operate under the US jurisdiction of the Nuclear Regulatory Commission (NRC). The NRC is responsible for ensuring that all of the federated states continue to adhere to the standards that have been established which regulate the use of radiopharmaceuticals in Veterans' Affairs (VA) hospitals and under the Department of Defense Hospitals. Provisions of the Radiation Safety Officer (RSO) are also properly empowered as the custodian of the radiopharmaceuticals in the NRC rule, which is the same as what is observed in the AERB regulation in India. The RSO is legally responsible for enforcing laws and ensuring the safe management of radioactive materials that are in the hands of the institutional facility. They are also responsible for ensuring the safety of employees and members of the general public.

Sites of usage and transportation of radioactive materials are required to display a notice indicating that the materials are radioactive and to be captioned in bold with the word "Danger." NRC, which originates in the US, was established in accordance with the rule of the Code of Federal Regulations (CFR) Title 10, Chapter I, Sections 1–199, which is embodied in the practice of nuclear medicine. Comparable to, for instance, Part 20 of the standard for operational procedures for protection against radiation, Part 35 of the standard describes the byproduct of radiopharmaceuticals that are used for medical purposes.

- The standard for protecting oneself from radiation is outlined in CFR Part 10, Sections 20.1001–20.2402.
- The medical uses of the radiopharmaceuticals material that was produced as a byproduct are defined in CFR Part 10, Sections 35.1 to 35.4002.

Transport of hazardous materials, such as radiopharmaceuticals and oil, is governed by CFR Part 49, Sections 100 to 185, and this section is overseen by the Department of Transportation (DOT). The DOT is given the authority to regulate the carriage of any sort of radioactive material that falls under the special category of hazardous materials ("hazmat"), as well as to establish safety guidelines for the transport of radioactive material in cargo. The international standard for the transportation of hazardous materials is specified in the Hazmat regulation. The NRC is an independent agency of the US government with the mission of promoting the secure and useful use of radioactive materials. Even though the NRC faces the greatest difficulty in finding a better strategy to protect radiation employees, the general public, and the environment from unsafe disposal, they are working hard to find a solution. Most of the time, the NRC has been responsible for regulating and implementing rules regarding medical applications of radioactive materials, nuclear power plants, and other establishments that made use of radioactive materials. The NRC is also responsible for forming the Advisory Committee on the Medical Uses of Isotopes (ACMUI) and establishing the specialised medical isotopes that are utilised for medical purposes.

24.9 IMPLEMENTATION OF GOOD MANUFACTURING PRACTICE FOR RADIOPHARMACEUTICALS

It was mentioned earlier that, after 1989, the FDA began to rigorously enforce and regulate the manufacturing of radiopharmaceuticals in accordance with the GMP. In 1989, the CFR began enforcing the implementation of the GMP under the designated

Title 21, Parts 210, 211, and 212, whereas the regulation of *in vivo* radiopharmaceuticals began in the CFR 21 of Part 315, 601 of Subpart 601.30 to 601.35. The radiopharmaceuticals can be given in a single dose unit as a colloidal solution, sterile liquid, capsule, or tablet. These different delivery methods are referred to as the route of administration. With the advancement in formulation technology in recent years, patient compliance has also grown with low radiation exposure. For example, a patient's own autologous cells may be radio tagged in order to obtain a diagnosis. Improving the greater stability of radiopharmaceuticals can sometimes be accomplished through the use of kits. These kits contain carrier molecules that have been tagged with the radiolabelled substance, while also including radioactive precursors that have been made into generators; both of these components are required to be assembled before being given to patients. More than sixty percent of kits on the market are radionuclide-based, while the remaining forty percent are offered in kit format. This is done commercially to ensure better stability compliance or to get around problems with the half-life. According to their half-lives, radiopharmaceuticals can be divided into three primary types. One of the first categories is radiopharmaceuticals, which are radioactive substances with a short half-life (less than 20 minutes) that need to be prepared at the bedside of the patients. The second categories of radiopharmaceuticals have a higher half-life and can only be distributed in restricted areas which include F-18 and Tc-99m, whereas the third category of radiopharmaceuticals have a lengthy half-life and are disseminated to all marketing channels. Examples of these include Y^{90} and I^{131}.

In the preparation phase, all of the procedures involved in the dispensing of the target radiopharmaceuticals must be documented. There should be no ambiguity regarding the process control, process variable, purity, percentage yield, or any of the other requisites. Because of their short half-lives, radiopharmaceutical preparations and positron emitters need to be produced in a controlled environment and their preciseness must be maintained.

Radiopharmaceutical preparations must be able to pass stringent quality controls before they can be distributed to patients. These controls ensure that the products are sterile, free of heavy metal contamination, and do not include any other intermediate isotopes, among other things. Patients must also be protected from radiation exposure.

Assuring the quality of a radiochemical product by ensuring its purity is essential for its application as a drug. This necessitates the adoption of effective separation methods for the purpose of separating the chemical that contains the radionuclide, and it is also necessary in order to determine the proportion of radioactivity. Paper chromatography, electrophoresis, thin-layer chromatography, gas chromatography, high pressure liquid chromatography, and liquid chromatography are some of the techniques that are described in the monographs as being applicable to the separation of pure radiopharmaceutical compounds. Other applicable techniques include liquid chromatography and high-performance liquid chromatography. A radiopharmaceuticals counter or an automatic-plotting apparatus are typically utilised for the measurement of radioactivity.

Packaging and Labelling: Notification is necessary for the container to be labelled clearly with readable writing including the radioisotope symbol to highlight that the product is radioactive. This requirement applies to both printed and written labels. Along with the identification bar code, the container needs to include the brand name of the radiopharmaceuticals, the name of the company that made them, and their chemical formula. Along with the date and time of manufacturing, the radioactivity was measured in concentration, either per millilitre or per milligram. Additionally, the conditions of storage, the antimicrobial that is contained within, and the method of administration should all be indicated on the label.

24.10 GMP FOR POSITRON EMISSION TOMOGRAPHY (PET) DRUGS

In the United States of America, the regulatory requirements of the PET pharmaceuticals were made mandatory by the law of Modernization Act, 1997, also known as Public Law 105–115, 1997. Before 1997, medicines used in PET scans were not required to meet certain standards set by the FDA. In the Modernization Act of 1997, Section 121 directed enforcement to be carried out by the FDA in order to adopt and comply with the GMPs for the PET medicines. The FDA began enforcing the regulations on December 10, 2009, which included the minimum requirement for GMP standards and inclusion of 21 CFR Part 212 for PET medicines. The regulatory guidelines also set required contents and formats for New Drug Application (NDA) and Abbreviated New Drug Application (ANDA) pertaining to PET medicines and these rules were enforced by the government. PET drug regulation is incorporated in 21 CFR Part 212 guideline, which was notified on December 10, 2009, and went into effect in June 2012. This guideline stipulates the provisions of current Good Manufacturing Practices (cGMP) for PET pharmaceuticals. The legislation is applicable to PET medicines that are currently being used in clinical practice. It is now required to file an application for a NDA or an ANDA, and this requirement has been extended to all PET medications that have been approved by the FDA, such as ^{18}F FDG, ^{18}F sodium fluoride, and ^{13}N ammonia, etc.

There is a modest or no change to the rule that all PET drugs should be made in a stringent GMP plant according to CFR Part 212. The Radioactive Drug Research Committee (RDRC), which is duly authorised by the FDA, should give their approval to any and all PET drugs. It is recommended that all IND PET radiopharmaceuticals be successful in the clinical trials for Phases 0-1-2, and that approval to sell the PET radiopharmaceuticals on the market be approved only after the conclusion of Phase 3 clinical trial.

24.11 EUROPE'S REGULATORY FRAMEWORK FOR THE RADIOPHARMACEUTICAL INDUSTRY

The European Union (EU) has a variety of regulatory frameworks that are implemented to cover radiopharmaceuticals, and these frameworks can be found across Europe. The European Medicine Agency, or EMA, is a delegate agency operating under the auspices of the EU. It is entrusted with the responsibility of scientific review, supervision, safety monitoring, and authorisation of radiopharmaceuticals distributed within the EU. The Committee for Medicinal Products for Human Use (CHMP), which operates within the confines of the European Medicines Agency (EMA), is responsible for establishing the uniform guideline of radiopharmaceuticals across Europe. The regulatory guidelines include similarities with those of the United States of America and India regarding the enforcement of GMP, or good radiopharmacy practice, clinical studies, and authorisation to release on the market as approved medications. In 1991, the EU harmonised and brought in the legal formats by enforcing Directive no. 91/356/EEC, which regulates the manufacturing of pharmaceutical products for human use under GMP conditions. This directive also brought in the legal formats. The scope of radiopharmaceuticals as medical products was expanded according to Directive 89/343/EEC of the European Union, which also raised the scope of the scope of Directives 65/65/EEC and 75/319/EEC, which govern the regulations connected to medicinal products and the permission of marketing, respectively. Even if Directive 89/343/EEC expanded the number of radiopharmaceuticals and tried to establish them as a special class, the problem that still emerges is the short life of radiopharmaceuticals and the special class of the nature that has radioactivity. The individual protection from radiation was disclosed in the Directive of the EU 97/43/EURATOM a, whereas the protection from radiation was given in the Directive of the EU 96/29/EURATOM.

The GMP guidelines for radiopharmaceuticals are disclosed in Annexure 3 of the same regulation. These guidelines cover areas such as production, installation, equipment, market authorisation, and distribution. In contrast to the regulations in place in the United States and India, the European Union possesses sole jurisdiction and power in matters pertaining to radiopharmaceuticals. The European Union has founded the European Association of Nuclear Medicine (EANM) group and oversees the production, use, and distribution of radiopharmaceuticals, including any types of lyophilised reagents or PET radiopharmaceuticals and all exclusivity of the PET radiopharmaceuticals. There is no leeway given for applications of INDA, ANDA, or NDA concerning radiopharmaceuticals, and all radiopharmaceuticals are required to go through the clinical trial process as outlined in the EU Clinical Trial Directive 2001/20/EC regulation. Under the mandatory clinical study of Investigational Medicinal Products (IMP), including radiopharmaceuticals, the UK legislature acknowledged the EU clinical regulation as well.

24.12 OTHER COUNTRIES' APPROACHES TO THE REGULATION OF RADIOPHARMACEUTICALS

The Australian Radiation Protection and Nuclear Safety Agency (ARPANSA) is the enforcing agency for Australia for any radiation, including radiopharmaceuticals, for regulatory actions for licensing, inspection, compliance, and enforcement. This includes sole regulatory activities. The Australian Radiation Protection and Nuclear Safety Agency (ARPANSA) provides advice to the Nuclear Safety Committee and the Radiation Health Committee of Australia regarding the development of standards and guidelines for the protection and safety of radiopharmaceuticals across the country.

Health Canada (HC) is the regulatory organization that enforces the rules governing the use of pharmaceutical products in Canada. It is responsible for putting national and public health policies into effect. Radiopharmaceuticals are subject to the control and regulation of the Health Product and Food Branch (HPFB).

24.13 ASSESSMENT OF THE RADIOPHARMACEUTICALS' SAFETY PRIOR TO CLINICAL USE IN OTHER COUNTRIES

Radiopharmaceuticals make up a unique subcategory within the pharmaceutical industry, and the term "radiopharmaceutical" was first coined to represent this category. These radiopharmaceuticals are required to adhere to a certain set of guidelines, which are outlined in various national regulations. EU, US, and Japan have all brought up concerns about the safety of radiopharmaceuticals and imaging agents. India has also taken steps for radiopharmaceuticals as drugs to follow the DCGI standard for the clearance procedure. In the US, the FDA has taken the necessary steps to ensure the safety of radiopharmaceuticals, and, in 2014, they published a guideline that categorizes these medications. Part 1 of the created guideline addressed the prerequisites for the safety evaluations, Part 2 addressed the clinical indications, and Part 3 addressed the analysis and interpretation of clinical studies. The process of clinical trials and the investigation do not undergo any kind of relaxation. It wasn't until much later, in 2012, that Japan regulated the clinical safety assessment and approved diagnostic radiopharmaceuticals. As a consequence of this, a regulation was established, and the normal evaluation technique of the clinical study was put into place, in order to determine the safety criteria. Radiopharmaceuticals are classified into one of three distinct groups in Japan. According to the classification, the class 1 categories are the radiopharmaceuticals that have the minimum pharmacological response and are administered as a tracer quantity; the class 2 categories classification of radiopharmaceuticals are tagged with trace amounts of the biological materials and having the allergic type reaction; and the class 3 categories classification of radiopharmaceuticals, having the pharmacological response and having the specific activity and dose selection, is very important for this type of radiopharmaceuticals. Radiopharmaceuticals, such as kits, radionuclide precursors, radionuclide generators, and industrially manufactured radiopharmaceuticals, all require the completion of a safety study.

24.14 THE EUROPEAN UNION NEEDS PRECLINICAL STUDIES FOR RADIOPHARMACEUTICALS AS EXPERIMENTAL MEDICINAL PRODUCTS

In order for any radiopharmaceutical precursors to be considered an experimental medicinal product, safety studies are a condition that must be met. It is necessary to have the specific facts, such as whether or not any free radionuclide poses any danger to patients, as well as information regarding occupational dangers and other toxicities.

24.15 RADIOPHARMACEUTICALS FOR "MICRO-DOSING" AND EVALUATION OF NON-CLINICAL SAFETY STUDIES

In June 2004, the European Medicines Agency highlighted the way to efficiently identify radiopharmaceuticals with little resources, and the microdosing concept provided a graphical explanation of the relationship between preclinical toxicity and human clinical trials. The selection of the microdose is based on the minimal dose being less than one-hundredth of the reported dose in the pharmacologic or pharmacodynamics response to *in vitro* and preclinical studies.

The US published a guideline in 2006 for single-dose acute toxicity studies for the investigator, the industry, and reviewers. In addition, the concept of a microdose was validated, as was mentioned earlier, and up to a maximum dose of 100 mg or less, depending on the substance's protein or antigenic nature, the dose of microdosing is capped at 30 nmol or less. This idea served as a foundation for the exploratory novel drug trials (eIND) conducted on human subjects. The eIND conducted research on a restricted number of human volunteers during either Phase "0" or the early stages of Phase 1. In the name of the trial, no diagnostic or therapeutic investigation of any kind is permitted to take place in this study.

Utilizing the eIND for first-in-human research is the option that makes the most sense. A preliminary clinical evaluation of the mechanism of action and pharmacokinetics of an investigational radiopharmaceutical can be carried out with its help. An exploratory investigational new drug, or eIND, is a more streamlined alternative to the IND, which is a process that can be somewhat time-consuming. An eIND can help researchers better understand pharmacokinetics, and it only requires a single set of pharmacology and toxicology investigations to determine whether or not a molecule is safe. Furthermore, eIND studies make strategic use of preclinical safety and pharmacology discoveries, while reducing the amount of money spent on human testing and studies.

24.16 EIND VS. IND: COMPARING RADIOPHARMACEUTICALS AND REGULATION IN THE UNITED STATES

The Radioactive Drug Research Committee (RDRC) is the authority for the approval of eIND radiopharmaceuticals for limited use in the delegated power as per the Title 21 Code of CFR Section 361.1. This approval must be submitted to the FDA. The eIND application is based on the concept of microdosage as well as acquired clinical information to assess the safety of the molecule. As a result, only the data obtained from Phase 0 through the early stages of Phase 1 investigations can be used to choose the radiopharmaceuticals with the greatest potential for success in a manner that is both economical and expedient. Monitoring for safety before its first use on humans is of the utmost importance. In order to monitor the mechanism of action, pharmacokinetics, biodistribution, dosimetry, dose determination, image quality with validation, efficacy, and the continuous safety test battery is necessary. An eIND application is the sole thing that sets it apart from a standard investigational new drug application in terms of the pre-clinical study going directly to limited volunteer use on a microdosing basis. The traditional IND applies to the other necessary data for the need, such as the manufacturing, quality control, chemical, process variable, and validation data. Studies using pharmacology are absolutely necessary for validating the target and mapping the receptors. Because of the microdosing and the design of the experiment, the toxicological evaluation has less significance in the eIND. This is because the experiment was planned so that it would not affect any pharmacological response. In eIND investigations, the necessity of toxicological research is restricted to only a single species of mammalian subject, in contrast to the IND studies, which mandated the use of two species of mammalian subjects. During the eIND investigations, clinical participants were evaluated all at once by a select group of volunteers in order to determine the metabolism. Distribution, pharmacology, pharmacokinetics, and pathophysiology of radiopharmaceuticals are important in eIND investigations. Both eIND and IND investigations meet the requirements of 21 CFR Parts 211 for SPECT or 21 CFR Part 212 for PET, respectively. The regulation known as 21 CFR Part 212 applies to radiopharmaceuticals that are specifically intended for use in investigations falling within Phases 1 or 2 of PET examinations, as well as those that have been approved by RDRC. The GMP implementation of trial radiopharmaceuticals must be properly adhered to in both the eIND and the IND, as required by 21 CFR Part 210. The eIND has carried out research to understand the toxicity to the animals in a single dosage for a period of fourteen days to observe acute toxicity, and it may also evaluate the possibility of conducting a trial on humans. As a cited example, the radiopharmaceutical's interactions with liver microsomes or cytochome can be easily studied, as can their effectiveness or any potential hepatic toxicity. The benefit of using an eIND is that only a limited number of non-clinical investigations are necessary, and these studies can be structured in a logical manner. In order to conform to acceptable laboratory practice, each and every toxicity study needs to be conducted.

The traditional IND is a more investigative, standardised written process where the pre-clinical to clinical research are to be completed over the course of three phases. The part of 21CFR that discusses IND investigations of radiopharmaceuticals can be found at Part 312.23. Traditionally, large and numerous doses are given to the animals at more than one hundred times the amount that would be given to humans in the recommended dose. There are times when the noticeable adverse effects or the not observable effective adverse effects are also the factors that are unfavourable criteria to the toxicological test. If there were any negative effects seen, the organ that was supposed to be affected should have been identified in the experimental animals. When we investigated the radiopharmaceuticals' dosimetry estimation with correlation from large animal studies to the human, the traditional IND are more acceptable. An IND investigation, where every step of the experiment must be thoroughly documented and validated, the investigator brochure is the most crucial component. At some point throughout the clinical study or during post-marketing surveillance, any clinically relevant adverse data must be disclosed.

BIBLIOGRAPHY

American Society of Radiologic Technologists. *Computed Tomography in the 21st Century—Changing Practice for Medical Imaging and Radiation Therapy Professionals.* Albuquerque: American Society of Radiologic Technologists, 2008.

EANM Radiopharmacy Committee. Guidelines on Current Good Radiopharmacy Practice (CGRPP) in the Preparation of Radiopharmaceuticals. 2007. Available from: http://www.eanm.org/scientific_info/guidelines/ gl_radioph_cgrpp.pdf.

F. No.29/Misc./4/2016-DC (101), Government of India, Director General of Health Services, Central Drug Standard Organization, New Delhi, India.

F.No. DCG(I)/Misc/2017 (11), Directorate General of Health Services, Office of Drug Controller General, India (Import and Registration).

Features of IP-Addendum-2015 to IP-2014. Available from: https://ipc.gov.in/images/pdf/File282.pdf. Accessed 21 June 2019.

Features of IP Addendum. 2016. Available from: https://ipc.gov.in/mandates/indian-pharmacopoeia/indian-pharmacopoeia-2014-and-its-addenda/8-category-en/444-features-of-ip-addendum-2016.html. Accessed 15 June 2019.

File No. DCG (I)/Misc/2017 (11), Directorate General of Health Services, Office of Drug Controller General, India.

Final Position Paper on Non-Clinical Safety Studies to Support Clinical Trials with a Single Microdose (EMEA/CPMP/SWP/2499/ 02/Rev1). Available from: http://www.emea.europa.eu/pdfs/human/swp/249902en.pdf.

Gamboa MML, Roesch HRM, Lemos VPA, RochaBO, Oliveira RS. Obligations, Precautions and Pending Issues in Regulatory Development for Radiopharmaceuticals in Brazil. *Brazilian Journal of Pharmaceutical Sciences* 2014, April/June, 50(2), 285–290.

Huang Y-Y. An Overview of PET Radiopharmaceuticals in Clinical Use: Regulatory, Quality and Pharmacopeia Monographs of the United States and Europe, Nuclear Medicine Physics, Aamir Shahzad and Sajid Bashir, IntechOpen. doi: 10.5772/intechopen.79227. Available from: https://www.intechopen.com/books/nuclear-medicine-physics/an-overview-of-pet-radiopharmaceuticals-in-clinical-use-regulatory-quality-and-pharmacopeia-monograp.

Indian Pharmacopeia. Available from: https://ipc.gov.in/mandates/indian-pharmacopoeia/about-ip.html. Accessed 15 June 2019.

Indian Pharmacopoeia. 2014. Available from: https://ipc.gov.in/mandates/indian-pharmacopoeia/indian-pharmacopoeia-2014-and-its-addenda/8-category- en/235-highlights -of-ip-2014.html. Accessed 19 June 2019.

Indian Pharmacopeia. Available from: https://ipc.gov.in/mandates/indian-pharmacopoeia/about-ip.html. Accessed 15 June 2019.

Lodha S, Patel H, Joshi S, Kalyankar G, Mishra A. Chapter 6 - Regulatory Requirements of Regulated Market. In Ali Javed, Baboota Sanjula (Eds) *Regulatory Affairs in the Pharmaceutical Industry.* Academic Press, 2022, pp. 113–161.

Lucignani G, Del Sole A. Nuclear Medicine: What Kind of Quality Would We Want If We Were the Patient? *European Journal of Nuclear Medicine and Molecular Imaging* 2010 November, 37(11): 2194–2198. doi: 10.1007/s00259-010-1595-x. PMID: 20838996.

Meher BR. Inclusion of Radiopharmaceuticals in the Indian Pharmacopeia: A Step Forward. *Indian Journal of Nuclear Medicine* 2020 January–March, 35(1): 1–3. doi: 10.4103/ijnm.IJNM_133_19. Epub 2019 Dec 31. PMID: 31949360; PMCID: PMC6958968.

Mehta S, Maheshwari D. An Insight on the Emerging Regulations for Radiopharmaceuticals by Europe and India. *Asian Journal of Pharmaceutical Technology & Innovation* 2017, 5(23): 86–96.

Pal R, Popli H, Randeo S. Radiopharmaceuticals - Regulatory Framework and Market Authorization Process in us and India. *International Journal of Current Advanced Research* 2019, 8(04): 18407–18411. doi: 10.24327/ijcar.2019.18411.3518.

Release of Indian Pharmacopoeia (IP). 2018. Available from: https://ipc.gov.in/mandates/indian-pharmacopoeia/indianpharmacopoeia-2018-and-its-addenda/8-category-en/557-release-of-indian-pharmacopoeia-ip-2018.html. Accessed 19 June 2019.

Salient Features of Addendum 2019 to IP 2018. Available from: https://ipc.gov.in/images/Salient_Features_of_Addendum_2019_to_IP_2018.pdf. Accessed 29 June 2020.

Sandeep S, Ashish B, Rakesh KS. Radiopharmaceuticals Regulations on Bioavailability and Bioequivalence: Present Status and Future Requirements. *Modern Applications of Bioequivalence & Bioavailability* 2017, 1(4): 555567. doi: 10.19080/MABB.2017.01.555567.

The Drugs & Cosmetics Act 1940 and Rules 1945. Delhi (India): Ministry of Health and Family Welfare (Govt. of India), 1945.

US Food Drug Administration. *PET DRUGS—Current Good Manufacturing Practice (CGMP).* Rockville: US Food Drug Administration, 2009.

Vallabhajosula S. *Molecular Imaging: Radiopharmaceuticals for PET and SPECT.* 2009, 197. doi: 10.1007/978-3-Springer-Verlag Berlin Heidelberg.

25 Abbreviated New Drug Application (ANDA) or Generic Drug Approval Process

25.1 INTRODUCTION

A drug that has been approved under an ANDA is a generic version of an existing drug, whose safety and clinical efficacy have been established. Because preclinical (animal) and clinical (human) evidence to show safety and effectiveness are typically not necessary, generic drug applications are referred to as "abbreviated" applications. Instead, generic applicants must prove, through scientific evidence, that their medication works in the same way as the innovator drug. The biological equivalence of generic medications, also referred to as "bioequivalence," means that they function in the same way as innovator drugs or established drugs in terms of absorption, bioavailability, and elimination rates. For a number of years, Indian pharmaceutical companies have taken the lead in filling out ANDA in the US and providing affordable, high-quality drugs to the general public. In particular, Indian pharmaceutical businesses improved and focused on research and development (R&D), which led to a rise in the popularity of generic segments with the highest level of FDA approval in ANDA sectors. After any patent's period of exclusivity expires and the pricing wars heat up, the ANDA filing process begins. India comes in third place overall and third in terms of the volume of pharmaceuticals it produces. Because the clinical trial step was skipped, while it was still determined that the ANDA drug was similar to or equivalent to previously approved or commercially available drugs, the ANDA or generic drug was made accessible at a more affordable price. Before the Kefauver-Harris amendments went into effect in 1962, the FDA's decision to approve a new drug for marketing was based mostly on its safety profile. However, once those amendments took effect, the FDA began to examine new drugs based on their "proof-of-efficacy."

25.2 THE HATCH-WAXMAN ACT (HWA)

The HWA was put into place in the USA in 1984 to speed up the USFDA's medication approval procedure. It also made it easier for generic drugs to enter the market quickly, provided for market exclusivity, and promoted ongoing innovation. Whereas post-HWA authorised the generic approval and did not require clinical trials and

DOI: 10.1201/9781003397854-9

tests, pre-HWA definitively expected the generic branded drug to prove safety and efficacy studies like the branded drug businesses.

Implementing Section 505(j) of the ANDA approval procedure, the approval of ANDA is based on the patent infringement of the innovator drug and claims of New Drug Application (NDA). The FDA publishes the Orange Book, a list of approved pharmaceuticals that are therapeutically equivalent to branded pharmaceuticals. The Orange Book listing may be inclusive or exclusive, and FDA has the legal right to approve ANDAs, market exclusivity, patent term extensions, and other terms.

It takes a long time and much money to complete the rigorous process of developing a New Drug Application (NDA), which includes four rounds of clinical studies to evaluate the safety and efficacy of the new pharmaceuticals. Branded drugs are those that have received NDA approval. As a result, it maintains the cost of medication development implemented to the patent period where investments are recovered. The monopoly of the patent holders or the monopoly of the branded drug, on the other hand, is the product of that one market participant. Generic medications could not access the market until the patents on branded pharmaceuticals expired, which restricted the development of generic medicine. In order for pharmaceuticals to be accessible to the general public at comparably cheaper pricing once they lose their patent protection, ANDA encouraged fair drug prices and the availability of branded drugs to the general public at reduced cost when they go off-patent. There are four different forms of ANDA submissions, and it is necessary to certify for each patent with a list of medications, when submitting a file.

Paragraph I: In the Orange Book, the drug's information is either not filed or no patent information is accessible.
Paragraph II: Patent expired.
Paragraph III: Patent that has not yet expired or that will do so very soon.
Paragraph IV: In case an ANDA is submitted, the patent must be invalid and won't be violated if the drug is used or sold.

The designations "Paragraph I," "Paragraph II," "Paragraph III," and "Paragraph IV" refer to each of these four categories of certificates. Any generic medication introduced after a branded or NDA drug's patent has expired is said to have violated the NDA patent. The Orange Book is essentially a comprehensive database of all patents, therapeutic equivalences, and licensed drugs.

Without a doubt, the HWA encouraged generic medications and their accessibility to regular people at substantially reduced costs. Prior to that, any generic medication used for the experiment was regarded as a patent infringement because it violated the extended patent of the drug's inventor. As a result, the HWA is allowed to utilise the patented medicine in an early experimental phase without fear of legal repercussions for doing so before the patent expires. HWA encouraged the development of generic medications and granted a 180-day period of profit-making exclusivity to the generic medicine company that submitted the initial application for the sale of the generic version of the innovator drug.

To make up for the time-consuming NDA process, the HWA legislation allows for a provisional extension of the patent period for branded medicine manufacturers of up to five years.

25.2.1 The Hatch-Waxman Act's Significance

Branded pharmaceuticals conduct the clinical trials, and ANDA pharmaceuticals are approved in accordance with the branded drug and clause. The lawsuits brought about by patent owners who attempt to protect their monopoly by *de facto* enforcing injunctions on the grounds of infringement suits of the patented drug against the generic drug are presented in Paragraph IV. When a district court judgment is issued about an ANDA medicine that is included in the Orange Book and under Paragraph IV's provisions, only a single 30-month *de facto* stay by using an injunction is allowed.

Once more, it is noteworthy that any ANDA that requests approval under the terms of Paragraph IV must notify the appropriate authorities within 20 days of filing. If the owner of the branded medicine company does not respond to the notification by putting on the notice about an infringement proceeding within 45 days, the declaratory judgement favours the ANDA-filled medications. The applicant was not sued, and the patent owner filed an extra counterclaim to enforce modifications to the Orange Book listings without facing legal action. Due to this simple process, which requires no money and has no time restriction rider, the original patent holder preferred changing the Orange Book entry. Acts pertaining to generic medications, procedures, FDA clearance processes, patent rights, extended patent rights, and Orange Book listing have been made mandatory by the Hatch-Waxman Act.

25.3 REGULATION OF SHORTENED NEW DRUG APPLICATIONS IN INDIA

The regulatory body responsible for approving and maintaining the ANDA medicine or generic drugs in India is the Central Drugs Standard Control Organization (CDSCO), which is part of the Ministry of Health and Family Welfare.

25.3.1 A four-year strategic medicine that has been approved for use for more than four years. If the drug has been approved for use for longer than four years, the applicant must provide the information to the State Licensing Authority (SLA) with the approval status from CDSCO sites before receiving permission. For the sale, distribution, and storage of medications other than those listed in Schedules C, C (1), and X, such as gels, fluids, oral dosage forms, and gels, the application may be made using Form 24, whereas Form 27 is used for applications for new licences or renewals for medications listed in Schedules C, C(1), and Schedule X.

25.3.2 A drug that is less than four years old. According to Rule 122-E of the 1940 and 1945 Drugs and Cosmetics Act and Rules, respectively, any drug that receives its first authorisation must be approved within four years. The central regulatory authorities are the only agency with the authority to grant such approval. After the New Drug Advisory Committee (NDAC) makes a recommendation for a new drug category, the applicant submits Form 44 to CDSCO, and Form 46 can then be used to request permission or approval for the manufacture of a new drug formulation.

25.3.3 A new drug is not approved for domestic use in India. Generic medications are subject to the same restrictions as the aforementioned new drugs.

25.3.4 New drug are approved/unapproved for export. By submitting Forms 25 and 28, CDSCO Zonal/Sub-zonal offices can grant No Objection Certificate (NOC) for the export of India's approved/unapproved new drugs.

Only when the safety and efficacy of the same active ingredient, or one that is similar, is established, then only ANDAs are considered for approval. Generic medications are those that are biologically and pharmaceutically equal to the approved product in terms of dose form, potency, mode of administration, use, and labelling. Because of this, any ANDA filing the medicine must have the same active ingredient(s), method of administration, dosage form, strength, and other substances that have already received identical NDA approval.

25.4 DOCUMENTS NEEDED IN INDIA FOR THE APPROVAL OF A BRIEF NEW MEDICATION/DRUG APPLICATION

1. Complete Application Form:
   Fill out the prescribed application form provided by the CDSCO.
2. Table of Contents:
   Provide a detailed table of contents outlining the structure of your application.
3. Justification for ANDA Application:
   Clearly state the reasons for submitting an ANDA, including details on the reference drug.
4. Conditions of Use:
   Describe the conditions of use, including indications, contraindications, warnings, and precautions.
5. Information About Active Components:
   Provide detailed information about the active pharmaceutical ingredients (APIs) in the drug.
6. Dosage Form, Strength, and Administration Method:
   Describe the dosage form, strength, and recommended method of administration.
7. Bioequivalence:
   Include data demonstrating bioequivalence if submitting an ANDA for a generic drug compared to a reference listed drug.
8. Labeling and Section:
   Present labeling information as per regulatory requirements.
   Include details on sections such as storage conditions, shelf life, and special precautions.
9. Chemistry, Manufacturing, and Control (CMC) Information:
   Provide detailed information on the chemistry of the drug, manufacturing processes, and quality control measures.
10. Pharmacokinetics and Bioavailability in Humans:
    Include data on the pharmacokinetics and bioavailability of the drug in humans.
11. Quality Control Techniques and Analytical Techniques:
    Detail the quality control techniques and analytical methods used for testing the drug's quality.
12. Case Report Forms:
    If applicable, include case report forms for clinical trials conducted as part of the drug development process.

13. BE Investigations - Bioequivalence Investigations:
    Provide comprehensive data on bioequivalence investigations, especially for generic drug applications.
14. Clinical Study Reports:
    Include reports of clinical studies conducted during the drug development process.
15. Stability Data:
    Submit data on the stability of the drug product under different storage conditions.
16. Regulatory Commitments:
    If any regulatory commitments were made during the development process, ensure they are documented.
17. Declaration of Compliance:
    Include a declaration of compliance with regulatory requirements.
18. User Fees:
    Pay applicable user fees as per regulatory guideline

BE studies are conducted to demonstrate that a generic drug product is equivalent to the reference listed drug (RLD) in terms of safety, efficacy, and pharmacokinetic parameters. These studies are an integral part of ANDA submissions, and their approval is necessary for the generic drug to be considered equivalent to the innovator product. The CDSCO is responsible for approving BE studies conducted for generic drug products in India. The approval process involves the review of the study design, methodology, and results to ensure that the generic product meets the required bioequivalence standards.

The amount of data required for BE study approval may depend on whether the New Drug Submission (NDS) approval for the innovator product has expired or is still valid. If the NDS approval has expired, there might be a need for additional data or information to support the BE study. In the case of a BE study application submitted for a novel chemical that was allowed in other countries but not in India, the applicant would typically need to provide comprehensive documentation. This documentation may include study protocols, methodology, analytical data, and other relevant information to support the bioequivalence claim.

Application is submitted when properly signed with the applicant's name, designation, and application Form 44.

25.5 APPROVAL OF BIOEQUIVALENCE (BE) STUDY

Study centre of BE studies requires approval from CDSCO. Approval of any study to be conducted in an approved BE study centre required authorisation from the sponsor, duly signed with the appropriate title and letter of designation with prescribed fees as challan as per The Drugs and Cosmetics Rules, 1945. The undertaking is taken as required by Appendix VII of Schedule Y of The Drugs and Cosmetic Rules, and this document has been signed by the principal investigator (PI).

The study's endpoint and voluntary recruiting have to be mentioned in the study's description.

- Pre-clinical research: Data on toxicity based on a single dosage or repeated doses.
- Clinical trial data on healthy volunteers' and patients' pharmacokinetic and pharmacodynamics have been published in reputable publications.
- Regulatory status: Whether the medication has received approval from another nation must be mentioned.
- If the medication is being marketed to foreign nations, that information should be mentioned. Package literature: information on the drug that will be included in the package.
- Analysis certificate: Report on the bioequivalence analysis of the reference and test formulations.
- Multiple doses: A BE trial using multiple doses must have sufficient safety data to support it. Before beginning the BE injectable formulation, the sub-acute toxicity of two species must be determined.
- Special type of drug: BE studies on healthy volunteers/patients or male/female subjects should be presented. Justification is necessary for medications like hormonal preparations and cytotoxic agents. The medication is produced as a generic after the patent for an original or branded medication expires. When the drug's patent expired, the brand's exclusivity was broken. The cost-effective generic medicine requires submission of the ANDA approval application before it may be sold in the US.

The generic medication is the more affordable alternative medication that is also safe and efficient. The Orange Book or FDA-approved drug therapeutic equivalence studies include branded drugs that have dosage, administration method, strength, and other criteria that are the same as or comparable to those branded drugs.

The Hatch-Waxman Act (HWA) is the law that strengthens the drug's ANDA filing. Furthermore, the Hatch-Waxman amendment created a new law known as the "Drug Price Competition and Patent Term Restoration Act of 1984," which introduces the bioequivalence concept. In accordance with the bioequivalence or similar effectiveness, the generic drug approval process becomes simple because it no longer necessitates repeating expensive and duplicative clinical trials to prove the ANDA drug is similarly effective and safe. Additionally, the statute enforced marketing exclusivity and the terms of the branded drug's patent to some extent. Additionally, the rule gives generic medication manufacturers the ability to legally challenge patents.

25.6 SUBMISSIONS OF ANDA IN THE US

The application must be submitted exactly as mentioned in the application.

1. Review and submit the ANDA in accordance with the filing checklist and the manual of policies and procedures.
2. Form FDA-356h required to be submitted to the FDA, a specific form for approving the sale of human-use biologics, novel drugs, and antibiotics.
3. Form FDA-3794: The cover sheet and instructions for utilising Form FDA-356h must be created in accordance with the revisions to the Generic Drug

User Fee Act (GDUFA). The GUDFA agreement is the result of negotiations between the FDA and a generic drug manufacturer's representative for better generic drug production and regulatory issues.
4. Form FDA-3674: Certificate of compliance is necessary, as said earlier.
5. Drug Master Files (DMFs): A Drug Master File (DMF) is a submission to the U.S. Food and Drug Administration (FDA) that provides detailed information about the manufacturing, processing, packaging, and storing of active pharmaceutical ingredients (APIs), excipients, or finished drug products.

DMFs are typically submitted by manufacturers, suppliers, or other entities as a means of providing confidential information to the FDA, without disclosing such information to the public (Table 25.1).

25.7 APPROVAL OF COMMON TECHNICAL DOCUMENT (CTD) FOR ANDA

An application must have a distinctive six-digit application number in order to be identified in the future. This number is a standard reference number for eCTD applications.

1. **Module I:** Administrative and prescribing data is required as per Form FDA-356h, which is one of the designated forms for approving the sale of novel medications, antibiotics, and biologics for human use. Furthermore, as said earlier, Form FDA-3794 is equally important to the consideration of the application.

Understanding the application's foundation—including any changes to the dosage form's strength, the parenteral dosage's concentration, the size of the vial or package, or the total amount of the drug—requires reading the cover letter. Additionally, oral liquid, ophthalmic, transdermal, or topical medication formulations must bc informed of any changes in the active drug concentration. By applying through Form 19-A, prescription drug goods can be switched to over-the-counter drugs (Rx-to-OTC changeover). The "Orange Book" also includes any inexpensive medications. Therapeutic equivalence with brand-name medications is also included there.

The administrative component of the ANDA file is a rigorous process, and Form 356h must be submitted in order to appoint the agent in the United States. The application must also include a statement that no debarment certification exists under the Generic Drug Enforcement Act of 1992, as well as a list of all convictions that may be listed under sections 335a(k), 335a(a), 306(k)(1), and 335a(b) of the Food Drug and Cosmetic Act. Five components make up the Common Technical Document (CTD), which is separated as previously explained in the preceding section.

2. **Module II:** The document comprises summaries and overviews of the following information.
    - Index of Contents:
        - A detailed listing of the contents of Module II, providing a quick reference for regulatory reviewers to locate specific information.
    - Overview of All Documents:

TABLE 25.1
Compression of ANDA Filing between India, the US, and Europe

Sl no.	Parameters	India	US	Europe
1	Authorities for regulatory approval	Central Drugs Standard Control Organization (CDSCO): CDSCO is the national regulatory authority for pharmaceuticals and medical devices in India. It operates under the Ministry of Health and Family Welfare "India"	EMEA European Medicines Agency (EMA): Location: European Union (EU) Role: EMA is the regulatory agency responsible for the scientific evaluation, supervision, and safety monitoring of medicines in the European Union.	FDA
2	Applicable regulation	According to The Drugs and Cosmetics Rules Section 122A, 122B, Appendix I, IA of Schedule Y	According the USFDA- (CFR) Section 505 (j) for ANDA	Directive 2001/83/EC-Article 8(j)
3	Submission format	CTD – Hard copy	Mandatory- e CTD /Paper CTD	e-CTD is not fully mandatory and submitted along with the paper
4	Procedure	Simple and straightforward	Simple and straightforward	Four procedures: Centralised, Decentralised, National, and Mutual recognition
5	Application	M&M	ANDA	MAA
6	Requirement for submission	on CD, one hard copy and three soft copies (PDF) format	Three copies for archival, review and field application	One Copy
7	Timeline for approval	One year	18 months	One year
8	License Validity	Three years	Five years	Five years
9	Exclusivity for the data	Approved drug in India in three categories: the drug is 4 years old, less than 4 years old, and unapproved.	Require approval of patent certification as per Paragraphs I, II, III, and IV of the Orange Book.	10 years or 8+2+(1)

    - A comprehensive overview summarizing the key points and contents of all documents included in the submission.
  - Overviews and Summary Statements:
    - This section includes summaries and statements related to various aspects of the submission.
  - M4Q - Quality of the CTD:
    - M4Q likely refers to Module 4 Quality, which provides detailed information about the quality aspects of the pharmaceutical product. This includes data on manufacturing, specifications, stability, and quality control.
  - M4S - Safety of the CTD:
    - M4S likely refers to Module 4 Safety, which focuses on safety-related information. This may include preclinical and clinical safety data, summaries of adverse events, and other safety-related aspects.
3. **Module III:** About the product quality
   - Table of Contents
   - Data

   Literature Reference
4. **Module IV:** About Non-clinical study

   Not applicable in an ANDA Filing.
5. **Module V:** Clinical study reports
6. Table of Contents.
7. Reports and Case Report and Tabulations.

   The FDA accept eCTD format which is described in the ICH M2 technical specification.
8. **Paragraph IV Patent Certifications and Paragraph IV Provisions**

Regulatory investigations ensure that parameters such as effectiveness, safety, and bioequivalence criteria are met before an ANDA drug is approved under Paragraphs I and II. When the original drug's patent expires and it is no longer patentable, approval of clause III is applicable. Therefore, the main component of the approval process for generic or ANDA is the patent restoration and validation of the branded medicine or original drug. Since both cases involve expired patents for the original or branded medications, determining the patent in Paragraphs I or II is quite simple, whereas Paragraph III ANDA drug approval is postponed until the branded medicine's patent has expired.

Abbreviated New Drug Application (ANDA) submissions are categorized into different paragraphs, but these are typically Paragraph I, Paragraph II, and Paragraph III. This refers to the situation where there is no patent information listed for the reference listed drug (RLD). The generic applicant may submit a Paragraph I certification, asserting that there is no unexpired patent for the listed drug. This is applicable when the patent for the reference listed drug (RLD) has expired. The generic applicant may submit a Paragraph II certification, indicating that the patent has expired. There is no specific provision or certification called Paragraph III in the context of ANDA submissions. It might be a reference to Paragraph IV certification, which is filed when the generic applicant challenges the validity or enforceability of the listed patent for the RLD.

Generic drugs are typically approved once the patents associated with the reference listed drug have expired, allowing for the introduction of generic versions. The ANDA approval process involves rigorous regulatory investigations to ensure that the generic drug meets the required standards for safety, efficacy, and bioequivalence compared to the reference listed drug.

A "Paragraph IV certification" is a legal document that states that, when a brand-name drug's patents expire, the generic drug will be approved under the "certification" clause if the generic applicant can attest that the patent for the generic drug is invalid, unenforceable, or won't be violated. Following the ANDA's approval, the medication is added to the therapeutic equivalence evaluations, which are documented in the Orange Book, which was first published in 2004. This book contains information on the drug's name, strength(s), dosage form, reference listed drug (RLD), new drug application (NDA) number, and the first ANDA(s) that were substantially complete or the agency that contained a Paragraph IV certification.

The Paragraph IV certification was implemented in accordance with Section 505(j)(2)(B)(i), 2157 CFR, and the NDA patent holder was notified that the conformity had not violated any patents. Under the "Drug Price Competition & Patent Term Restoration Act" of 1984, the USFDA may suspend approval of an ANDA applicant if the original patent owner files a notice of claim or makes allegations of patent infringement against the applicant within 45 days of the ANDA applicant receiving notice under the clause of the Paragraph IV certificate.

It appears there might be a reference to Paragraph IV or a similar provision in the context of ANDA (Abbreviated New Drug Application) filings. Paragraph IV certification is a crucial aspect of the ANDA process, where a generic drug applicant challenges the patents associated with the brand-name drug. The 30-month stay refers to the period during which the FDA may delay the approval of an ANDA if a Paragraph IV certification has been submitted, and the patent holder initiates a lawsuit for patent infringement. This period allows time for the court to adjudicate patent disputes.

The 180-day exclusivity period is granted to the first generic drug applicant that successfully challenges a listed patent via a Paragraph IV certification. This exclusivity period provides the first filer with a competitive advantage, allowing them a period of exclusivity to market their generic version before other generic competitors can enter the market. This section of the Federal Food, Drug, and Cosmetic (FD&C) Act outlines the provisions related to generic drug approvals, including the Paragraph IV certification process, exclusivity, and other regulatory aspects.

2019's Drug Competition Action Plan (DCAP) includes updated and retrospectively certified Paragraph IV practical information that is more exclusive than that found in the Orange Book. The "Guidance on Statistical Procedures for Bioequivalence Studies Using a Standard Two Treatment Crossover Design," published by the Division of Bioequivalence's Office of Generic Drugs of CDER directed the process and validation of the legitimate statistical analysis for bioequivalence assessment.

Paragraph IV certification is a component of the Abbreviated New Drug Application (ANDA) process in the United States, particularly related to generic drugs. When a generic drug manufacturer seeks approval for a drug that is still under patent protection, it can submit a Paragraph IV certification as part of the ANDA filing.

1. Name of the active ingredient

   The recognized or non-proprietary name of the drug product's active ingredient(s) is required.
2. Dose form and strength

   All dosage forms, including liquid, solid, injectable, and others, must be displayed together with the strength.
3. RLD name and NDA number

   The proprietary name must be reflected together with the RLD or NDA number.
4. First PIV "Post-Implementation Verification" submission

   The initial application must have a certification under Paragraph IV and at least one patent mentioned in the Orange Book. The first filing of the ANDA and the first submission of Paragraph IV are both referenced in the Prescription Drug Improvement and Modernization Act of 2003. (pre-MMA) The individual dates of pertinent submissions under the pre-MMA statutory regime and the grant of the 180-day exclusivity under patent verification are not practicable.
5. 180-day decision status

   The FDA has approved four different types of ANDA drug products, and the choice of whether a therapeutic product qualifies for 180 days of exclusivity is significant. First, when the FDA authorised at least a portion of the ANDA application for a 180-day exclusivity at the time of approval, the application is considered "eligible." Second, "delayed" refers to the first receipt of FDA approval. Third, a condition known as "non-forfeiture" was discovered and tentatively granted, based only on the first applicant's eligibility for exclusively for 180-day reasons for forfeiture. Fourth, if all of the first applicants have voluntarily surrendered or renounced eligibility for 180-day exclusivity, the clause of "extinguished" is applicable. However, related to obtaining approval after the maximum 30-month approval for exclusivity, the FDA often encounters challenges in making forfeiture decisions within the framework of the statutory provision for 180-day exclusivity
6. 180-day decision posting date

   The 180-day decision status of the month and year was updated by the FDA in the IV Certification List, and the column is cumulative, with the most current decision date represented first.
7. Date of "First Applicant's" First Approval, ANDA

   The initial date when an ANDA for a first applicant gained final approval is shown in this column. Only the first approval date is posted if there are several first applicants.
8. First commercial marketing

   The FDA updates the "Orange Book" date of the first commercial marketing of any first applicant, and ANDA(s) are eligible for 180-day exclusivity. Additionally, the Orange Book displays a Patent Challenge (PC) code under "Exclusivity Data."

TABLE 25.2
Requirement of Common CTD for ANDA Filing and Comparison among India, the US, and Europe

	Module 1 (Administrative)			
	Parameters	**India**	**US**	**Europe**
1	Cover letter, table of contents, and details relevant.	Relevant	Relevant	Relevant
2	The method of application	Application Form 44 and the required fees must be submitted in order to obtain authorisation to manufacture, import, or conduct clinical studies for new medications.	Application Form 3794 applicable for generic drug Application Form 356h applicable in order to seek approval for the marketing of a New or Abbreviated New Drug for biological or human use, the application process must be undertaken.	Application through the prescribed forms and prescribed fees.
3	Important legal documents needed for marketing, importing, and manufacturing	BE/NOC certificate from CDSCO (Central Drugs Standard Control Organization) A licence to sell drugs in forms 20B and 21B. Batch release certificate and free sale is required. Add a copy of Form 11 and the Form 25/28/25's current manufacturing licence.	Demand the field copy, the financial certification, and the debarment certification. Information about patents.	Not- applicable
4	Product information that has been authorised in the Nation	Regulations that apply to other nations	Relevant	Relevant
5	Agent mandated or national authorisation	Not applicable	Applicable	Not applicable

(Continued)

TABLE 25.2 (CONTINUED)
Requirement of Common CTD for ANDA Filing and Comparison among India, the US, and Europe

6	Categorisation of risk management	Not applicable	Risk management and classification are mentioned in the Policy Management System (PMS). It is also necessary to mention the mitigation plan.	Applicable
7	Information of drug product	Applicable	Applicable	Applicable
8	Exclusivity of data	Not applicable	Certification of Paragraph IV or patent clause	Not applicable
9	Braille-formatted name of a pharmaceutical product	Not applicable	Applicable	Not applicable
10	Draft labelling with annotations (side by side)	Require of specimen label on the primary package, second package. A summary of the packaging requirements for shipments from India with proposed draft cartons and labels are required	The strength and packaging size are mentioned in the labelling details and suggested draft label. Drug product package inserts is required.	Product characteristics label samples, quick packaging, and carton packaging are all necessary.
11	Test Protocol executive summary	Not applicable	Not applicable	Not applicable
12	Request for waiver	Not applicable	Not applicable	Not applicable
13	Environment Assessment Statement (EAS) and Risk	Not applicable in GMO or Non-GMO	Compliance with the law of Environmental Protection	The US Environmental Protection Agency's (EPA) agreement on environment risk certification applies to genetically modified organisms (GMOs).
14	Draft labelling with annotations (side by side)	Not applicable	Applicable	Nothing needs to be annotated, but the packaging insert must have all necessary information.

(Continued)

TABLE 25.2 (CONTINUED)
Requirement of Common CTD for ANDA Filing and Comparison among India, the US, and Europe

15	Information about experts	Required along with the *curriculum vitae*	Not applicable	Name. address and signature of all non-clinical and clinical experts shall be included.
16	Agent authorisation	Not applicable	Not applicable	Applicable
17	Other requirements	This study focuses on the research activities and market presence of manufacturers in both domestic and worldwide markets. The acquisition of drug product samples necessitates the provision of a deposit.	Pharmacovigilance information required	If required, petition of approval suitability is required.
		Module 2 (Summaries and Overviews)		
1	Quality-based evaluation	Not applicable	Not applicable	Not applicable
		Module 3 (Product quality)		
1	Justification of specification	Not applicable	Not applicable	Applicable
2	Regional information	Not applicable	Batch and blank master batch record of entire manufacturing process including the packaging is to be provided. The declaration of residual solvents limits or impurities in drug substances and excipients, in accordance with the limits set by the United States Pharmacopeia (USP), is required. Suppliers and applicant declared about the drug substance including the lots, package material etc. Comparability protocols are provided.	Process validation process to be mentioned. Impurities declaration in Q3C(R3) format as per ICH guideline including mention of the residual solvent's limits or presence of any impurities in drug or excipient Certificate of suitability obtained from EDQM is required.

(*Continued*)

TABLE 25.2 (CONTINUED)
Requirement of Common CTD for ANDA Filing and Comparison among India, the US, and Europe

			Packages for comparing protocols and validating procedures are included. Bovine Spongiform Encephalopathy (BSE) and Transmissible Spongiform Encephalopathy (TSE) are to be tested for.	Packaging validity, components, compatibility of the ingredient data are not required. Bovine Spongiform Encephalopathy (BSE) and Transmissible Spongiform Encephalopathy (TSE) certificate are not required.
		Module 4		
Pre-clinical Study Reports on ANDAs application are not required.				
		Module 5 (Clinical Trial)		
1	Number of volunteers/ subjects participating	Not less than 16	Sufficient to achieve statistically analysis with variance to the power analysis	More than 12
2	Study dose along with the test /reference	Made by the manufacturer in or outside India	Produced by a company in or outside of India.	Manufacturing with manufacturer RLD in EU
.3	Criteria for BE	90% confidence index, 80.00–125.00% for C_{max},	90% confidence index, 80.00–125.00% for C_{max} AUCt, $AUC_{0-\infty}$	90% confidence index, 80.00–125.00% for C_{max}, AUCt, $AUC_{0-\infty}$. For highly variable drugs, the range is wider, i.e., 75.00– 133.00%
4	Good Clinical Practices (GCP) requirements	Applicable CDSCO GCP guidelines	Applicable ICH GCP guidelines	Applicable ICH GCP guidelines
5	Pharmacokinetics Parameters	C_{max}, T_{max}, $AUC_{0-\infty}$, AUC_{0-t} for steady state: $AUC_{0-\tau}$, C_{max}, C_{min}	C_{max}, T_{max}, AUC0-∞, AUC_{0-t}, $t_{1/2}$, λz	C_{max}, T_{max}, AUC_{0-t}, $AUC_{0-\infty}$, $t_{1/2}$, λz

(*Continued*)

TABLE 25.2 (CONTINUED)

Requirement of Common CTD for ANDA Filing and Comparison among India, the US, and Europe

6	Design of study	Two separate designs evaluated one in fasted state and other in the fed state. Followed by two-way crossover design and parallel design data generated	Randomised block, crossover design and non-replicated data generated	Randomised block, crossover design and non-replicated data generated
7	Fasting/fed state studies	Fasting and Fed conditions studies are required	Fasting and Fed conditions studies are required	Only fasting
8	Sampling points	12–18 samples are evaluated up to three or more half-lives. Minimum 3–4 samples should be collected at T_{max}	A total of 12–18 samples are assessed for a minimum of three or more half-lives. It is recommended to collect a minimum of three to four samples at the maximum temperature (T_{max}).	It is recommended to collect a minimum of three to four samples during the terminal log linear phase.
9	Analytical process validation parameters	Precision, Accuracy, Recovery, Range and Linearity, Stability of the drug, Specificity/ Selectivity, Sensitivity,	Accuracy, Precision, Reproducibility, Calibration curve, Sensitivity, Selectivity, LOQ and Stability	Accuracy, Repeatability, Detection, Precision, Intermediate precision, Limit of Quantitation (LOQ), and Linearity range
10	Analyte in plasma	Active drug/metabolite	Active drug/ metabolite if applicable	Active drug/ metabolite if applicable
11	Reserve sample	Not applicable	5 times require for each analysis	Not applicable
12	Retention of sample	Typically, a period of three years is observed from the date of priority, though no guideline established	Typically, a period of five years, though no guideline established	Typically, a period of three years, though no guideline established.

25.8 EUROPEAN UNION ANDA APPROVAL (EU)

The European Economic Area (EEA) was founded on January 1, 1994, between the 27 members of the European Community (EC), which eventually became the EU. The competent EEA authority must be consulted for the marketing of ANDA medications. After November 2005, orphan medical goods used to treat cancer, diabetes, cancer, and neurological disorders must use a centralised registration process. Decentralised/mutual recognition is also offered for innovations that are helpful in an emergency, for medical treatment, or that are advantageous to the patients or community. Through the decentralised process, ANDAs can be filed. The document must adhere to Modules 1 through 5 of the Directive CHMP/ICH/2887/99 (Table 25.2).

BIBLIOGRAPHY

ANDA Filing Checklist [Internet]. FDA, 2018 [cited 2018 May 15]. Available from: http://fdaguidance.net/anda-filing-checklist/.

Approved Drug Products with Therapeutic Equivalence Evaluations (Orange Book) [Internet]. U.S FDA, 2018 [cited 2018 May 17]. Available from: https://www.fda.gov/drugs/developmentapprovalprocess/howdrugsaredevelopedandapproved/approvalapplications/abbreviatednewdrugapplicationandagenerics/default.htm.

Approved Drug Products with Therapeutic Equivalence Evaluations (Orange Book) [Internet]. U.S FDA, 2018 Available from: https://www.fda.gov/drugs/developmentapprovalprocess/howdrugsaredevelopedandapproved/approvalapplications/abbreviatednewdrugapplicationandagenerics/default.htm.

Available from: http://www.ema.europa.eu/docs/en_GB/document_library/Scientific_guideline/2009/09/WC500002721.pdf.

Bhardwaj S, Budhwar V, Gupta VK. Comparative Study: Requirements for the Submission of Generic Drug Application across US and EU in CTD/ECTD Format. *AJPSR* 2011, 1: 1–14.

Bioequivalence and Bioavailability Studies. Central Drugs Standard Control Organization (CDSCO) under Directorate General of Health Services, Ministry of Health & Family Welfare, Government of India. Available from: http://cdsco.nic.in/html/BE%20Guidelines%20Draft%20Ver10%20March%2016,%2005.pdf. Accessed March 2020.

Common Technical Documents. Central Drugs Standard Control Organization (CDSCO) under Directorate General of Health Services, Ministry of Health & Family Welfare, Government of India, 2019. Available from: http://www.cdsco.nic.in/writereaddata/CTD%20Guidance%20Final.pdf. Accessed March 2020.

Detailed Information on Paragraph IV Challenges for Drugs Launched Since 1994 [Internet]. Cornerstone Research, 2018[cited 2018 May 09]. Available from: https://www.cornerstone.com/Publications/Research/Trends-in-Paragraph-IV-Challenges#.

eCTD Template [Internet]. FDA, 2018 [cited 2018 May 12]. Available from: https://www.fda.gov/drugs/developmentapprovalprocess/formssubmissionrequirements.

Electronic Submissions Modules in CTD [Internet]. ICH.Org, 2016 [cited 2018 May 13]. Available from: http://www.ich.org/products/ctd.html.

General Provisions of the Act Recent Additions to the Hatch-Waxman Act Under the "Medicare Prescription Drug and Modernization Act", 2003 [Internet]. Slide Share, 2012 [cited 2018 May 25]. Available from: hcopgnt.com/admin/uploads/anda%20filing.pptx.

Handoo S, Arora V, Khera D. A Comprehensive Study on Regulatory Requirements for Development and Filing of Generic Drugs Globally. *International Journal of Pharmaceutical Investigation* 2012, 2(3): 99–105.

Khatun MS, Katamreddy JD, Reddy PJ. A Review on ANDA Submission Requirements for Generic Drugs: "Paragraph IV Certification" as Per FDA CDER Guidelines. *International Journal of Drug Regulatory Affairs* 2018 September 15, 6(3): 5–12.

Module I. Administrative and Prescribing Information [Internet]. ICH.Org, 2016 [cited 2018 May 11]. Available from: http://www.ich.org/fileadmin/Public_Web_Site/ICH_Products/CTD/M4_R4_Organisation/M4_R4__Granularity_Document.pdf.

Module II. Summaries and Overviews and Module III: Information on Product Quality [Internet]. ICH. Org, 2002 [cited 2018 May 13]. Available from: http://www.ich.org/fileadmin/Public_Web_Site/ICH_Products/CTD/M4_R1_Quality/M4Q__R1_.pdf.

Module IV. Nonclinical Study Reports [Internet]. ICH.Org, 2002 [cited 2018 May 24]. Available from: http://www.ich.org/fileadmin/Public_Web_Site/ICH_Products/CTD/M4__R2__Safety/M4S_R2_.pdf.

Module V. Clinical Study Reports [Internet] ICH.Org, 2002 [cited 2018 May 14]. Available from: http://www.ich.org/fileadmin/Public_Web_Site/ICH_Products/CTD/M4E_R2_Efficacy/M4E_R2__Step_4.pdf.

Neetu SA, Thakur M. Critical and Comparative Analysis of ANDA Filling of Tablets in India, Europe and US. *Pharma Tutor* 2017, 5: 17–27.

Paragraph IV Certification Section & Patent Challenge Successful [Internet]. Slide Share, 2014 [cited 2018 May 22]. Available from: https://www.slideshare.net/anthonycrasto64/nda-anda-ind-by-anthony-crasto.

Patent Certifications, Paragraph IV Certifications List [Internet]. FDA, 2018 [cited 2018 May 27]. Available from: https://www.fda.gov/drugs/developmentapprovalprocess/howdrugsaredevelopedandapproved/approvalapplications/abbreviatednewdrugapplicationandagenerics/ucm047676.htm#p.

Pingle S. Indian Pharma Companies Grab 290 Final ANDA Approvals from US FDA in 2018. *Pharmabiz* 2019, 8. Available from: http://pharmabiz.com/ArticleDetails.aspx?aid=113233&sid=1. Accessed February 2020.

Requesting a Pre-Assigned ANDA Number [Internet]. FDA, 2018 [cited 2018 May 12]. Available from: https://www.fda.gov/drugs/developmentapprovalprocess/howdrugsaredevelopedandapproved/approvalapplications/abbreviatednewdrugapplicationandagenerics/ucm120955.html.

Sokal AM, Bart A. Gerstenblith Article About the Hatch-Waxman Act: Encouraging Innovation and Generic Drug Competition Hatch-Waxman Act [Internet]. Finnegan, 2018 [cited 2018 May 23]. Available from: https://www.finnegan.com/en/insights/the-hatch-waxman-act-.

Submitting Marketing Applications According to the ICH/CTD Format: General Considerations. U.S. Food and Drug Administration. Available from: http://www.fda.gov/downloads/drugs/guidancecomplianceregulatoryinformation/guidances/ucm073308.pdf. Accessed March 2020.

Swapna G, Bindhu MC, Anusha P, et al. Comparative Study of Dossier Submission Process for Drug Product in USA, EU & Indian Regulatory. *WJPR* 2014, 3(6): 406–411.

26 Biological Licence Application (BLA) Procedures

26.1 INTRODUCTION

Biologicals are substances that were derived from live organisms with the intention of being used for medical, diagnostic, or disease preventative purposes. These substances were originally developed for use by humans. Vaccines, serums, monoclonal antibodies, antigens, therapeutic proteins, antitoxins, DNA vaccines, fusion proteins, and antitoxins are all examples of biotechnology-based drugs. In India, biological products are regulated by the Central Drugs Standard Control Organization (CDSCO). In the US, biological products are regulated by the US Food and Drug Administration (USFDA). The Drugs and Cosmetics Act, 1940 and Rules, 1945, as well as the Rules for dangerous microorganisms/genetically engineered organisms or cells, 1989, as notified under the Environment (Protection) Act, 1986, regulate the making, storing, distributing, exporting, and importing of biologicals.

As more than 300 biological novel medicines and vaccines are accessible for the treatment of a wide variety of ailments, and as with an Abbreviated New *Drug* Application (ANDA) or generic medications, some biological molecules are recognized as "biological similar" and are marketed after the patent of the innovator has expired; the phrase "biological similar" refers to biologically similar products. In the production of biologically related products, India is widely regarded as one of the world's leading producers.

The manufacturing of advanced, large-scale biologicals is facilitated by recombinant DNA technology. This class includes vaccines, blood components, stem cells, and other things derived from DNA. Biological therapies are crucial for the treatment of numerous diseases and conditions.

A vaccine is a biological preparation intended to build protective immunity against a particular pathogen by stimulating the immune system to recognise and destroy that pathogen and any future microorganisms that might be related to it. The infectious microorganisms that cause disease are imitated in vaccines by utilizing weakened or dead forms of the pathogen, one of the pathogen's surface proteins, or one of the pathogen's toxins.

A kit is a substance made from a living organism or its products that is used to diagnose or alleviate symptoms of a disease.

DOI: 10.1201/9781003397854-10

A biological similar product is a type of medical product that exhibits pharmacological activity or other direct effects that are comparable with those of the biological reference medical product in the context of disease diagnosis, cure, mitigation, treatment, or prevention.

But they also implemented the related rules, which are:

- Import and Export of Micro-organisms and Genetically Engineered Organisms, 1989.
- Recombinant DNA Safety Guidelines, 1990
- Guidelines for Gathering Pre-clinical and Clinical Data for rDNA Vaccines, 1999.
- Instructions and a Manual for the Institutional Bio-Safety Committee
- Advice from CDSCO for Business, 2008

26.2 CONSIDERATIONS RELEVANT TO MOLECULAR BIOLOGY

26.2.1 Clearly Specify the Strain(s) of Bacteria Used in the Production

Provide details on the source and characterization of the bacterial strain. Clearly state the biological origin of the product.

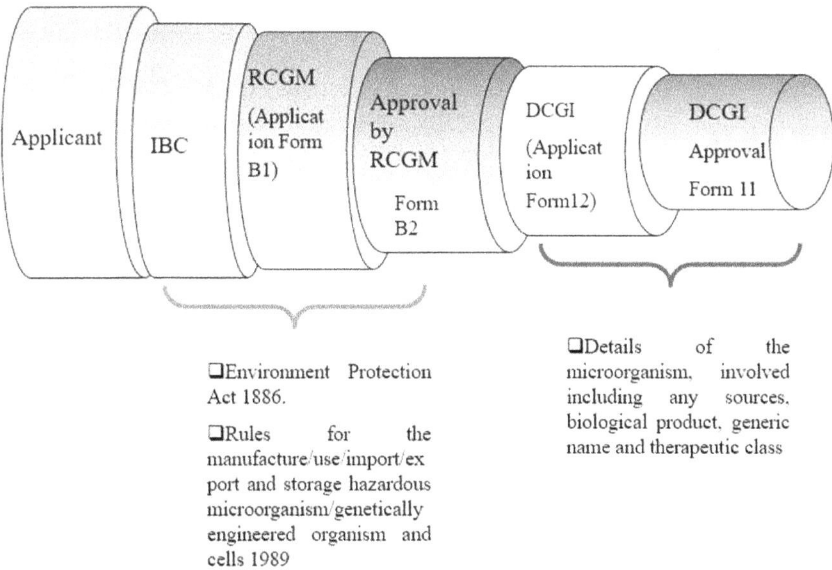

FIGURE 26.1 Process initialization of the regulatory process of research and development of biological products or imported biological products.

Include information on any biological materials used in the manufacturing process.

If a cell culture is involved, provide detailed information about the host cell line. Include information about the origin, characterization, and handling of the cell culture. If embryonated eggs are used, provide information on their source and handling. Detail the cell substrates used, specifying their origin and characteristics. Clearly describe the gene sequences, vectors, and promoters used in the production process. Provide information on their source, design, and any modifications. Specify any translational modifications that occur during the manufacturing process. Address considerations such as oxidation, glycosylation, and other modifications. If there are different forms or substituted products, clearly outline them. Describe how variations in the manufacturing process may result in different product forms. Ensure that all the information provided aligns with regulatory requirements. Follow guidelines from regulatory bodies pertaining to the manufacturing of biological products. Implement robust quality assurance measures throughout the manufacturing process. Document quality control checks and validations. Keep comprehensive records of the manufacturing process. Document any deviations from standard procedures and corrective actions taken.

26.2.2 Recombinant Products

Recombinant technology (r-technology) makes up for the development of the vast majority of biological products. Since a gene from a foreign source was used in r-technology, the safety and quality control of the technology need to be looked at more closely. The processes for clone production and nucleic acid sequences are vital, and if any vector is used, the name, source, map of the vector, and information about the host(s) that contain the vector(s)/target gene must be provided. Characterising and establishing the purity of the recombinant protein is a challenge. Here are the standards we use to ensure our peptides are of the highest quality:

Sodium dodecyl-sulphate polyacrylamide gel electrophoresis (SDS-PAGE) analysis for determination of the relative purity of proteins in comparison to a reference standard (if there is one).

- Peptide mapping of the protein.
- Analysis of amino acids, in particular the N-terminal part.
- A preliminary study of the interaction between the protein of the host cell and the DNA of the host cell in regard to the product.
- Neutralisation Assays
- The quality controls of the conventional products are similar to the recombinant protein.

26.2.3 Biological Characterisation

It is essential to have an in-depth knowledge of both the *in vitro* and the *in vivo* tests for safety and effectiveness of the biologicals. When it comes to conventional products, inactivation, detoxification, stereotyping, attenuation, and neutralisation assays, as well as neurovirulence testing, are necessary. Recombinant proteins require careful characterisation of Master Cell Banks (MCB), Working Cell Banks (WCB), and End-of-Production Cells (EPC) or Cells At the Limit (CAL), with regard to sterility, viability, purity, bacteriophages, and plasmids, among other factors.

Also, the purity of the cell substrate of the product is required. In addition, the assessment of product purity, which encompasses the absence of contaminating cells, microbiological contaminants, and adventitious viruses, is conducted by the application of SDS-PAGE., whereas the detection of toxins is performed using Western blotting. The uniformity of the inactivation procedure as well as the immunogenicity of the result also needs to be documented. The selection of analytical procedures is considered an important parameter for demonstrating product assessment of quality control and comparability in case of similar biologicals. In advanced analytical procedures, there are many complementary methods for the purpose of characterisation of biologicals. In order to identify "slight differences" in any of the important quality characteristics, it is necessary to identify a comprehensive set of modern analytical methods and follow the monograph from the Indian Pharmacopoeia subject availability of the monograph. The utilisation of adequately qualified assays, that are capable of reproducibility and dependability, is required for the measurement of quality attributes during the characterisation process. The validation of the analytical procedure is necessary to ensure its accuracy and reliability. It is important to adhere to the applicable *International Council for Harmonisation* of Technical Requirements for Pharmaceuticals for Human Use (ICH) principles while conducting attribute testing for batch release, stability studies, and in-process controls, specifically ICHQ2, Q5C, and Q6B guidelines. The analysis for characterisation investigations of r-DNA-generated product, the reference biologic as the control, also known as the positive standard, and a negative control should also be included. The appropriate statistical analysis should be followed for presentation like the expression of mean and the standard deviation, and, at a minimum, triplicate experiments should be carried out.

26.2.3.1 Product Characterisation

Characterization investigations pertaining to comparable biologics encompass an assessment of their physicochemical attributes, biological efficacy, immunological characteristics, functional assays, purity (including impurities associated with the manufacturing process and final product), contamination, potency, and content. Similar biologics are also referred to as biosimilars. It is important to adhere to the principles that are defined in the ICH Q6B guideline. If it is available, the Indian Pharmacopoeia Monograph should be used as the standard.

26.2.3.2 Physicochemical and Structural Qualities

The establishment of main and higher order structure of biological substances, as well as other key physicochemical qualities, are necessary to understand the functionality or pharmacologic response. Amino acid sequence similarity with reference to a biological is an important parameters of any class of similar biological (protein). As said earlier, the biological and functional assay processes are to be validated with statistically satisfactory levels of precision and accuracy. Furthermore, post-translational modifications are to be explored thoroughly by both preclinical studies and clinical trials.

26.2.3.3 Biological Assays

When applicable, biological assays should be confirmed against a national or international reference standard. When external reference standards are unavailable, an internal one must be developed in accordance with ICH regulations. Bioassay(s) can be performed in accordance with the documented procedures as described in the specification. There could be a wide variety of biological activities and, in such cases, it is recommended that the appropriate biological tests for characterisation of the activity, identification of the product's mechanism of action, and evaluation of the product's clinical effects be conducted.

26.2.3.4 Immunological Properties

It is well known that the manufacturing method of similar biologics can influence the number of process-related contaminants as well as post-translational modifications that are present in the final product. The immunogenicity of the product might be altered as a result of these changed properties. Therefore, evaluation of similar biologicals is to be done by comparison to the reference biological in terms of specificity, affinity, binding strength.

26.2.3.5 Quality Comparability Study

It is necessary to evaluate the quality of similar biologics in relation to reference biologics. An extensive quality dossier that complies with CDSCO guidance for industry, 2008, must be submitted, so that a comparable information exercise between the similar biologic and the reference biologic is taken in account for clinical development. In order to demonstrate that the production process is reliable, it is necessary to make use of the first three consecutive batches that have been standardised. At the level of the active drug product, comparisons between the comparable biologic and the reference biologic require head-to-head characterisation and investigations to be carried out. It is important to carry out a molecular structural comparison between the active drug substance contained within the reference biologic and the active drug substance contained within the similar biologic. If the requisite quality attribute assessments of the active substance of the reference biologic can be performed on the finished product, then it is possible that testing the isolated active ingredient is not required. It is possible that more characterisation studies will be necessary in order to assess the influence that any differences between the reference biologic and the similar biological have on the efficacy and safety of the similar biological.

Similar biologics may deviate slightly from the reference biologic in a number of ways. However, appropriate information must be provided to guarantee that these adjustments do not affect safety or efficacy. High-resolution analytical techniques and processes are available to detect the possibility of modifications to the product. The similar biologic should be compared with the reference biologic using Quality Attributes (QAs). The Quality Attributes of a comparable biologic can be categorised into two broad categories from the perspective of establishing consistency, namely Clinical Quality Attributes (CQAs) and Key Quality Attributes (KQAs), standing for "critical" and "key" quality characteristics, respectively. First, CQAs are those that directly affect patient clinical safety or treatment success in the clinic. All molecular features that affect the established mechanism(s) of action fall within this category. CQA limits must be established in relation to the reference biological. KQAs are quality attributes that are important from a product and process consistency perspective but are not known to affect clinical safety and efficacy. In this category, we find molecular features that do not influence the molecule's established mechanism(s) of action. Although it's crucial that KQAs stay within acceptable bounds, modest deviations from the reference biologic might be allowed. Because of their focus on molecular structure, function, and heterogeneity, QAs provide a useful foundation for identifying areas of analytical differences.

26.3 PRECLINICAL TOXICITY STUDY REQUIREMENT FOR A BIOLOGICAL

It is necessary to do pre-clinical toxicity testing on a biological drug in order to gain an understanding of both its pharmacologic and toxicologic effects. Biological products are required to be tested in accordance with the ICH for Pharmaceuticals for Human Use (ICH) S6 guideline. In India, the review committee on genetic manipulation (RCGM) is the authority that has the power to authorize any pre-clinical toxicity testing. In India, applications are submitted using Form C3a, and permission is approved using Form C5a. The pre-clinical testing required for the safety characteristics of biologically derived medical products was recommended in this guideline. The guideline is an all-encompassing instruction regarding the general toxicity in animal species, with the choice of species being either rodents or large animals. In accordance with the recommendations laid out by the ICH M3, there is a requirement for a collection of data about the safety pharmacology and biologics. This includes the immunogenicity of monoclonal antibodies as well as the absorption, distribution, metabolism, and excretion (ADME) characterisation of the biological product.

26.3.1 Species Selection

Choose species in which the compound demonstrates pharmacological activity. Assess whether the physiological response in the chosen species is relevant to the intended therapeutic effect in humans. Evaluate cross-reactivity of the compound across different species. Ensure that the compound interacts with the target molecule in a manner similar to its interaction in humans.

Examine whether the epitopes recognized by the compound are expressed in the chosen species. Verify that the biological activity is elicited through interactions with relevant epitopes.

Select species that exhibit similarity in terms of physiological processes, organ systems, and responses to the compound. Ensure that the chosen species mimics human biology to a reasonable extent.

Consider the relevance of the chosen species to the therapeutic indication of the drug. Evaluate whether the chosen species reflects the disease or condition being targeted in humans.

Assess the pharmacokinetics of the compound in the selected species. Ensure that the absorption, distribution, metabolism, and excretion (ADME) characteristics align with those in humans. Conduct toxicology studies in species that are sensitive to the toxic effects of the compound. Identify potential adverse effects and determine their relevance to humans. Recognize species-specific differences in physiology, anatomy, and metabolism. Adjust study parameters accordingly to account for these differences. Follow regulatory guidelines for the selection of relevant species in preclinical studies.

Different regulatory authorities may have specific recommendations for species selection. Adhere to ethical considerations when selecting and conducting studies on animals. Minimize the use of animals and employ humane practices. Evaluate the translational potential of findings from animal studies to predict responses in humans. Consider the predictability of efficacy and safety outcomes.

In recent years, with the help of molecular biology techniques, it has become possible to study antibody binding with animal cells using flow-activated cell sorting (FACS) or microarray technology. These methods have largely supplanted the more conventional immunohistochemistry experiments. It is possible to investigate amino acid sequences and DNA target antigens in order to have a better understanding of the similarity that exists between species and epitopes or antigens.

When attempting to comprehend human risk assessment or predictive toxicology, the selection of the appropriate species is essential, particularly in cases where antigen tissue distribution or target-biology toxicities play a major role. Therapeutics, such as Natalizumab (4-intergrin) for the treatment of multiple sclerosis while TGN1412 (anti-CD28) for the treatment of B cell chronic lymphocytic leukaemia (B-CLL), have been withdrawn from the market because of severe toxicities including fatal viral demyelinating disease, progressive multifocal leukoencephalopathy (PML), and a storm of cytokine activity as a result of a mass release of proinflammatory cytokines. Primate studies using TGN1412 demonstrated that human T-cell biology is distinct from primate biology, and that primate responses to TGN1412 are distinct from human responses. Consequently, the antigen similarity and distribution of animal models must be equivalent to that of humans, and the regulatory documents must include the species that were chosen, based on their relevance to toxicity.

There are two ways to conduct animal experiments for biological purposes: either using transgenic animals, in which the animal's genes have been modified so that they express the human target antigen, or using human therapeutic antibodies to surrogate antibodies, which may react with homologous antigens. Cell-based toxicity assays are tested as off-target toxicity investigations when the toxicity models are unavailable. Studies of this type provide evidence that human exposure to risk is relevant.

26.3.2 Immunogenicity

Immune responses are a common outcome observed in preclinical studies of biological therapies like vaccines, yet immunogenicity can bring a storm of cytokine activity that might be deleterious. Anaphylaxis is a life-threatening allergic reaction caused by the body's immune system mistakenly attacking its own tissues instead of the injected or used material.

Since the objective of the immune response is to counteract the effects of the biologic, it is important to confirm its pharmacokinetic (PK), pharmacodynamic (PD), and adverse event prediction (AE) characteristics.

Finally, sponsors should know that immunological responses in animals do not necessarily reflect those in humans. Conventional preclinical studies and plasma distribution (PD) studies, including *in vitro* binding assays and *in vivo* investigations, are typically required of sponsors in order to evaluate the product's pharmacologic activity and establish its mechanism of action. As was previously mentioned, it is common practice for biologics to perform single and repeat dose toxicity studies with appropriate species.

26.4 SAFETY PHARMACOLOGY STUDIES OF BIOLOGICAL PRODUCTS

Acute single toxicity, sub-acute toxicity, and repeated toxicity studies are used in safety pharmacology to determine the functional effects on individual organs of the main systems in the body. The concept of biological route of administration, dosage response absorption and rate of elimination, therapeutic index, etc., is derived from pre-clinical toxicity studies. Understanding the absorption, disposition, and clearance, and evaluating the exposure consequences requires knowledge of the plasma kinetics or toxicokinetic.

The therapeutic dose of the biologic should be used as the basis for the calculation of the dose. Prior to beginning the toxicity research, it is recommended that a pilot dosage response study be carried out on a large number of animals. In animal toxicology studies, there are often three different levels of doses employed, referred to as low, medium, and high, corresponding to one, two, and five times the human equivalent dose, respectively, or a larger test dose when it comes to repeated-dose toxicity studies. During the toxicity test, the biologics have to be contrasted with one another at a dose that is at least one times the human equivalent dose (HED). Any significant discrepancy in the dose levels should be adequately explained and sanctioned before the studies begin, in terms of the schedule for the administration of the medication.

The step required to induce euthanasia was one of the components of the protocol, along with the activities and observations that took place before and after the euthanasia was carried out. Other toxicity studies, such as safety pharmacology, reproductive toxicity, mutagenicity, and carcinogenicity investigations, are typically not necessary for the evaluation of a comparable biological, unless the results of repeated-dose toxicological studies indicate that they are necessary. All of the components that were approved in the protocol should be included in the final report of the study, as well as any extra sections or documents, such as approval from the RCGM (Recombinant DNA Advisory Committee) for the protocol, the defined test centre, approval from the *Institutional Biosafety Committee* (IBC) for the report, and approval from the Institutional *Animal Ethics* Committee (IAEC) for the use of animals and the procedures. It is important to provide further additional documentation in the form of a quality management statement, approvals from the study's director, all investigators involved in the study, and quality analytical results pertaining to both the test material and the vehicle. Animal feed and animal health certifications, as well as any experimental protocols and any deviations from those protocols, must be mentioned. The findings are to be summed up, along with a description and a discussion of the findings, as well as data on individual animals, summary data, and any other relevant data, such as the results of computer analysis, etc.

In order to have a deeper understanding of the formulation's toxicity compared with protein-based vaccinations, numerous adjuvants needed to be tested separately. Additional information and procedures are necessary, such as collecting and analysing blood, measuring body weight, documenting the amount of food consumed, and so on, before euthanasia. The events that took place immediately after euthanasia are determined, as well as the necropsy, gross description, organ weights, and organs that were sampled for histopathology. In order to maintain Good Laboratory Practices (GLP) compliance during the toxicity testing, any changes to the biochemical parameters, specifics of the equipment, and the protocol that was followed, units of measurement, and expressions must be reported. Haematology procedures are equally essential to understanding any consequences that the toxic substance may have, and in such circumstances, the reports contain all relevant parameters, details regarding the methodology, and information regarding the instrument that was used, regardless of whether it was automated or manually operated. Bone marrow was examined using either an aspirate or a smear, or it was studied using histopathology or necroscopy. Each histopathological or necropsy observation that deviates from the described normal histology must be recorded, and the frequency of each must be indicated across the various groups, because this information is crucial to understanding the changes at the cellular level that occur because of any toxicities.

Confirming whether such a feature is significant or not can be decided on review of statistical significance or dosage response data, or whether it falls within or outside the normal range of values in the case of biochemical and haematological observations. It is also necessary to determine whether such a characteristic is related to the observed dose response. If there is an unnaturally early death or morbidity, the suggested course of action is to be stated in the protocol. Additionally, in these kinds of situations, necroscopy of all animals must be performed and recorded.

In addition, the reported toxicities have been documented. in addition to this systemic toxicity, the following toxicities studies are required to also complete the listed studies as follows:

- Fertility Study and Female Fertility Study (Segment I)
- Teratogenicity Study (Segment II)
- Perinatal Study (Segment III)
- Female Reproduction and Developmental Toxicity Studies
- Local Toxicity
- Allergenicity/Hypersensitivity
- Genotoxicity

26.5 CARCINOGENICITY STUDIES OF BIOLOGICAL PRODUCT

The standard carcinogenicity bioassays used to evaluate risk have been approved by the S6 guideline. These tests involve exposing a substance to both carcinogenic and healthy human cells, as well as to other relevant animal species. To evaluate the safety of a novel medicine, it is necessary to employ non-human primate species that are susceptible to both the expected and unexpected side effects, such as a high abortion rate and a small litter size.

The route of administration, dosage form, vehicle, dose calculation, and method of administration must all be covered in pre-clinical toxicity protocols. The experiment location's accredited status, containment facilities, and institutional biosafety permission are all necessary.

26.6 COMPLIANCE OF PURITY OF EXCIPIENTS FROM ANIMAL OR HUMAN ORIGIN

Any biologicals, such as FCS, gelatine, vitamins of animal origin, or antibodies, that are derived from humans or animals must be certified by the Department of Animal Husbandry of the state in which they were produced to be free of Transmissible Spongiform Encephalopathies (TSE) and Bovine Spongiform Encephalopathies (BSE). In most cases, the development of biological agents requires the use of meat as a medium. This meat must be free of both TSE and BSE, and certificates must be shown from the Animal Husbandry Department of the relevant state.

26.7 VALIDATION STUDIES (ANALYTICAL METHODS) OF BIOLOGICAL PRODUCTS

In order to submit a Biologics License Application (BLA), application, investigators are required to conduct analytical and validation investigations, which cover topics such as precision, accuracy, and others. The method of analysis and validation is responsible for attributing the essential quality of the product. The methodology of the analysis conformed to the indicated International Standard (IS) techniques or the standard guideline. The following analytical procedures can be used in the following manner.

26.7.1 Limit of Detection and Limit of Quantification

The limit of detection, abbreviated as LOD, is specified as 3.3 × σ /S, while the limit of quantification, abbreviated as LOQ, is 10 × σ/S.

σ = Standard deviation of the intercept of the calibration curve

S = Slope of the curve

26.7.2 Linearity

The standard deviation of identical results indicates that the test is linear. In the event that xs out of n attempts are successful, the fraction of successes is denoted by x/n. The theory of the binomial distribution provides the following formula to calculate the standard deviation, which is then used to measure the degree of variation that exists within the testing.

26.7.3 Accuracy

Accuracy of any biological product is the range of success after multiple use and is determined as per the guideline ISO 5725-2:1994 Part II.

According to the ISO 5725 accuracy can be determined as follows:

m: general mean (expectation)

B: laboratory component of variation (under repeatability conditions)

e: random error (under repeatability conditions)

26.8 STABILITY STUDIES OF BIOLOGICAL PRODUCTS

The efficacy of a drug product ingredient during storage is measured by its stability studies, also known as its shelf life. To ensure accuracy, studies on drug substances and products should be conducted in containers and under conditions that mimic those used in actual storage. Data on accelerated stability must be collected for three months on pilot-scale batches, and data on real-time stability must be collected for the same amount of time on pilot-scale batches.

26.9 ACCELERATED STABILITY STUDIES OF BIOLOGICALS

Accelerated stability studies of biological studies could be done in three ways, as follows.

(1) Long-term (12 months) 25°C ± 2°C / 60% RH ± 5% RH; or 30°C ± 2°C/65% RH ± 5% RH

(2) Intermediate (6 months) 30°C ± 2°C / 65% RH ± 5% RH

(3) Accelerated (6 months) 40°C ± 2°C / 75% RH ± 5% RH

The ICH guideline divides products and applications into six distinct categories. Chosen guideline:

ICH guideline Q1A (R2): Stability Testing of New Drugs and Products (Revised Guideline)
ICH guideline Q1B: Photostability Testing
ICH guideline Q1C: Stability Testing of New Dosage Forms
ICH guideline Q1D: Bracketing and Matrixing Designs for Stability Testing of Drug
Substances and Drug Products
ICH guideline Q1E: Evaluation of Stability Data
ICH guideline Q1F: Stability Data Package for Registration in Climatic Zones III and IV (Table 26.1).

It is recommended that real-time stability tests be utilised in order to identify the optimal shelf life and storage environment for the drug substance and drug product. Guidelines like ICH Q1 A(R2), ICH Q5C, and WHO TRS 822 indicate that when testing the stability of drug substances and drug products, it should use cases and storage conditions that are like the real ones.

26.10 INFORMATION ON BIOLOGICAL DRUG PRODUCT FOR APPROVAL

At the time of application, information about biological drug products must be provided in accordance with the guideline of ICH Q6B for international references or monographs, such as the Indian Pharmacopoeia for India. This information must include the physicochemical qualities, immunological properties, biological activity, functional analysis, purity, contamination, strength, and content of the biological drug product. It is important to understand the critical quality which attributes to the product in order to assure consistency in product quality and comparability. Specifications play a significant role in this understanding of the biologicals. Recent

TABLE 26.1
The Climatic Zone May Classify According to the Temperature Zone I to Zone IV

Sl no.	Climatic Conditions	Zone I Temperate	Zone II Sub-Tropical	Zone III Hot dry/Hot Moderate	Zone IV Very Hot/ Humid
1	Mean annual temperature	<20°C	20.5-24°C	> 24°C	> 24°C
2	Kinetic mean temperature	21°C	26°C	31°C	31°C
3	Mean annual relative humidity	45%	60%	40%	70%

directives issued by the CDSCO stipulate that the following information must be provided in conjunction with the application:

1. Mass analysis and mapping of peptides, including a description of N-terminus amino sequencing data.
2. Secondary structure of biologicals by CD spectroscopy, including in the near- and far-UV/visible spectra, and each batch product's quality parameters are to be overlayed onto the spectra.
3. The fluorescence spectroscopy spectra and the quality parameters for each batch of goods are going to be overlaid on the spectra.
4. Information on disulphide bonds, if the structure has any.
5. Evaluation of the heterogeneity of the charge distribution utilising techniques such as isoelectric focusing and cation exchange chromatography, etc.
6. Carbohydrate and glycan analyses, as well as the information of composition, if present.
7. The presence of aggregation has been verified by several methods such as dynamic lighting scattering (DLS), size exclusion chromatography, and so on.
8. Testing for pyrogenicity as well as endotoxins.
9. Host cell protein and DNA content.
10. A functional bioassay in accordance with a standard or the ICH guideline
11. A functional test is necessary for the binding of the receptor, the activation of signal transmission, the anti-proliferation cell assay, apoptosis, neutralisation, and tissue-specific actions, such as the reduction of glucose and cytotoxicity, among other things.
12. The presence of high- or low-molecular-weight proteins, as well as impurities associated with protein presence.

26.11 IMPORTANCE FORM 29 FOR APPROVAL OF BIOLOGICAL PRODUCTS

The completion of Form 29 is required in order to obtain approval to make biological products, which is done for the purposes of testing and analysis. According to the innovator's claim, a test licence can only be provided for the purpose of conducting an examination, test, or analysis of biologicals. The CDSCO is authorised to proceed with testing and analysis on test batches supplied by the company. A Form 30 signed off on by a director of the firm or company must be submitted to the State Licensing Authority (SLA). According to the SLA, the act assigned four drug inspectors to carry out inspections of locations where biological products are manufactured, either with or without prior notice. These inspections may take place either with or without prior notice. Under the licence that is given to the producer in order to conduct an examination, test, or analysis, all parties involved are required to keep a record of the quantity of drugs that are manufactured.

26.12 PROTOCOL OF CLINICAL TRIAL OF BIOLOGICAL PRODUCTS

The writing of a clinical trial is a highly technical art where the primary goal is to demonstrate that the benefit-to-risk ratio is favourable. The following components were essential to the success of an ideal clinical trial.

26.12.1 Trial Objective

One of the most crucial steps in designing a study is formulating a statement regarding the null hypothesis, which defines the need for clinical trials, the feasibility of conducting a population-based trial, and so on.

26.12.2 Study Design and Duration of the Trial

The research design is essential for gaining an understanding of the practicality of the clinical trial, the results of which must be free from bias. A variety of trial designs, including randomisation, blinding, and the use of a comparable agent, are used. Any assertions that are connected to the planned study need to be related to the study's designs and substantiated in order to provide support. The expected start and end dates of the study, as well as the total number of volunteers, should be specified.

26.12.3 Total Number of Sites and Multicentric Trial

A total number of trial sites have been allotted across the globe, and sites in India that correspond to geographical areas are to be included.

26.12.4 List of Investigators

Investigators' detail at each site of the trial is to be mentioned.

26.12.5 Sample Size and Patient Population

Any clinical trial requires careful planning, including estimations of the necessary sample size, the likely attrition rate, and other factors. Indications, conditions, treatments, disease stages, and other relevant diagnostic criteria should all be mentioned as they pertain to the study participants. There is a need for specific approval to include some trial volunteers, such as members of the armed forces, soldiers, children, pregnant women, and members of minority groups.

26.12.6 Inclusion and Exclusion Criteria

Conditions of the inclusion and exclusion of any volunteers recruited for any trial in the proposed clinical trial.

26.12.7 Drug Formulation

There should be a clear discussion of the drug(s) and formulation(s) that will be utilised in the clinical trial, as well as evidence supporting the formulation(s) that were employed in any relevant preclinical or other clinical trials. There must be full transparency on the commercial formulation and the corresponding clinical trial.

26.12.8 Dosage Regimen

Schedule(s) dosage including escalations, maintenance, reductions, or withdrawal needs to be described, if relevant, as is the rationale for dose selection. It is important to note any potential toxicities or adverse medication reactions, as well as any specific antidotes or supportive care that should be taken. There should be discussion of washout periods before and after the study.

26.12.9 Data Generation

Clinical confirmation of the event schedule and monitoring of baseline data from the volunteer are both required. All procedures, visits, and visits that are part of the clinical study should be mentioned, and data can be collected even if concurrent medicine is used.

26.12.10 Risk Management

The provision of withdrawing from the trial and receiving the necessary treatment in the event that an adverse reaction should be available, as well as the requirement that any necessary antidotes or supportive measures be mentioned, along with the ongoing obligation to do follow-up evaluations.

26.12.11 Consent from the Volunteer

This is an important document to grasp in order to realize that the volunteer's rights are maintained during any clinical experiment. The Form has to specify both the risk and the benefit.

26.12.12 Discontinuation Criteria

The patient has the right to discontinue or withdraw from the clinical trial whenever they feel it is necessary, regardless of whether or not any adverse reactions were detected in the volunteer or other subjects during the clinical trial.

26.12.13 Efficacy Variables and Safety Variable Analysis

The responses to the treatment or variations from the baseline data are to be noted and validated following treatment. In addition, the secondary alterations or endpoints that were determined by the clinical trial need to be described in detail. Validation and monitoring are to be performed on any adverse reactions or events, including toxicities that are related to the clinical trial.

26.12.14 Statistical Analysis

It is essential to do statistical analysis in order to have a proper understanding of the trial parameters, such as the endpoint, efficacy, safety, pharmacokinetics, and pharmacological or biochemical reaction. Additionally, the statistical data are essential in order to comprehend the demographic dynamics of the population as well as the interim analysis of the safety data monitoring.

26.13 ACCELERATED CLINICAL TRIAL OF BIOLOGICAL PRODUCTS

In the event of a medical emergency in India, Schedule Y, Clause 1(3) of The Drugs and Cosmetics Rules, 1945, allows for some leeway in terms of toxicological and clinical data requirements. These requirements can be postponed or even eliminated altogether, if necessary. The Drugs and Cosmetics Act,1940, and its implementing rules do not recognise "life-threatening diseases" or "serious diseases" as legitimate disease categories. On the other hand, diseases like cancer and AIDS are almost always seen as being extremely serious and potentially fatal. Form 40 is used to submit applications, whereas Form 41 is used to issue licences after those applications have been processed.

26.14 MARKETING AUTHORISATION OF THE BIOLOGICAL PRODUCTS

A new biologic molecule must go through a regulatory process that is very similar to that of a novel drug, and it is necessary to fill out Form 44 in order to be approved as a new biological substance in accordance with The Drugs and Cosmetics Act of 1940 and the Rules of 1945. After analysing the five modules that the innovator or applicant has provided, the Central Drug Standard Control Organisation, also known as the CDSCO, is the authority that decides whether or not to grant approval for marketing. These modules are Administrative/Legal Information, Summaries, Quality Information (Chemical, Biological, and Pharmaceutical), Non-Clinical Information, and Clinical Information. In Form 46, the CDSCO indicates that it has granted approval or authorised marketing.

26.15 POST-APPROVAL CHANGES TO BIOLOGICAL PRODUCTS

Post-approval changes to biological products are considered to be the same as changes made to an approved product if they have an effect on the product's safety, effectiveness, or other regulatory standards. According to The Drugs and Cosmetics Rule (Rule 122E), it is against the law to make such changes without first informing the licensing authority. Such modifications are regarded as New Drug 122E, which necessitated obtaining a new authorisation from the CDSCO and calling for the collection of supporting evidence. The study and the categorical statement are required in order

TABLE 26.2
CDSCO Has Mandated that the Following Forms be Filled Out

Sl	Subject	Authority	Specified Forms	Approval
1	A manufacturing licence for the purpose of inspection, analysis, and testing	State FDA	Form 30	Form 29
2	Obtaining a licence to import for the purpose of inspection and analysis.	Zonal FDA	Form 12	Form 11
3	The importing, exporting, or transferring of any cell bank-related means	RCGM	Form B1/B3/B5 and B7	-
4	The investigation and creation of any biotechnological product or genetically modified micro-organism	RCGM	Form C1	Form C2
5	Authorisation for Preliminary Clinical Trials	RCGM	Form C3	Form C4
6	Submission of Preclinical Study Results	RCGM	Form C5	Form C6
7	Authorisation for the Conduct of Clinical Trials	CDSCO	Form 44	CT permission letter
8	Approval for Importing, Manufacturing, and Distribution	CDSCO	Form 44	Form 45A/46A for bulk product and Form 45/46 for finished product
9	Licence to Manufacture	State FDA/ CDSCO	Form 26D	Form 28D
10	Submission of an application for an import certificate	CDSCO	Form 40 with schedule DI and DII and Form 44	Form 41 and 45
11	Authorisation or a licence to import a product.	CDSCO	Forms 8 and 9	Form 10

to determine how post-approval alterations influence the quality of the product, as well as its validation, animal toxicity, stability, and clinical (safety and efficacy) status. Changing the production premises and the licence requires an application to be submitted to the respective state licensing authorities, zonal offices, or sub-zonal offices of the Central Licensing Approval Authority (CLA), together with the necessary payments.

26.16 IMPORT LICENCE OF BIOLOGICAL PRODUCTS

In India, obtaining an import licence for biological products is governed by The Drugs and Cosmetics Act and Rules. The Environment (Protection) Act of 1986 includes provisions for the regulation of the production, use, import, export, and storage of genetically altered organisms or cells, as well as potentially harmful microorganisms. Therefore, an application for an import licence must be submitted after obtaining a certificate of no objection from the Ministry of the Environment and Forest and Climate Change. This is then followed by the submission of an application for an import licence for biological materials using Form 8, with the licence being granted using Form No. 10, and for the Schedule X category, the licence being granted using Form 10A. The import licence for biological products is issued and remains valid for a period of three years, until it is cancelled in accordance with Rule 24 of The Drugs and Cosmetics Rules.

26.17 BIOLOGICAL REGISTRATION FOR MANUFACTURING AND IMPORT

To register biological products in India under the rules of Section 3b of The Drugs and Cosmetics Act (1940) and Rules (1945) under Rule 26A, We need to follow a systematic process. The registration process typically involves providing evidence of the safety and effectiveness of the biological product. Here is a general guide on the steps need to take:

1. Preparation of Documentation:
   Prepare a comprehensive set of documents providing detailed information about the biological product.
   Include data on safety, efficacy, manufacturing processes, quality control, and any other relevant information.
2. Appoint an Authorized Agent:
   If a foreign manufacturer, appoint an authorized agent in India. The authorized agent serves as a liaison between the regulatory authorities and the foreign manufacturer.
3. Local Testing and Clinical Trials:
   Conduct local testing or clinical trials in India if required. This is often necessary to provide evidence of the product's safety and efficacy in the local population.
4. Submit Application:
   Submit a registration application to the Central Drugs Standard Control Organization (CDSCO) in India.
   Include the required documentation, such as:
   Manufacturing details and compliance with Good Manufacturing Practices (GMP).
   Preclinical and clinical trial data.
   Stability data.
   Product labeling and packaging details.
   Pharmacovigilance plan.
5. Review and Evaluation:
   The CDSCO will review the submitted application and conduct an evaluation of the provided data.

This may involve inspections of manufacturing facilities to ensure compliance with GMP.

6. Expert Committee Evaluation:
   The CDSCO may refer the application to an expert committee for evaluation.
   The committee assesses the safety, efficacy, and quality aspects of the biological product.
7. Granting of Registration Certificate:
   If the CDSCO and expert committee are satisfied with the submitted data and compliance, a registration certificate for the biological product is issued.
8. Post-Marketing Surveillance:
   After registration, continue monitoring the safety and efficacy of the product through post-marketing surveillance.
   Adverse events should be reported to the regulatory authorities as required.
9. Renewal and Updates:
   Renew the registration certificate as per the specified timelines.
   Submit updates to the regulatory authorities if there are changes in manufacturing processes, labeling, or any other relevant information.
10. Compliance with Regulatory Changes:
    Stay informed about changes in regulatory requirements and ensure ongoing compliance.

BIBLIOGRAPHY

Available from: http://cdsco.nic.in/writereaddata/bio_div_vacc/check_tl_form_11.pdf.

Available from: https://en.wikipedia.org/wiki/Vaccine.

Central Drug Standard Control Organization Directorate General of Health Services Office of Drugs Controller General (India), Biological Division. Checklist for Pre-Screening of Applications for Variations Under Post Approval Changes as Per CDSCO Guidance for Industry. Available at: https://cdsco.gov.in/opencms/opencms/system/modules/CDSCO.WEB/elements/industry_download.jsp?num_id=MzY=. Accessed 11 June 2016.

Checklist for Registration Certificate of Biologicals, Form 41. Available from: https://cdsco.gov.in/opencms/export/sites/CDSCO_WEB/Pdf-documents/biologicals/Biologiclas_Checklist_Oct2018.pdf. Accessed 11 June 2016.

Checklist for Import Licence (Form 10). Available from: https://cdsco.gov.in/opencms/export/sites/CDSCO_WEB/Pdf-documents/biologicals/Biologiclas_Checklist_Oct2018.pdf. Accessed 12 June 2016.

Clini Experts. Available from: https://cliniexperts.com. Accessed 3 October 2023.

Guidance Document on Grant of Licence in form 11(Test Licence) for the Purpose of Examination Testing and Analysis as Per Rule 33 of Drugs and Cosmetics Acts and Rules 1945. Central Drugs Standard Control Organization Directorate General of Health Services Ministry of Health and Family Welfare Government of India. http://www.cdsco.nic.in/writereaddata/GUIDANCE%20DOC.pdf.

The Drugs and Cosmetics ACT, 1940 and Rules 1945. Available from: https://cdsco.gov.in/opencms/export/sites/CDSCO_WEB/Pdf-documents/acts_rules/2016DrugsandCosmeticsAct1940Rules1945.pdf. Accessed 13 June 2016.

The Drugs and Cosmetics ACT, 1940 and Rules 1945. Available from: https://cdsco.gov.in/opencms/export/sites/CDSCO_WEB/Pdf-documents/acts_rules/2016DrugsandCosmeticsAct1940Rules1945.pdf. Accessed 13 June 2016.

27 Regulatory Approval of Biosimilars Including Nucleic Acid-based Recombinant Products, Recombinant Therapeutic Enzymes, and Protein

27.1 INTRODUCTION

The process of developing biologics and biosimilars is difficult due to the enormous complexity of the molecules involved. The guidelines for biosimilar pharmaceuticals have been thoroughly defined in the United States (US) and the European Union (EU); more recently, India framed the regulatory guidelines and data necessary for the approval of biosimilar drugs. The name reflected the fact that biologicals had reference molecules, or molecules that have been approved, which established that they are safe and effective. In most cases, biosimilars are not an identical replica of the approved biologicals or "the twin but not the clone," having many similarities, treating the same condition with the same doses, but they cannot be said to be the generic medicine. The market for biosimilars is expanding at an exponential rate each day, and many different types of drugs are now being recognised to be in this category. Some examples of biosimilar drugs include recombinant granulocyte colony-stimulating factor (G-CSF), recombinant erythropoietin, human insulin, interferon alpha and beta, and human growth hormone.

Cancer, diabetes, infectious/inflammatory diseases, autoimmune diseases, growth deficits, and haematological abnormalities are just a few of the many conditions that monoclonal antibodies are used to treat. Pharmaceutical businesses that focus on research as well as those that produce generic drugs seize opportunities to produce "generic" versions of original biologics. In India, there are regulatory bodies controlling the development of biosimilars and they have definite roles.

DOI: 10.1201/9781003397854-11

27.2 WAIVER PROVISIONS OF THE SAFETY AND EFFICACY DATA

1. If the structural and functional high degree of similarity with the reference biological is demonstrated by physicochemical and in vitro procedures, then the biosimilar can be used interchangeably with the reference biological.
2. A comparable biologic was used for the preclinical studies, and this was compared with the reference biological.
3. It has been established that the clinical outcome is comparable with that of the pharmacokinetic (PK) or pharmacodynamic (PD) investigations when compared with the PD indicators, safety measurements, and immunogenicity assessment of the reference biological.
4. Additional safety data, with a focus on immunogenic data, must be provided, and the plan for managing risks after release to the public must be described in detail.
5. The study is linked with high-molecular-weight biologics, such as monoclonal antibodies, in which the conclusive clinical safety and efficacy study cannot be skipped.
6. If the immunogenicity data is successfully obtained during the PK/PD trial, and, more specifically, if such data shall be generated in the post-approval Phase IV study, then the Phase III could potentially be skipped in this situation.
7. The Phase I remaining risk for analogous biologicals is significantly lower than that for the reference biologicals, and the two have equivalent PK and PD profiles, as established by pre-clinical studies and in vitro characterisation. In these circumstances, the need for clinical trials can be waived.
8. If a reliable PD marker has not been validated in a clinical study, then the need for a clinical safety and effectiveness investigation cannot be avoided.

27.3 PRODUCT CHARACTERISATION

Regarding the purpose of characterisation of the biosimilar, either the ICH Q6B guidelines or the United States, European, or Indian Pharmacopoeia, or any official monograph, should be followed, if any are available.

1. Structural and Physicochemical Characterisation

In order to determine the majority of proteins or biosimilar pharmaceuticals, both the primary and higher-level structures, as well as the significant physicochemical properties, need to be known. The structure of the amino acid sequence, as well as its confirmation similarity, has to be comparable with that of the reference biosimilar. In addition, the target amino acid sequence of the biosimilar must be comparable to the sequence of the reference biologicals, and the validation of its biological, functional, and analytical methodologies must be measured. Any post-translational changes that were made must be specifically addressed, as well as how those changes affected the pre-clinical and clinical settings.

2. Biological Activity

The mechanism of the product's therapeutic effects is studied through the development of biological assays. If the unit is not universally recognised, the biological assay must be validated in accordance with ICH; otherwise, the assay may be created using internal references in accordance with ICH guidelines.

3. Immunological Properties

Post-translational modification occurs often during manufacturing and, in most situations, the modifications reflect directly on the product's immunogenicity. Specificity, affinity, binding strength, and Fc functions can all be compared to the reference biological by characterisation of the antibody or antibody-derived product. Characterizing the Fc region is essential for understanding the antibody's interaction with immune cells and other immune system components. Fc functions can influence the antibody's therapeutic efficacy.

4. Purity and Impurities

It is crucial to characterise a biosimilar through the use of analytical processes. If any impurities are found in the biosimilar, they must be reported, and it is also necessary to describe the biosimilar's level of purity. The biosimiliar's efficacy and safety must not be compromised in any way by impurities of any kind. There are many unwanted substances that are formed, such as variants of products (glycoforms, isomers, and so on), impurities (aggregated, oxidised, or deamidated product), contaminants related to the host cell (host cell protein, host cell DNA, and so on), and process-related contaminants (residual media components, resin leachates, and so on).

5. Quality Comparability of Biosimilar to Reference Biological

Choosing the appropriate analytical methods is necessary in order to ensure product comparability with respect to the essential quality characteristics of established reference biologicals. The comparison of the quality or its attribution of the same biologicals is to be compared with orthogonal methods for characterisation, such as the aggregation of products. State-of-the-art analytical procedures need to be utilised in order to identify even "slight differences" in all of the important quality criteria. The utilisation of adequately qualified assays that are also capable of reproducibility and dependability is required for the measurement of quality attributes that are included in the characterisation process. The Quality Attributes (QAs) clause is the part of the agreement in which the reference product and the biosimilar product are placed in the resolution to analytical similarities and the ability to detect any divergence from the reference products is required. Critical Quality Attributes (CQA) and Key Quality Attributes (KQA) are the two categories that are used to classify QA. If the Indian Pharmacopoeia monograph is accessible for the product or mentioned, it should be used. In the event that it is not available, the next best thing is to use the other pharmacopoeia monographs which are accepted in India. Regarding batch release, International Council for Harmonisation of Technical Requirements for Pharmaceuticals (ICH) recommendations (ICHQ2 or Q5C or Q6B) are to be followed, and stability studies and in-process controls should be validated accordingly. The quality attributes for characterisation are transmitted through the use of this method. As a form of control, reference biologicals are compared with both known positive standards and known negative controls. The point-to-point comparison of the biosimilar and the reference biologic is performed in accordance with the CDSCO recommendation for industry from 2008. In the beginning, the first three batches in succession are standardised, and they all exhibit the same level of consistency when compared with the reference biologicals. Because safety and efficacy are the most important parameters that are considered for the biologicals and biosimilar, any difference in the structure and bio-analytical characteristics from the reference biologicals are noted and accordingly assessed for additional research in order to understand how the safety and efficacy may deviate.

4.1. Critical Quality Attributes (CQA)

Accountability shall be within the limit of the reference authorised drugs, since this parametric assessment, where the safety and efficacy may directly impact the clinical safety, efficacy, and mechanism of action, is of extreme significance.

4.2. Key Quality Attributes (KQA)

Accountability shall be within the limit of the reference authorised drugs, since this parametric assessment, where the safety and efficacy may directly impact the clinical safety, efficacy, and mechanism of action, is of extreme significance.

Acceptable statistical significance needs to be expressed throughout the characterisation data, and, as a result, for the purpose of optimising the statistical data, each quantitative experiment must be carried out a minimum of three times, and data need to be expressed in terms of mean and standard deviation.

27.4 CHARACTERISATION, BOTH PHYSICOCHEMICAL AND BIOLOGICAL, OF NUCLEIC ACID-BASED RECOMBINANT PRODUCTS (INCLUDING, BUT NOT LIMITED TO, VECTORS FOR THE PRODUCTION OF RECOMBINANT PROTEINS, SIRNA AND SNRNA, ETC.).

1. The structure of the active substance is to be mentioned.

1.1. Identity Analysis

The sequence of the biosimilar product must be identical to that of the biological references being used, as this is a requirement for importation under the CQA.

1.2. Analysis of the Secondary Structures

In the event that the molecular structure of the reference biologicals is a restriction map for more than 1000 base pairs, then the structure must be comparable to the structure of the reference biologic. In addition, the circular dichroism (CD) spectra of the biosimilar and the reference biological must be identical throughout a wavelength range of 190 to 800 nm. Furthermore, the results of gel electrophoresis (agarose/acrylamide/urea PAGE) for a representative molecular weight as well as Southern/northern blot/hybridisation to the sequence of interest are to be compared with the reference biologicals. Since this is an importation attribution under CQA, no modification from the reference is permitted.

2. Product-related Impurities

Both the contaminant and the linked foreign protein could potentially acquire an unwanted activity or immunogenicity, both of which would reflect negatively on the product's overall safety. The nanodrop or reagent method was used to determine the impurities associated with RNA or DNA, whereas the high-performance liquid chromatography (HPLC) method was used to determine the purity. Under the KQA, this is an example of an importation attribution.

3. Process-related Impurities

Once mass manufacturing is underway, it is understood that some level of process-related impurity is unavoidable; nonetheless, it remains imperative that this level of impurity does not compromise the integrity of the biosimilar molecules' biological properties.

4. Biological Characterisation (Functional and Biological Activity)

The expression pattern of the biosimilar and the reference biological must be identical to that in the host cell target host cell and must not deviate from this pattern in any way. Expressions of both biosimilar and reference biological were determined to have taken place in the target cells and organs of the human and target species, with the vehicle control serving as the negative group. In addition to this, the efficiency of the biosimilar must be evaluated, as well as the positioning of the vectors and the activity of the promoters in the target cells. In comparison with the reference biological, the kinetics of the protection provided by the biosimilar, as well as its half-life, will need to be determined. Under CQA, all of this must be attributed properly, and deviations from the reference are not permitted.

5. Efficacy (*In Vitro*/*In Vivo*)

It is crucial to choose a species that is as similar as possible to the target population or human population in order to conduct a reliable assessment of efficacy of the biosimilar. Biosimilars and reference biologicals are to be compared for their therapeutic efficacy and adverse effects. Under CQA, all importation credits must be given in this manner.

6. Expression of Small Interfering RNA (siRNA)/ (Small Nuclear RNA(snRNA) in Vector

It is essential to compare the expression profile of the biosimilar to that of the reference biologicals when incorporated into the target host cell. In addition, the expression of the biosimilar into the target cells or organs of the biosimilar of a comparable species to humans or the target species is essential, and the study needs to be compared with the reference biologicals.

27.5 PHYSICOCHEMICAL AND BIOLOGICAL CHARACTERISATION OF RECOMBINANT THERAPEUTIC PROTEINS

It is essential to compare the expression profile of the biosimilar with that of the reference biologicals when incorporated into the target host cell. In addition, the expression of the biosimilar in the target cells or organs of the biosimilar in a comparable species to humans or the target species is essential, and the study needs to be compared to the reference biologicals. Comparisons with the reference biologicals have to be made regarding the vector position and promoter function inside the target cell, as well as the kinetics, therapeutic efficiency periods, or protection time. After obtaining the satisfactory results, research of a similar nature needs to be carried out on the closest species to human, or the target species; this is an essential component of the CQA.

1. Primary Structure Analysis

Biosimilars and reference biologicals should have similar complete amino acid sequences (including C and N terminals), intact mass assessments using Liquid Chromatography-Electrospray Ionization-Mass Spectrometry (LC-ESI-MS) or matrix-assisted laser desorption ionisation time-of-flight mass spectrometry (MALDI-TOF MS), and peptide mapping. This is an important CQA attribution.

2. Secondary Structure Analysis

UV circular dichroism spectrum/Fourier transform infrared spectroscopy (FTIR) analysis in the wavelength range 190–800 nm is required to compare and match the spectra of biosimilars and reference biologicals. In addition, the position of the sulphydryl groups and disulphide bridges between the biosimilar and reference biologicals, as well as the tryptic peptide map-1D and -2D for conserved secondary structure, must be determined. In terms of CQA, this is also a crucial attribute.

3. Tertiary Structure Analysis

It is under the important attribute of CQA that the spectra of biosimilars and reference biologicals are developed and matched using fluorescence spectroscopy, near-UV circular dichroism spectroscopy, and UV-VIS spectroscopy.

4. Isoforms of Active Substance

The biosimilar manufacturing process may involve isoform formation via post-translational modifications such as glycosylation, acetylation, methylation, PEGylation, phosphorylation, or esterification. Isoformation can alter the properties of the final products in a number of ways, including the formation of aggregates and clipped products, the reduction or modification of the N or C terminal, the formation of additional charge, and the alteration of the unexpected behaviours that switch the targets to the binding or other receptor-binding activities, all of which have an impact on the mechanism of action. Biosimilar isoforms can be detected using HPLC and MALDI-TOF, and their relative charges can be calculated using isoelectric focusing. Ion exchange chromatography is used to detect heterogeneity, and C-terminal sequencing verifies the development of isoforms. In terms of CQA, this is also a crucial attribute.

5. Host- and Process-related Impurities

Host cell proteins, protein A, host cell DNA, leachable protein, and other foreign proteins may affect product quality but have no effect on biological activity. Therefore, the presence of such alien artifacts must be within the allowable range, and such evaluations qualify as KQAs. Host cell DNA analysis, limulus amoebocyte lysate (LAL) test, bacterial endotoxin test (BET) for pyrogen content, and protein analysis are all possible.

6. Drug Product Characteristics

The quality attributes of the biosimilar should ideally be comparable with those of the reference biologicals. Protein content, pH, osmolarity, appearance, formulation of major excipients, including stabiliser and visible/sub visible particles, and pyrogen content are just a few examples of tests that can be used to establish similarities.

7. Product-related Impurities

Many analytical instruments and procedures are used to detect contaminants, such as reversed-phase high-performance liquid chromatography (RP-HPLC), inverted-phase high-performance liquid chromatography (IE-HPLC), SDS-polyacrylamide gel electrophoresis (SDS-PAGE), cerium elution chromatography (CE-IEF), and western blotting. Light and heavy chain separation, with reference to the antigenic recognition motif or the helix-to-coil transition profile, is also examined for quality control.

8. Functional and Biological Activity

Establishing that the target host cell, which should ideally be neutralised by the biosimilar, and further establishing the *in vivo* system of the species closest to the target species and evaluating the effectiveness of the vector/antibody, as well as the alteration of the promoter activity in the target organ/cells, is to be carried out *in vitro*. Biosimilars to commonly used Indian variant strains are evaluated for their therapeutic efficacy, half-life of protection, and biological activities, and the results are compared with those of the reference biologicals for purposes of attributing efficacy under CQA. In addition, the effects of the comparable biologic on proliferation, cytotoxicity, and neutralisation might be assessed by comparing them to the effects of the reference biological.

27.6 PHYSICOCHEMICAL AND BIOLOGICAL CHARACTERISATION OF RECOMBINANT THERAPEUTIC PROTEINS

Insulin is regarded as the most significant biosimilar product available on the international market and, along with human growth hormone, a significant number of chemotherapy drugs may be aimed towards the Indian market.

1. Primary Structure Analysis

These factors are deemed to be attributes under CQA, and, as a result, the biosimilar and reference biologicals are required to exhibit a similarity of primary structure by the amino acid sequence with the entire structure, N terminal assay, intact mass evaluation by LC-ESI-MS/MALDI-TOF-MS, and peptide map.

2. Secondary Structure Analysis

These parameters are also considered as attributes under CQA, and, as a result, the biosimilar and the reference biologicals need to establish a similarity of secondary structure by the absorbance spectra determined by the circular dichroism spectrum and the Fourier transform infrared analysis spectrum. Additionally, the secondary structure needs to be conserved and can be analysed by the tryptic peptide map in both 1D and 2D.

3. Tertiary Structure Analysis

These criteria are also taken into consideration as an attribute under CQA; therefore, a resemblance of tertiary structure must be established between the biosimilar and reference biologicals using absorbance parameters of fluorescence spectroscopy, near UV-circular dichroism spectroscopy, and UV-VIS spectroscopy.

4. Isoforms of the Active Substance

The biosimilar manufacturing process may involve isoform formation via post-translational modifications such as glycosylation, acetylation, methylation, PEGylation, phosphorylation, or esterification. Isoformation can alter the properties of the final products in a number of ways, including the formation of aggregates and clipped products, the reduction or modification of the N or C terminal, the formation of additional charge, and the alteration of the unexpected behaviours that switch the targets to the binding or other receptor-binding activities, all of which have an impact on the mechanism of action. Biosimilar isoforms can be detected using HPLC and MALDI-TOF, and their relative charges can be calculated using isoelectric focusing. Ion exchange chromatography is used to detect heterogeneity, and C-terminal sequencing verifies the development of isoforms. In terms of CQA, this is also a crucial attribute.

5. Product-related Variants and Impurities

5.1 Purity and Impurities

Characterisation of a similar biological involves evaluation by a combination of analytical processes and biological assays. Different parameters, such as the formation of the glycoforms, isomers, etc., must be taken into account during production in order to characterise a similar biologic. Other contaminants that may have been present during product manufacture include oxidation, dimidiation, and aggregate formation. Sometimes, contaminants from the host cell, including foreign DNA or protein that derived from the host cell, are found as well. Many contaminants, including residual medium components and resin, are produced as a byproduct of the intricate biological production process.

There should be no discernible differences between the similar biologic and the reference biologic in terms of purity or impurity profile. It is important to recognise and characterise any impurities present in the biosimilar. Safety and efficacy have not been compromised, either, according to both preclinical and clinical investigations of similar biologicals. During the manufacturing process, undesirable proteins can be developed, which can have a negative impact on the product's activity, immunogenicity, and, ultimately, its efficacy and safety. There are a number of instruments and procedures that can be used to detect impurities, including RP-HPLC, IE-HPLC, SE-HPLC, Western Blot, SDS-PAGE/CE-SDS-PAGE, and IEF/CE-IEF. In addition, the quality control was checked by separating the light chain from the heavier chain, and then comparing the results to an antigenic recognition motif or a helix-to-coil transition characteristic.

5.2. Specifications

In accordance with the applicable guideline (ICH Q6B), quality standards of similar biologics are also comparable with the reference biologic and such specifications are referred to as quality attributes (QAs). Methods of analysis are based on characterisation in the process of characterising a product and determining whether or not it is equivalent to the standards of other products. Acceptance limits should be set using reference biologic data and data from a sufficient number of batches from preclinical or clinical batches, and these limits should be consistent with international standards.

6. Process-related Impurities

The production of foreign proteins involves a careful analysis of various components, and the use of analytical methods such as host cell protein analysis, host cell DNA analysis, and pyrogen testing is essential for ensuring the quality and safety of the final product. Process controls and a robust analysis system are critical for maintaining consistency and adherence to regulatory standards throughout the production process. Analysis of host cell proteins, analysis of host cell DNA, and analysis of pyrogen content are the three methods that might be used to detect process controls and analysis system. Protein content, appearance, pH, osmolarity, and the formulation content of the excipient, comprising stabiliser or particle size distribution from visible particles, as well as the pyrogen content, are all considered to be attributes under KQA. Additionally, the pyrogen content is included in the category of process-related impurities.

7. Functional and Biological Activity

Once *in-vitro* and/or *in-vivo* data creation has been completed successfully, more validation is necessary to elucidate the drug's mechanism of action and the biosimilar's attachment to receptor-binding studies, both of which are indicative of the drug's safety. The pharmacokinetics of any biological presents a picture of protection periods, therapeutic time, *Km* (Michaelis constant), and *Ki* (inhibitor constant) with known inhibitors is contrasted with the reference biologicals. Biosimilar was also evaluated with regard to the target host cell and the animal species that is most closely related to humans, in addition to developing the appropriate disease and infection model in order to understand the mechanism of action, which included the interaction with the target organ as well as proliferation, cytotoxicity, and effects with neutralising in comparison to reference biologicals. The following are the details and data that need to be documented (Table 27.1).

27.7 RESEARCH AND DEVELOPMENT PROCEDURE FOR BIOSIMILAR

Any biosimilar developed is initiated with the regulation Environment (Protection) Act 1986 with the vested regulation of Guidelines for Research, Trials and Commercial Applications on Biotechnological Products, 1990. the IBC serves as a critical gatekeeper in the biosafety and ethical oversight of research involving biotechnological products. Its thorough review, facility inspections, and approval process are essential components of ensuring the safe and responsible conduct of such research.

The regulatory and permission required for importing any cell bank, export or transfer or exchange through the application B1/B3/B5/B7, and the RCGM is the authority to approve after the recommendation of IBC, whereas the licence is issued by CDSCO after obtaining the recommendation of the RCGM for import, test, analysis, and examination of any biological material through the application Form 12 and granted by Form 11 (Table 27.2).

TABLE 27.1
The Necessary Documents Required for Approval for Biosimilar

27.1.1 Overview of the biosimilar, their applications, and a brief description of their development.

- 27.1.1.1 Document Formatting: The documents must be page numbered, indexed, and printed on both sides, with all annexures(s)
- 27.1.1.2 RCGM approval(s) and IBC recommendation(s) included.
- 27.1.1.3 The selection of the reference biological, as well as its functionality and the specifics of its approval in India or any other country, are all required. The same levels of safety, efficacy, and quality must be present in imported versions of reference biologicals in order for them to be compliant with government regulations and eligible for import licences.
- 27.1.1.4 It is required that reference biologicals have a dose form, strength, and method of administration that are comparable to those of the reference biologicals.

27.1.2. Brief about the reference of biologicals including the mode of action, therapeutic indications, dosage and side effects, and animal toxicology. Furthermore, molecular similarity and dissimilarity between the biosimilar and reference biologicals are to be mentioned.

- 27.1.2.1 Status of approval and marketing of the reference biologic in the many other nations.
- 27.1.2.2 Status of approval for comparable biological products and biosimilars in India
- 27.1.2.3 Molecular characterisation of biosimilars, including GMOs and LMOs, is utilised in the development process
- 27.1.2.4 The genesis of the gene or genes and the process of molecular coding
- 27.1.2.5 Nucleotide and protein sequences that are biosimilar once they have been translated
- 27.1.2.6 If any change in the amino acid sequence occurred from the reference biologicals, such cases as the alignment or modifications at DNA and protein level and the gene sequence to be submitted to the gene bank and the accession number to be provided
- 27.1.2.7 The reference biologicals' amino acid sequence may have changed, in this particular instance, the alignment or changes at the DNA and protein levels may have changed. It is required that the gene sequence be submitted to the gene bank, and the accession number to be provided
- 27.1.2.8 Observable traits of the organism serving as host
- 27.1.2.9 Characterisation of the risk in the host organism
- 27.1.2.10 The consistency of the plasmid expression in the host cells both before and after the induction of the fermentation process of the microbes
- 27.1.2.11 Levels of plasmid-encoded protein expression
- 27.1.2.12 During both the research and production phases, significant measures are taken to ensure the biosafety and environmental safety of the process
- 27.1.2.13 Standardised procedures for fermentation and manufacturing
- 27.1.2.14 The fermentation process is broken down into its component parts, including the medium, composition, pre-inoculum, and production process media composition, as well as the feeding rate, which is measured in gram of nutrient per hour per litre of starting fermentation broth
- 27.1.2.15 The volume of liquid that can be fermented in a batch procedure expressed in litres
- 27.1.2.16 During the fermentation process, consolidated quality controls of cell growth, pH, temperature, product production, dissolved oxygen, nutrient intake, aeration rate, agitation rate, and CO_2 supplementation

(Continued)

TABLE 27.1 (CONTINUED)
The Necessary Documents Required for Approval for Biosimilar

27.1.3	Fermentation part: A percentage yield expressed as a volumetric productivity with regard to each respective concentration. Second, the stability of the specific protein yield, which can be defined as the protein concentration per unit of cell mass at varying cell concentrations while the protein is being fermented
27.1.3.1	During production, a focus is placed on the downstream processes and purification steps
27.1.3.2	During the manufacturing of biosimilar pharmaceuticals, the process of purification is one of the most important phases involved
27.1.3.3	Specific information regarding the reagents, resins, and membranes that are utilised throughout the process of purification, along with the qualities possessed by each of these components
27.1.3.4	The batch process of fermentation, including its operation and subsequent purification of biosimilar pharmaceuticals, as well as the consistency setup necessary to generate chromatograms for three batches of varying consistency, are described and explained in detail
27.1.3.5	Details about the recombinant protein, such as the formation of inclusion bodies, the process of refolding the protein, validation of the quality of the refolded protein, and confirmation that the protein is both soluble and free of any protein aggregation, must be provided.
27.1.3.6	SDS-PAGE analytical results and containing both reducing and non-reducing gels together with the appropriate molecular standard marker and the loading concentration of the isolated protein were included in the report. Additionally, the data is required to ensure the quality of the purified protein and conduct chromatographic analysis at each step of the purification process, taking into account the reference molecule and all batches
27.1.3.7	After the products have been purified, an overall recovery of at least three batches' worth of data is required
27.1.3.8	A synopsis of the consistency of the recovery of the biosimilar pharmaceuticals after each phase of the purifying process
27.1.3.9	A minimum of three batches of reference biologicals and biosimilar versions will need to compare have their physicochemical characteristics defined
27.1.3.10	Confirmation of the identical mass of the biosimilar pharmaceuticals, together with a comparison to the reference
27.1.3.11	Combine the results of peptide mapping performed on all batches of biosimilar pharmaceuticals with data obtained from the comparison of reference molecules and data obtained from the sequencing of -terminus amino acids
27.1.3.12	In order to access the secondary structures of reference biologicals and biosimilars, overlaying results of circular dichroism (CD) data, near- and far-infrared spectroscopy data, and ultraviolet spectroscopy data are necessary
27.1.3.13	In order to access structures that are similar to those of the reference biologicals, it is necessary to overlay the results of fluorescence spectroscopy over those data
27.1.3.14	In order to comprehend the charge heterogeneity, cation exchange chromatography and isoelectric focusing data are necessities for both the reference drug and the biosimilar drug
27.1.3.15	An analysis as well as the specifics of the components that make up the carbohydrate and glycoprotein content of biosimilar drugs

(Continued)

TABLE 27.1 (CONTINUED)
The Necessary Documents Required for Approval for Biosimilar

27.1.3.16	Biosimilar pharmaceuticals are proteins found in nature, and there is a possibility that they might aggregate, which is not acceptable. Such a quality control parameter can be calculated using contemporary analytical techniques like size exclusion chromatography (SEC) and dynamic light scattering (DLS), among others
27.1.3.17	Each batch should be tested for the presence of endotoxin and pyrogen
27.1.3.18	The amount of DNA and protein contained in the host cell will be measured and analysed for each consistency batch
27.1.3.19	Bioassay for determining the binding and functional properties of biologics that are very similar to one another.
27.1.3.20	Validation of biological assays to be carried out in accordance with the requirements of the international standard, and the selection of the internal standard ought to be carried out in accordance with the ICH guideline
27.1.3.21	A summary of the findings from the functional assays, including the binding to receptor, tissue-specific activities, activation of signal transduction, complement-dependent cytotoxicity (CDC), antibody-dependent cellular cytotoxicity (ADCC) apoptosis, neutralisation, cAMP level, glucose level, anti-proliferate cell assays, and *in vivo* assays
27.1.3.22	In the biosimilar, there are detectable levels of impurities with both high and low molecular weights
27.1.3.23	It is required that the formulation and stability studies of both the biosimilar and the drug product be submitted in three separate batches in accordance with the regulatory guideline
27.1.3.24	In order to comply with the regulatory requirement, consolidated batch data must be provided
27.1.4	Analysis Part : Analysis using size exclusion chromatography and superimposition of the biosimilar molecule on top of the reference molecule
27.1.5	Specific information regarding the bioactivity of the biosimilar in relation to the reference molecules.
27.1.6	Data on the accelerated and real-time stability of biosimilar molecules and final formulations compared to the reference biologic, determined using a functional bioassay to assess efficacy relative to the reference biologicals or reference biologicals.
27.1.7	In the formulations of biosimilar drugs, the specifics of the excipient and stabilisers that are used are described in extensive detail; in the event that the formulations differ, the excipient and stabilisers must be internationally approved
27.1.8	The biosimilar drugs are required to be accepted by a pre-clinical safety study and are required to be according to the data from the reference biologicals
27.1.9	A comparison of the biosimilar drug's specifications and quality criteria with those of the finished formed biologicals is required for attribution purposes
27.1.10.	A comparison of the resembles and the biosimilar drugs of the test findings between reference and the proposed similar biologic

TABLE 27.2
The Mandatory Application Permission for Biosimilar Research

Sl No	Stage	Authority	Application No.	Approval
1.	License for import, test, analysis and examination	CDSCO (zonal)	Form 12	Form 11
2.	Import or export or transfer or received of cell bank.	RCGM	Form B1/B3/ B5/B7	-

27.8 RESEARCH ACTIVITIES RELATED TO RDNA TECHNOLOGY

Any import of GMOs/LMOs/r-DNA, the investigator shall report to the IBS, after reviewing the same to recommend to RCGM through the application Form C1 and the RCGM approval by Form C2 with the strong monitoring and the conditions laid out as per recombinant DNA safety guidelines, DBT Guideline, 1990. Furthermore, the processing of the biosimilar drugs require the necessary approval from the RCGM/GEAC/DCGI as deemed to be applicable through the respective guidelines and forms. The major concern facing any biosimilar is when the end products are live microorganisms, where many legislations are implied (Table 27.3).

27.9 PRECLINICAL STUDY OF BIOSIMILAR

The therapeutic dose of the reference biologic should be used as the basis for the calculation of the dose. Prior to beginning the toxicity research, it is recommended that a pilot dosage response study be carried out with a large number of test animals. In animal toxicology studies, there are often three different levels of doses employed, referred to as low, medium, and high, corresponding to one, two, and five times the human equivalent dose, respectively, or a larger test dose when it comes to repeated-dose toxicity studies. During the toxicity test, the biosimilar and the reference biologic have to be contrasted with one another at a dose that is at least twice human equivalent dose (HED). Any significant discrepancy in the dose levels should be adequately explained and sanctioned before the studies begin. In terms of the schedule for the administration of the medication, the therapeutic schedules should be monitored strongly for up to 14 days.

Pre-clinical research is essential for determining whether or not a biosimilar is safe and effective for human use, and two statutory approvals are needed to begin such research. First, authorisation of a pre-clinical study from the RCGM is required. A detailed study is recommended by the IBC through the application of Form C3a, while permission is gained through Form C4, and the reports, when they are complete are provided by Form C5a. Second, in order to carry out the pre-clinical research, one needs to receive approval from the Institutional Animal Ethical Committee. In addition, all animal studies have to comply with the GLP norms and

TABLE 27.3
The Mandatory Application Permission for Recombinant DNA (Cloning) Technology for Biosimilar Development

S. No	Stage	Agency Involved	Application	Approval
1.	After NOC from CDSCO, the small batch manufacturing licence for test, analysis and examination purposes only (not mandatory GMP)	State FDA	Form 30	Form 29
2.	Research and Development involving r- DNA technology	RCGM	Form C1	-
3.	Permission for Preclinical Studies	RCGM	Form C3a	-
4.	Submission of Preclinical Study report	RCGM	Form C5a	-
5.	Marketing Permission for Import / Manufacturing	CDSCO	Form 44 (separate for DS and DP)	Form 45A/ 46A (Bulk product) and Form 45/46 (Finished product)
6.	Manufacturing Licence	State FDA/ CDSCO (counter signature)	Form 27 D	Form 27 D
7.	Registration for import	CDSCO	Form 40 (with schedule DI and DII) /Form 44	Form 41/Form 45
8.	Permission for Marketing/Licence for imported product	CDSCO	Forms 8 and 9	Form 10

disclose the required information about the test site and personnel, such as the director, principal investigator, pathologist, quality assurance officer, and other investigators that are going to be involved in the process of conducting the study.

In order to get approval from the RCGM for preclinical studies, the biosimilar drugs have to be fully described, including their molecular biology, used cell bank, origin of gene, gene sequences, cell culture/fermentation, harvest, excipient, formulation, purification, and primary packaging interactions. After the marketing approval has been received, each and every item of data is stored for a period of five years. During the study of gross anatomy and microscopy, photographs should be taken with appropriate shadow reduction under white light. The images should then be printed on photo grade, glossy ink jet paper with a dimension marker (scale) for valid documentation. The gathering of fundamental knowledge is essential prior to conducting any preclinical research on biosimilar.

Reference biologicals' data are essential for comprehending drug types, rates of absorption and excretion, routes of administration, dose-response relationships, established therapeutic indices, and bioequivalence intervals. The drugs caused a deposition that caused localised toxicities, particularly to the tissue-specific organs that were the target.

27.10 PHARMACODYNAMIC STUDY OF BIOSIMILARS

The methodologies to be used must be consistent with the goal of the pre-clinical studies, and the pre-clinical studies must be completed with the full formulation of the biosimilar, with the dose, mode of administration, and strength being comparable to the reference biologicals.

The pharmacodynamic studies are limited to in *vitro* bioassay data such as cell growth, cytotoxicity, neutralising, and receptor binding assays, whereas *in vivo* pharmacodynamic research provides for understanding the activities of biosimilars to different organisms or anatomy.

27.11 BIO-IMMUNE RESPONSES OF BIOSIMILARS IN ANIMALS

The safety of biosimilars is ideally evaluated both before and after it has been given regulatory clearance. Comparative pre-approval safety data, including immunogenicity data, is required for all biosimilars, including those for which confirmatory clinical trials have been exempted, as part of the pre-approval safety evaluation. The antibody response of the biosimilar and the reference biologicals can be understood by analysing host cell proteins. Although data on immune toxicity can be gleaned from acute toxicity studies, the most useful information comes from sub-acute repeated-dose studies. Immune complex development in the organ of interest is crucial to understanding during the safety analysis. The RCGM is required to provide the DCGI with safety data that are consistent with the reference biologicals, as well as product characterisation and specifications, along with opinions that are comparable with those of the reference biologicals. The immunogenicity and safety of the experiment can be deduced from the number of volunteers that were recruited. If the sponsor conducts pre-approval studies on the suggested similar biologic drug involving more than 100 patients, the number of patients in the Phase IV study can be adjusted so that the safety data (from both Phase III and IV) is derived from a minimum of 300 patients treated with the biosimilar.

27.12 TOXICOLOGICAL STUDIES OF BIOSIMILARS IN ANIMALS

Data on repeated toxicity of biosimilars are generated in an animal species that is pharmacologically relevant, and a dose and mode of administration that are comparable with reference biologicals. It is required that explanation for the animal selection be provided, and while new animal models are being developed, it is also required that non-availability of animal models be justified. In accordance with the requirements of Schedule Y of the Drugs and Cosmetic Act, 1940 and data on the biosimilar toxicities must be generated for a minimum of 28 days, and the recovery period must last for a minimum of 14 days. The biosimilar is used in the process of selecting the appropriate dose, and toxicity studies are carried out using low, medium, and high doses, respectively equating to one, two, and five times the HED of reference biologicals. Any changes to doses must first be deemed reasonable and receive approval from the institutional Animal Ethics Committee and followed by RCGM before implementation. In the event that numerous adjuvants are utilised in the formulations, the safety research must be carried out separately and without the active constituents to conclusively evaluate the toxicities of the adjuvant. The purpose of the investigations on local toxicity is to gain an understanding of the effects of the biosimilar that are linked to local tolerance and repeated-dose toxicity. The endpoints of any toxicity are frequent outcomes like behavioural changes, euthanasia, procedure blood drawing, body weight, biochemical parameters, haematology, histopathology necropsy, gross description, organ weights, and organs sampled for histopathology. In addition, there is an evaluation of the bone marrow, a micronucleus assay, and an investigation of the statistical approaches that were applied. Animal toxicity testing must comply with the requirements outlined in Schedule Y Appendix III, and, the majority of the time, data are collected using either a single dosage or repeated doses. Numerous studies, including those on male and female fertility, reproduction toxicity (Segment I), teratogenicity (Segment II), and perinatal development (Segment III), as well as essential studies on allergenicity/hypersensitivity, local toxicity, genotoxicity, and carcinogenicity, must be conducted in the test battery.

27.13 PHARMACOLOGY (NON-CLINICAL) OF SIMILAR BIOLOGICS

The specifics of the study must adhere to the guidelines outlined in Appendix IV of Schedule Y, of the Drugs and Cosmetics Act, 1940 and the therapeutic potential of the biosimilar drug must be equivalent to that of the reference product. It is necessary to determine the specific pharmacological activities, the target organ, and the safety pharmacology.

Most pharmacologists use their own innovative methods when writing the final report, but it's still important for the report to cover the protocols that were followed, the data from each animal, the results of any microscopy, the quality confidence study, the analytical reports, the animal feed, the health certification of animals, conclusion, and the laboratory's accreditation status (Figure 27.1).

27.14 DATA REQUIREMENT OF PRECLINICAL STUDY FOR THE APPROVAL OF THE BIOSIMILAR DRUGS

For the approval of biosimilar medications, the preclinical studies need to meet certain data requirements. After the pre-clinical study has been finished, the application must be sent to the DCGI through the RCGM, together with Form 44 and any other necessary data. These data are listed below.

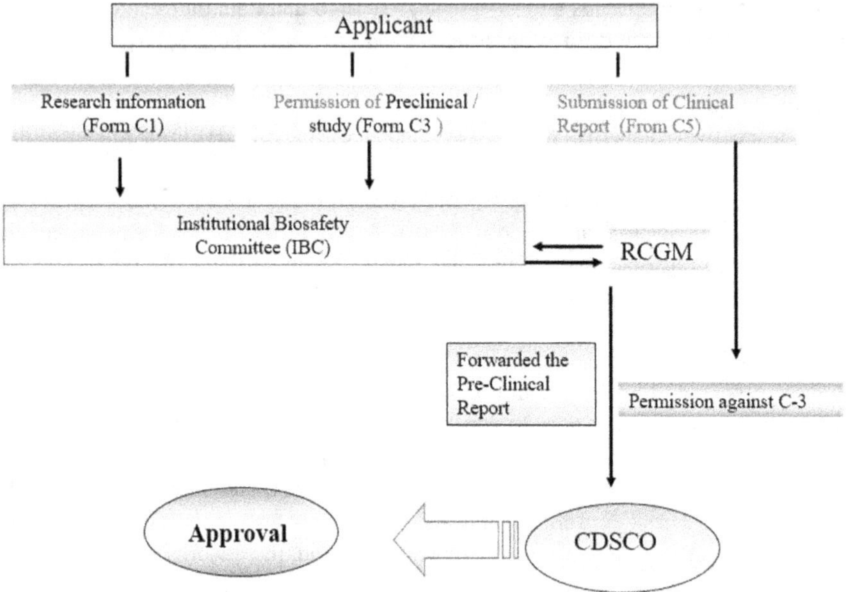

FIGURE 27.1 Process of the research and development of biosimilar drugs.

---

1. Studies in pre-clinical toxicity of biosimilar that are being proposed, together with a condensing of the biological references
2. If the RCGM has not approved the toxicity data for the batch after production of biosimilar, it is necessary to view the whole comparison data of the batch whose consistency has been accepted in the past, if any.
3. Reporting of any adverse reactions or toxicity that is known to have occurred with the reference biologicals.
4. Study in detail of the preclinical toxicity test battery that is required as per Schedule Y of biosimilar-treated group, as well as investigations on immunogenicity
5. Animals were divided into groups based on predetermined selection criteria.
6. Data on the immunogenicity and toxicity of biosimilar from preclinical studies are to be reported. The procedures need to include information of biosimilar regarding the specifics of the formulation, such as the active molecules, their exact sequences, any other proteins they do not specifically target, and the adjuvant. In addition, the protocols should include information regarding the mode of administration, vehicle, basis of dose calculation, and route of administration.
7. The accreditation status and address of the laboratory at the facility where the studies are going to be carried out were also examined.
8. A declaration regarding the correctness of the containment facility's procedures. Precautions taken in an emergency.
9. Statement about decontamination and disposal mechanisms.
10. Precautions taken in an emergency.
11. The approval of the study was included in the minutes of the IBC meeting.
12. Letter of undertaking or declaration with signatures.
13. Evaluations and studies in a pre-clinical setting of biosimilar-treated group, including a reference biological
14. QA declaration.

15. The signatures of each investigator who contributed to the study, along with the approval of the project's director.
16. Plan out the details of the study, such as when it will start, how long each experiment will last, and when the study will be over.
17. An analysis or summary of the findings from the pre-clinical study of the biosimilar-treated group.
18. Any discrepancies from the pre-clinical study of the biosimilar-treated group as well as any necessary modifications.
19. Details on the euthanasia, body weight, blood drawing, organ weights, and histology of the organs are to be recorded of the biosimilar-treated group, together with the equipment used, technique details, and assessment of the endpoints with the units.
20. If there is a significant difference between the quantitative results of biosimilar and the reference biologicals, it must be explained. This includes data like food intake, body weight, haematological, organ weight, and biochemical markers.
21. The results of the experiments conducted with the biosimilar at the low dose
22. Smears of bone marrow of the biosimilar-treated group.
23. Gross necropsy results from the biosimilar-treated group.
23.1. Weights of the major organs are listed quantitatively in a table, either as absolute weights in gram or as weights in gram per kilogramme of body mass.
23.2. Any variations from normal appearances and abnormalities must be recorded in the picture of the biosimilar and reference biologicals or any other group when it comes to the qualitative parameters of the primary organ.
23.3. Parenterally dosed forms of biosimilar of administration must be photographed, and photographs of the injection sites themselves must be taken if there is any noticeable abnormality observation that has to be reported. Comparable vehicle control of the injection site must also be documented.
23.4. If the injection site does not display any obvious signs of abnormalities, then one photo of the vehicle control and one of the maximum doses must be documented.
24. Histopathology studies
24.1. Notification of changes and the histology of the major organs of the biosimilar-treatment group are to be mentioned. An evaluation of the data against the reference biologicals is required.
24.2. Both the normal histological specification and the explanation for it must be provided for the biosimilar treatment in comparison with reference biologicals.
24.3. In the event of any adverse reaction of the biosimilar group at the high dose, organs will be subjected to gross microscopy. Histopathology of reference biologicals at the low dose are compared with the control and reference biologicals.
24.4. In the event that any anomalous findings become apparent in histopathology in the biosimilar treatment group, a comparison with the reference biologicals along with the documentation and photographing of the findings is essential.
24.5. Any morbidity or mortality that is noticed after dosing with biosimilar must be included, as well as the necropsy, histology, and status of the major organs are to be reported.
25. Animal health certifications as well as quality certification of animal feed should be communicated.
26. It is important to mention the findings as well as the discussion and the conclusions.

27.15 EXTRAPOLATION OF EFFICACY AND SAFETY DATA TO OTHER INDICATIONS

Once quality similarity to reference biologicals of the biosimilar has been established, safety and efficacy data from clinical studies and other clinical indication can potentially be extrapolated to data from studies of other clinical indications with comparison of reference biologicals. In addition, it has been demonstrated that there is a similarity between the preclinical assessment of the reference biological and the biosimilar, as well as an indicator of clinical safety and efficacy that is confirmed to be biosimilar to the reference biologicals. The mechanisms of action and receptor selection, as well as clinical indications, which are comparable to those of the reference biological, are taken into consideration when extrapolating data (Figure 27.2).

27.16 STABILITY STUDIES FOR THE APPROVAL OF BIOSIMILAR DRUGS

According to the ICH QI A (R2) guideline, the stability studies or shelf life of the biosimilar are assessed. According to the guideline, any product that goes through significant change that is related to failing to meet its specifications is considered to have failed to satisfy its specifications. Because of this, the biosimilar loses its potency, and the data collected are compared to those of the reference biological, particularly if we take into account the fact that India is located in the climate zone IV b as per ICH classification, and that the data are produced under accordingly extreme conditions (Table 27.4).

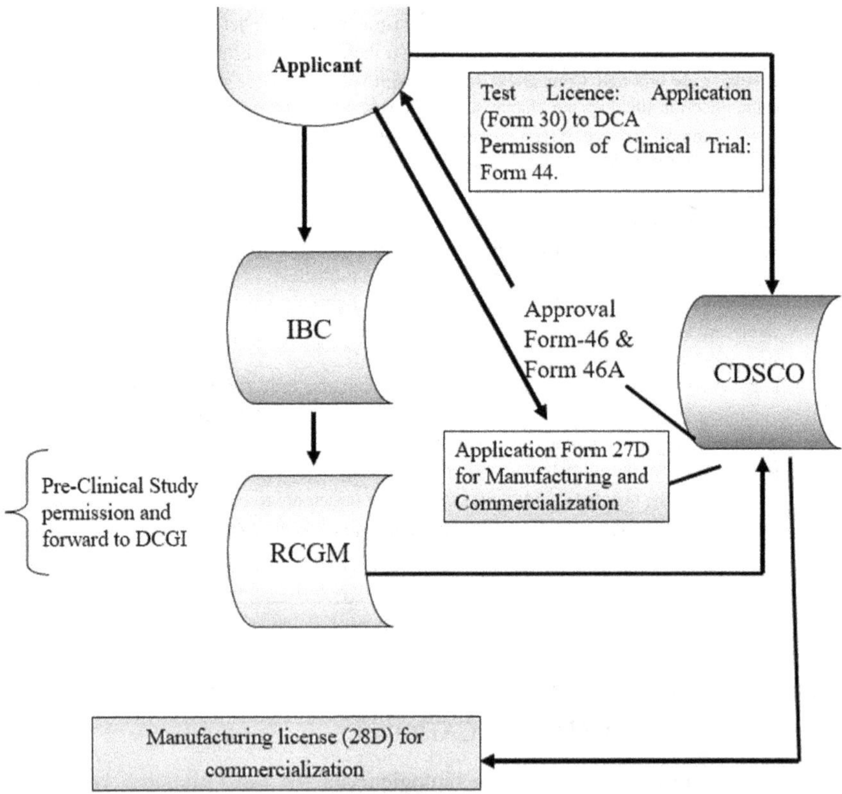

FIGURE 27.2 Approval process of the biosimilar drugs and involvement of DCGI.

TABLE 27.4
The Stability Studies of Biosimilar Drug Development

S. No	Type of Drugs	Condition of Storage	Test Period or Shelf life	Study	Minimum Time Period (rnonths)	Frequency of Test Details
1.	Biosimilar	5±3°C (Condition-1)	Less than 1 year	Real time: at the claimed actual circumstances of the storage temperature	12	Tests are to be run at real-world storage conditions for at least three months at monthly intervals (the first, second, and third months) and then every three months (6th, 9th, and 12th months). After that, data will be collected once a year, then every six months during the second year, and finally once a year thereafter if stability is asserted across consecutive years.
				Accelerated: 30°C ± 2°C/70± 5% R.H	3	The data relating to the tests are to be gathered at intervals of 0, 1, 2, and 3 months.
				Stress: 40/50/60°C ± 2°C/60± 5% R.H	1	The data from the tests are to be collected at intervals of 0, 1, 2, 3, and 4 weeks respectively.
			Greater than 1 year	Real time: at the claimed actual circumstances of the storage temperature	12	The data from the tests are to be collected at the 0, 3-, 6-, 9-, and 12-month intervals, and after the first six months of the second year, the tests are to be performed annually until the end of the planned re-tests period.
				Accelerated:30°C ± 2°C/70 ± 5% R.H"	3	The data from the tests are to be gathered at intervals of 0, 1, and 3 respectively.
				Stress: 40/50/60°C ± 2°C, 60 ± 5% R.H	4 weeks	The test data are to be collected at intervals of 0, 2, and 4 weeks.

(Continued)

TABLE 27.4 (CONTINUED)
The Stability Studies of Biosimilar Drug Development

S. No	Type of Drugs	Condition of Storage	Test Period or Shelf life	Study	Minimum Time Period (rnonths)	Frequency of Test Details
2.	Biosimilar	−20±5 °C (Condition 2)	Less than 1 year	Real time: at the claimed actual circumstances of the storage temperature.	12	To be carried out in real time storage conditions for a minimum of three months at monthly intervals (0, 1st, 2nd, and 3rd month and at three-month intervals thereafter (6th, 9th, and 12th month). After thereafter, statistics are collected every six months during the second year, and after that, data are collected annually if stability has been asserted over consecutive years. Then, every six months during the second year, and finally, once a year if stability is claimed for at least that many years in a row.
				Accelerated:30°C ± 2°C/70± 5% R.H"	3	At intervals of 0, 1, and 3 months, the data from the tests need to be collected.
				Stress: 40/50/60°C ± 2°C/60± 5% R.H	4 weeks	The data from the tests are to be collected at intervals of 0, 1, 2, 3, and 4 weeks respectively.
			Greater than 1 year	Real time: at the claimed actual circumstances of the storage temperature	12	To be carried out in real time storage conditions for a minimum of three months at monthly intervals (0, 1st, 2nd, and 3rd month and at three-month intervals thereafter (6th, 9th, and 12th month). After thereafter, data are collected every six months during the second year, and after that, data are collected annually if stability has been asserted over consecutive years.
				Accelerated:30°C ± 2°C/70 ± 5% R.H"	3	Data for the tests must be gathered at intervals of 0, 1, and 3 months. After three months, data were obtained at the six-, nine-, and twelve-month intervals.

(Continued)

TABLE 27.4 (CONTINUED)
The Stability Studies of Biosimilar Drug Development

S. No	Type of Drugs	Condition of Storage	Test Period or Shelf life	Study	Minimum Time Period (rnonths)	Frequency of Test Details
				Stress: 40/S0/60°C ± 2°C, 60 ± 5% R.H	4 weeks	The data from the tests are to be collected at intervals of 0, 1, 2, 3, and 4 weeks respectively.
3.	Biosimilar	−20±5°C (Condition 3)	Less than 1 year	Real time: at the claimed actual circumstances of the storage temperature.	12	To be performed at real time storage conditions for at least 3 months at a monthly interval (0, 1st, 2nd, 3rd month and at 3-month intervals thereafter (6th, 9th, 12th month). Followed by every 6 months over the second year and further the annually data collected if stability claimed over consecutive year.
				Accelerated: 5±3°C	3	The test data shall be collected at 0-, 1-, 2- and 3-months intervals.
				Stress 30 ± 2°C, 70 ± 5% R.H.	4 weeks	The test data shall be collected at the 0-, 2-, and 4-weeks intervals.
4.	Biosimilar	5±3°C, (Condition - 4)	Greater then 1 year	Accelerated: 5±3°C Stress: 30± 2°C, 70± 5% R.H.	4 weeks	At the conditions of 5±3 °C for three months, with data collected at 0, 1, and three months; this was then followed by testing under conditions of 30±2 °C and 70% ±5% relative humidity, with data gathered at 0, 2, and four weeks.
				Real time: at the claimed actual circumstances of the storage temperature.	12 months	To be carried out in real-time storage circumstances for a minimum of three months at regular intervals of one, two, and three months respectively month as well as in three-month intervals following that (the sixth, ninth, and twelfth months). Thereafter, data analysis is collected every six months during the second year, and after that, data are collected annually if stability has been asserted over consecutive years.

(*Continued*)

TABLE 27.4 (CONTINUED)
The Stability Studies of Biosimilar Drug Development

S. No	Type of Drugs	Condition of Storage	Test Period or Shelf life	Study	Minimum Time Period (rnonths)	Frequency of Test Details
				Accelerated: 5±3°C	3 weeks	The data relating to the tests are to be collected at intervals of 0, 1, 2, and 3 weeks.
				Stress: 30± 2°C, 70% ± 5%R.H.	4 weeks	The data relating to the tests are to be gathered at intervals of 0, 2, and 4 weeks.
5.	Biosimilar	5±3°C (Condition-5)	Less than 1 year	Real time: at the claimed actual circumstances of the storage temperature.	12	For at least three months, at monthly intervals (the first, second, and third months), and then every three months (the sixth, ninth, and twelfth months), under real-world storage circumstances. After that, data will be collected once a year, then every six months during the second year, and finally once a year thereafter if stability is asserted across consecutive years.
				Accelerated: 30 ± 2°C/70 ± 5% RH	3 weeks	The data relating to the tests are to be collected at intervals of 0, 1, 2, and 3 weeks
			Greater than 1 year	Stress: 40/50/60°C ± 2°C/65 ± 5% RH	4 weeks	The data relating to the tests are to be gathered at intervals of 0, 2, and 4 weeks.
				Real time: at the claimed actual circumstances of the storage temperature.	12	For at least three months, at monthly intervals (the first, second, and third months), and then every three months (the sixth, ninth, and twelfth months), under real-world storage circumstances. After that, data will be collected once a year, then every six months during the second year, and finally once a year thereafter if stability is asserted across consecutive years.
				Accelerated: 30 ± 2°C/70 ± 5% RH	3 weeks	The data relating to the tests are to be collected at intervals of 0, 1, 2, and 3 weeks.

(Continued)

TABLE 27.4 (CONTINUED)
The Stability Studies of Biosimilar Drug Development

S. No	Type of Drugs	Condition of Storage	Test Period or Shelf life	Study	Minimum Time Period (rnonths)	Frequency of Test Details
6.	Biosimilar	−20±5°C, (Condition -6)	Less than 1 year	Stress: 40/50/60°C ± 2°C/65 ± 5% RH	4 weeks	The data relating to the tests are to be gathered at intervals of 0, 2, and 4 weeks.
				Real time: At actual conditions of storage temperature as claimed	12	To be carried out in real-time storage conditions for a minimum of three months at a monthly schedule (0, 1st, 2nd, and 3rd month and at three-month intervals thereafter (6th, 9th, and 12th month).
				Accelerated: 5±3°C	3 months	The data relating to the tests are to be collected at intervals of 0, 1, 2, and 3 weeks.
				Stress 30 ± 2°C, 70 ± 5% R.H.	4 weeks	The data relating to the tests are to be gathered at intervals of 0, 2, and 4 weeks.
			Greater then I year	Real time: At actual conditions of storage temperature as claimed.	12	To be carried out under real-time storage conditions for a minimum of three months at monthly intervals (months 0, 1, 2, and 3), and then at three-month intervals thereafter (month six, month nine, and month twelve). Thereafter, data are taken every six months throughout the second year, and after that, data are gathered annually if stability is reported over consecutive years.
				Accelerated: 5±3°C	3 months	The data relating to the tests are to be gathered at intervals of 0, 1, 2, and 3 months.
				Stress: 30 ± 2°C, 70 ± 5%R.H.	4 weeks	The data relating to the tests are to be gathered at intervals of 0, 2, and 4 weeks.

27.16 CLINICAL STUDIES OF BIOSIMILAR DRUGS

1. Clinical Trial

It is necessary to conduct clinical investigations (trials) of the biosimilar in order to gain an understanding of its safety and efficacy and to reach a conclusion regarding its risk to benefit ratio. In order to initiate the clinical research, the findings from the pre-clinical toxicity tests must first be provided. Comparative pharmacokinetics in the form of a single parallel or crossover design is used in the process of evaluating biosimilar pharmaceuticals in relation to reference molecules. The comparative pharmacodynamics must also be established, and this can be done by experiments using parallel arms or crossover designs. As a result, the pharmacokinetic and pharmacodynamics tests are carried out with the biosimilar version, which is comparable with both the biologic and the reference biologic.

2. Phase I Trial

The Phase I clinical study, which should be submitted simultaneously with the application along with all requisite documents, can be carried out in India or other nations according to where the substance was discovered or being to be use. The Phase I study must only be carried out at one or two locations, and it must be performed by trained professionals who have received approval from an Institutional Ethical Committee. In order to compare the outcomes, each dose needs to be administered to a minimum of two different groups of peoples and conclusive statistical procedures are to be used.

3. Phase II Trial

After receiving clearance from the CDSCO, the Phase II trial should be carried out on at least 10–12 people across each dose level. The trial ought to be carried out at three to four distinct locations by therapeutics-trained staff.

4. Phase III Trial

After receiving approval from the CDSCO, pharmaceutical companies in India are obligated to carry out Phase III tests on developed biosimilars before receiving authorisation to market them. In order to determine whether or not the biosimilar is both safe and effective, the Phase III trial needs to be carried out on at least one hundred participants across three to four different locations. However, if the biosimilar has been discovered in India, then it needs to be tested on at least 500 patients across 10–15 different locations.

5. Regulatory Documents

If the biosimilar needs to be imported, then Form 44 must be submitted, and the licence is provided by the Form 45/Form 45 A. However, Form 44 is necessary for the application of a clinical trial, and the CDSCO must grant permission for it.

6. Global Clinical Trial (GCT)

When organising a clinical trial, it is essential to keep ethnic aspects in mind because, in contrast to a domestic clinical study, a global clinical trial is conducted across a wide variety of areas and ethnic groups. Therefore, taking into consideration the difficulties that are outlined in the ICH E5 Guideline is also helpful when conducting a worldwide clinical study. A "global clinical trial" is a trial established to test the efficacy of a novel biosimilar that aims for global development and approval. A single clinical trial will be conducted in this trial with participants from multicentric institutes from various nations, areas, and academic medical centres, and it will be conducted concurrently in accordance with a clinical trial protocol that is standard. In order to be approved, the application for the GCT must include a significant amount of documentation, particularly regarding the new biosimilar. Essential information must be shared, including the name of the biological, a synopsis of its chemical and pharmacological qualities, and information on how it can be administered, including dosage forms and stability data like melting point, stability conditions, and reactivity. The safety studies of the summary Phase 0 clinical study or pre-clinical studies, as well as the summary of clinical studies such as Phase I/II/III trials, including the place of study and study protocol, along with the arguments for the planned research and how they will assist patients. The proposal is structured in accordance with the objective of the study, and it contains characteristics like the patient population, the study design (such as randomised controlled or double-blind studies), and subject selection criteria, which explain how patients were chosen to take part in the study. In addition, the evaluation of the experiment's safety and effectiveness, as well as the total number of subjects in India or around the world, as well as the permission forms used to ensure that patients were treated in an ethical manner during the trial. The sites of the trials, the quality of care for patients experiencing adverse effects, and the regulatory status of the biological by the Government of India must all be mentioned.

27.17 MANUFACTURING PROCESS

It is necessary to use a reference biological as a standard when conducting comparability studies with a biosimilar in order to demonstrate that both biologics are comparable with regard to their levels of safety, efficacy, and overall quality. The reference biological should be licensed and approved on the CDSCO basis of full safety, effectiveness, and quality statistics. So, a biosimilar can't be a marketed as the reference biological until the user country has cleared or accepted it. The manufacturing process is a significant parameter since biosimilar products are required to be made in a manner that result in comparable quality products in terms of their identity, purity, and potency in comparison with the reference biological. It is necessary to confirm the manufacturing process for biosimilar and demonstrate that it maintains its consistency throughout the production phase, utilising the same host cell line for the production of both reference biologicals and the biosimilar, provided that the host cell line is disclosed. Cell lines could be one of the alternatives for evaluating the properties of the biosimilar, which could be evaluated to reduce clinical toxicities and immunity and be considered as quality attributes (QA). The ICH's Q5A, Q5B, and Q5D guidelines should be consulted as a guide for the characterisation of cell banks.

Complete information about the manufacturing process, including characterisation of cell banks, clone stability, cell culture/fermentation, harvest, excipient, formulation, purification, and primary packaging interactions, must be made public in order to pass regulatory review. In addition, information regarding host cell cultures (including viral clearance), vectors, gene sequences, promoters, and other components utilised in the manufacture of identical biologics should be provided alongside the required drawings and figures. The specifics of post-translational changes, such as glycosylation, oxidation, deamidation, and phosphorylation, among others, need to be clarified.

1. Process Development in the Upstream Stage

The validation procedure takes into account the medium components utilised for cell development throughout the fermentation process, as well as the data from three batches of reproducible fermentations performed at the pilot scale. The data that are provided include the procedure, the batch size, the purification process, and the product that is used to generate preclinical data. The upstream process also generates the production kinetics data from the consistency batches, which influence various aspects like cell growth, pH, temperature, dissolved oxygen, major nutrient consumption pattern, agitation rate, and product formation. The ultimate outputs in terms of product/litre, yield, and volumetric productivity are considered. Reports on active protein yield (the amount of protein produced per unit of cell mass), productivity that can be replicated, and scalability are required.

2. The Development of the Downstream Process

In this process, detailed description of the methods, steps, and reagent quality are followed for the cell harvesting and extraction of the protein. Furthermore, the process of protein purification is to be described.

27.17 PHARMACOKINETIC (PK) STUDIES OF BIOSIMILAR DRUGS

In order to support using the PK data from the reference biologicals, the biosimilar may advance forwards into Phase III clinical development. Normal healthy volunteers and/or patients are recruited for the data development from a comparative pharmacokinetic PK study of the biosimilar after extensive essential physiochemical and biological characterisation, pre-clinical study, and quality attributes, as was stated before. This is done in preparation for the study of the biosimilar. The essential information is generated through the PK study, such as the biosimilar half-life, the linearity of its PK parameters, the diurnal fluctuations of those parameters, the methods of administration, the indications for doses, and the diseases. The design of the PK research is determined by the data that is necessary in order to understand the efficacy of the treatment; the single-dose PK studies may be comparative, parallel arm, or crossover multiple dosage comparisons between reference biologicals and the biosimilar.

27.18 SINGLE-DOSE AND COMPARATIVE PK STUDIES OF BIOSIMILAR DRUGS

The dose selection of the biosimilar is essential, and it must be rationalised in comparison with the biological references. The selection of volunteers needs to follow a logical order for the study to be considered statistically significant. In this kind of investigation, having a good understanding of the study design is also crucial. If the biosimilar in question has a lengthy half-life, or is a protein found in nature, or results in the production of antibodies, then a parallel arm research design would be effective. On the other hand, a crossover study design would be acceptable for biosimilars that have a short half-life. The PK study can employ any dose selection, but the dose must fall within the therapeutic dose range. The analytical methodologies, the validation of the procedures, and having the specificity and sensitivity to differentiate the metabolites, degradation products, and protection time relative to the same biological and the reference biologicals are all highly important aspects. It is important to investigate any differences in the kinetics of elimination that exist between the biosimilar and the reference biological, such as clearance and elimination half-life. The degree of similarity between the two substances in terms of their ability to be absorbed and used by the body should not be the only measure of relevance. When investigating a biosimilar with a lengthy half-life or proteins in patients in which it is anticipated that antibodies would be formed, research with a parallel arm design is the most appropriate method to use. In the event that the half-life is somewhat short, a crossover design might be something to explore with a scientific justification.

27.19 MULTIPLE-DOSE COMPARATIVE PK STUDIES OF BIOSIMILAR DRUGS

The PK investigations of several dosing regimens of the biosimilar and the reference biologicals are relevant to the impacts of the steady state of the biosimilar, where the protection time, degradation, and metabolites could be examined in a time-dependent manner. The majority of the time, a study design known as a parallel arm study, is used when conducting multi-dosage research. One important thing to think about when figuring out a biosimilar dose sequence is the PK parameter. It has been seen that after a single-dose study, the PK parameter is not as strong or lower as thought. To get a more accurate picture of the PK parameter, more than one dose is used for the steady-state study. While multi-dose comparative PK investigations are often integral to biosimilar development, providing acceptable reasons for their omission is a critical aspect of the regulatory submission. A thorough scientific justification, adherence to regulatory guidelines, and transparent communication with regulatory agencies are key components of demonstrating biosimilarity when multi-dose studies are not feasible or appropriate.

27.20 PHARMACODYNAMIC STUDIES OF BIOSIMILAR DRUGS IN HUMAN VOLUNTEERS

Studies of the pharmacodynamics (PD) of the biosimilar, in addition to comparisons with reference biologicals, are carried out using a study design that is either parallel arm or crossover. In the PD study, the detection of the marker or the validation of the marker is the most crucial part. Monitoring the availability of the PD marker to the healthy volunteer is done, or alternative markers, known as surrogate markers, are produced or evaluated for the data analysis. The ethical side of PD studies is important, just like it is for any disease that has ended, like tertiary cancer, where harmful side effects of treatment are predicted, and such monitoring is seen as unethical. The PD study may be conducted in conjunction with the Phase III clinical trials or in combination with the PK study. Comparative pharmacodynamic (PD) studies are only effective when the markers are established with the reference biologicals. Also, it is required to understand the correlation between dosage and pharmacodynamic marker(s) and the response and effectiveness of the reference biologicals. This correlation should be employed to substantiate the design of the study.

It is important that the acceptability ranges for demonstrating similarity in PD parameters be set and well justified. Studies on pharmacodynamics (PD) and pharmacokinetics (PK) might be integrated; in this case, the PK/PD connection should be characterised. In the event that there is no PD marker available, and the PK study can be done on patients, then the PK study can be integrated with the Phase III clinical investigation. Additionally, where appropriate, the PD research can be included into ongoing Phase III clinical studies.

27.21 WAIVER OF SAFETY AND EFFICACY STUDY

There is the possibility of skipping the confirmatory clinical safety and efficacy study, and it had a set of parameters. The structural and functional comparability between a biosimilar and reference biological entities can be reliably assessed by the application of physicochemical *in vitro* techniques. These approaches can be used to study the similarities and differences between the biosimilar and reference biologicals. The biosimilar is comparable with the reference biological in each and every preclinical evaluation that was carried out. Then, the PK/PD study must have demonstrated the comparability of PD markers that have been validated for their clinical outcome. Additionally, the structural and functional comparability between the biosimilar and the reference biological entities can be reliably assessed by the application of physicochemical *in vitro* techniques. A detailed post-marketing risk management plan has been presented, and it has been said that it will be used to collect additional safety data, with the primary focus being on the collection of immunogenicity data. It is not possible to skip the confirmatory clinical safety and efficacy study, particularly not for a biosimilar with a high molecular weight, such as monoclonal antibodies. In the event that the safety and effectiveness trial is not performed, it is possible that all of the indications that were approved for the reference biologicals will be given based on equivalent quality, convincing PK/data, and on-clinical evidence. The immunogenicity should have been gathered during the PK/PD study, and it will also need to be created during the post-approval Phase IV research. This is true regardless of whether or not the Phase III trial is skipped. It is impossible to avoid conducting the confirmatory clinical safety and efficacy trial if there is no reliable PD marker that has been validated for clinical outcome. If PK and PD equivalence is confirmed in a Phase I investigation for a product that has been determined to be similar in pre-clinical, *in-vitro* characterisation using recognised PK methodologies and a PD marker, that is an equivalent of efficacy, the residual risk is greatly decreased. In situations like this, it is possible to forego conducting clinical tests.

1. Safety and Immunogenicity Data of Biosimilar Drugs in Human Volunteers

Concerns regarding the safety of the approval process for biosimilar medications are among the most significant, and it is desirable to conduct safety evaluations both before and after the products is approved. Even if clinical trials could be skipped, safety data on biosimilar pharmaceuticals must still be provided. The reference biological must guarantee the absence of any unanticipated safety issues and emergence of any unanticipated safety risks. Pre-approval studies in 100 individuals must demonstrate safety and non-immunogenicity before biosimilar medications can be used on more than 300 patients in Phase IV research.

2. Extrapolation of Efficacy and Safety Data

Extrapolation in biosimilars is a scientifically supported regulatory approach that allows for the extension of indications based on the similarity demonstrated in a well-characterized indication. It requires a comprehensive understanding of the biosimilar's characteristics and performance across multiple dimensions. Furthermore, reference biologicals and biosimilar drugs generate similar data like preclinical, clinical safety, efficacy, mechanism of action, and receptor bindings. The new indications or new claims are to be applied to separate applications.

27.22 APPROVAL OF THE MARKET AUTHORISATION

The CDSCO has the jurisdiction to issue authorisation for the commercialisation of any biosimilar medications once it has been satisfied that all of the necessary data, including the results of clinical trials that have been properly authenticated by the primary investigator, have been submitted. In addition to the two hard copies and two soft copies, i.e., CDs (PDF format), the sponsor/institution must also take the pre-permission for the clinical trial as previously indicated. The clinical data that were reported to the CDSCO must be archived for a period of five years by the sponsor or the institution. The CDSCO granted an authorisation of approval for the biosimilar through the Form 46/46 A after a thorough review of the data provided. After the manufacturing industry has been granted a licence by the CDSCO, they are required to submit Form 27D to the State Licensing Authority (SLA) in order to manufacture biosimilar products. Approval for these products will be granted using Form 27D and all biosimilar products must be produced in GMP-certified facilities.

The following information must be sent to the CDSCO in order to receive approval for the biosimilar:

1. Module I: General Information Administrative/Legal Information
2. Module II: Summaries
3. Module III: Chemistry Manufacturing Quality Information (Chemical, Pharmaceutical, and Biological)
4. Module IV: Non-Clinical Information Animal Pharmacology, and Animal Toxicology
5. Module V: Clinical Information Phase I, II, & III Studies

Furthermore, the following documents are required in addition to the modules.

5.1. Form 44, complete with all of the necessary information.
5.2. A synopsis of any relevant pre-clinical safety information, the investigator's brochure for the clinical research, standard operating procedures, etc.
5.3. Case report form in accordance with the trial procedure outlined in Appendix X of Schedule Y
5.4. Clearance from the Ethics Committee in accordance with the requirements of Appendix VIII of Schedule Y of the Drugs and Cosmetics Act, 1940
5.5. Copies of patient information sheets, informed consent forms, and other documents required by the Drugs and Cosmetics Act of 1940, as specified in Appendix V of Schedule Y.
5.6. Investigation carried out in accordance with Appendix VII of Schedule Y of the Drugs and Cosmetics Act of 1940
5.7. It is necessary to disclose the regulatory status of biosimilar drugs or inventor drugs from other countries.

27.23 POST-APPROVAL CHANGES OF BIOSIMILAR DRUGS IN HUMAN VOLUNTEERS

Post-approval changes are modifications that are made to biological products after they have been granted approval. These modifications are made to provide data regarding a change that is considered adequate to allow an assessment of the impact that the change will have on the quality of the approved products in terms of their safety, effectiveness, and/or effective use of the products. These modifications are known as post-approval changes. The applicant is allowed to make post-approval revisions once their application has been approved, so long as those changes are notified to the CDSCO under one of the appropriate categories. In the event that post-approval modifications are made, it is essential to submit fresh biological or manufacturing licences for biological products, as per the latest amendment that was introduced by the CDSCO. In the event that any changes are made to biological products after approval, the CDSCO needs to be informed.

If a change made to a biological product after it has been approved would make it a new drug under the definition of Rule 122E of the Drugs and Cosmetics Rules, the applicant for the biosimilar must apply for new drug authorisation. In the event that the manufacturing premises are relocated, the licensee is responsible for submitting an application for additional product permission to the appropriate state authorisation authorities, zonal offices or sub-zonal offices, and the Central Licensing Approval Authority (CLA), in accordance with the requirements of the Drugs and Cosmetics Act and Rules, as well as the necessary fees, in accordance with the usual procedures. In the event that there is a significant change in the product's quality, the applicants are required to submit a new biological application. In the event that there is only a moderate change in the product's quality, the applicants are required to submit filings such as an additional manufacturing licence. These filings must include explicit statements of the change regarding procedural, qualitative, and quantitative modifications in the form of a comparative table. Because of any alterations which may put the integrity or safety of the approved biosimilar at risk, the terms of the post-approval challenges have been severely restricted. Furthermore, the sponsor is required to be informed of any post-approval changes made to the biosimilar, including those made to its purity, strength, dose, performance, and efficacy, as well as any changes made to the impact that these post-approval alterations may have on its safety or efficacy, if any such changes are made. The biosimilar molecules are the ones that were derived, and since there is a significant threat to their safety, there needs to be a mention of an emergency plan, a pharmacovigilance adverse drug reaction monitoring plan, and post-marketing monitoring. The following documents must be submitted to DCGI in order for post-approval revisions to be considered.

1. A covering letter includes a brief explanation of the changes and a mention of the list of revisions.
2. A comparison of the information on the biosimilar that has been approved and the information that has been altered.
3. An overall summary of the quality of the biosimilar following post-approval modifications.

27.24 PROVISIONS OF FORM 44 AND FORM 46

One of the most important and significant achievements of contemporary medical research is the development of biopharmaceuticals. Since the past few years, India's biopharmaceutical industry has seen significant expansion. It is made up of both innovator biologics and biosimilars, the latter being biologics that are quite similar to one another. Biosimilars are new versions of pioneering biopharmaceutical products that are typically brought to market after the original patents on such pioneering products have expired. It is anticipated that similar biologics would emerge as a significant economic and therapeutic driver in the Indian pharmaceutical business.

Included in the category of biologics are therapeutic proteins, monoclonal antibodies, DNA vaccines, and fusion proteins. A regulatory process of biosimilars that is comparable to that of any other novel medicine is followed by an innovative biologic molecule. As a means of streamlining the submission process and making requirements simpler to comprehend, the CDSCO established the format for the information that must be provided in order to obtain market approval for novel biological drugs like any biosimilar. As earlier mentioned, Form 44, an application for permission of new drug approval, must be submitted by the producer or sponsor in accordance with the requirements outlined in The Drugs and Cosmetics Act of 1940 and the corresponding Rules of 1945. The completion of Form 44 is required in order to submit an application for authorisation to import or manufacture a novel drug. Furthermore, as stated earlier, the requirements for chemical and pharmaceutical information are in accordance with the International Submission requirements of the Common Technical Document (CTD). As previously stated, the set of requirements comprises four modules, namely administrative/legal data, summary quality information, non-clinical data, and clinical data.

In India, marketing authorisation for biosimilars must comply with a different set of rules. A biosimilar product is one that, in terms of quality, safety, and efficacy, is comparable to an approved innovative biological product or reference biological. Comparability is the basis for determining a biosimilar product. Before obtaining permission to be sold on the market, biosimilars must go through a process that consists of multiple steps and involves a number of different Government agencies which includes CDSCO, RCGM, DCGI, IBC, GEAC, and the Institutional Animal Ethics Committee (IAEC). In order for the biosimilar to be developed in India, the reference inventor must first be registered in the country. In any other case, in order to receive marketing authorisation, it must first be sold on the market for a minimum of four years in a market that is highly controlled. The corporation must first provide the relevant authorities with comprehensive product data before they will provide their permission. These data must include the production process, product attributes, pre-clinical research, and fundamental clinical information. In the second step, approval is given for the pre-clinical trial, and, in the third step, the clinical trial actually takes place. After this, the company is able to submit an application to the DCGI for market authorisation of the biosimilar. In addition, the post-marketing surveillance data submission requirement must be met.

Because of the vast, detailed, and even excessive degree of information that is required for the description of a biological product, there are a number of obstacles that must be overcome in order to receive clearance for biologics. Marketing permission for import /manufacturing are granted through Form 46 which is issued by DCGI against Form 45 for application for approval of the biosimilar.

27.25 BIOSIMILAR APPROVAL IN USA

The biosimilar is "highly similar" to the reference product and the ultimate objective is to ensure that there are no significant clinical disparities between the biological product and the reference product with regards to their safety, purity, and potency as mentioned in Section 351(k) of the Public Health Service Act (PHSA) and 21 CFR Parts 600 to 680 pertaining to Biologics Licence Applications (BLA). According to the Food, Drug, and Cosmetic Act (FD&C Act) of the United States of America, the biosimilar should have the same dosage, mode of action, reduced adverse reactions such as immunogenicity/PK, PD, and should be comparable with the reference molecules in terms of purity, safety, and potency. According to the FD&C Act, the term "biosimilar" refers to any protein, toxin, virus, vaccine, therapeutic serum, blood, blood component or derivative, antitoxin, allergenic product, or analogous product.

Insulin, glucagon, and human growth hormone products are all regulated by Section 505 of the FD&C Act, which does not fall under the biosimilar clause. This regulation applies to items that contain cells or microbes, among other things. The Biologics Price Competition and Innovation (BPCI) Act was passed by the United States Congress in 2010 under the section 351(k) of the Public Health Services Act under an abbreviated approval pathway known as "biosimilar" or "interchangeable" FDA-approved biological product. This Act was the impetus for the development of biosimilars, which began with the goal of providing protection to the average person while also maintaining an affordable health care system. In addition, a provision was made for the category of biosimilar pharmaceuticals that falls under both 35 U.S.C. 271 (patent infringement) and 27 U.S.C. 2001 (declaratory judgement) (Tables 27.5, 27.6, and 27.7).

27.26 FDA APPROVAL PROCESS OF BIOSIMILAR DRUGS

According to the FDA, a biosimilar product need not have the same structural characteristics as the reference product; however, it must have the same functionality, safety, and clinical efficacy as the molecule that was previously approved. Instead of depending on repeating clinical trials, which are seen to be superfluous, the goal is to employ direct comparisons on a smaller scale in conjunction with extrapolation.

TABLE 27.5
Important Format for Approval of the Institutional Biosafety Committee in India

		Institutional Biosafety-related Documents
27.5.1	Form A1	Submission of an Application to Register an Institutional Biosafety Committee (IBC)
27.5.2	Form A2	Submission of an Application in Connection with the Renewal of an Institutional Biosafety Committee (IBC)
27.5.3	Form A3	Report presented annually to the RCGM by the Institutional Biosafety Committee
27.5.4	Form A4	Medical Surveillance Report
27.5.5	Form A5	Confidentiality Agreement Regarding Medical Surveillance Reports Concluded Between the IBC Members and the DBT Nominee

TABLE 27.6
Important Format for Approval of Import, Export, Transfer, and Receipt of Biological Material

Approval of Import, Export, Transfer and Receipt of Biological Material		
27.6.1	Form B-1	Approval of import: RCGM is the authority for permission of import of GMOs/LMOs and product(s) for research and development purposes. Applications are made through the Form B-1 following approval, and they are forwarded by IBC.
27.6.2	Form B-2	Permission of import: Letter of authorisation or permission to import GMOs/ LMOs and products thereof for the purposes of research and development, issued by the RCGM using Form B-2.
27.6.3	Form B-3	Approval of export: RCGM is the authority for permission of export of GMOs/LMOs and product (s for research and development purposes, and application is made using the Form B-3 following the approval and provided by the IBC.
27.6.4	Form B-4	Permission of export: Letter of authorisation or permission to import GMOs/ LMOs and products thereof for the purposes of research and development, issued by the RCGM using Form B-2.
27.6.5	Form B-5	Receive of LMO/GMO: Letter granting permission to receive GMOs, LMOs, and goods derived therefrom for the purpose of research and development in India, issued by the RCGM using Form B-5.
27.6.6	Form B-6	Authorisation letter for receipt of LMO/GMO: The RCGM Form B-5 is an authorisation letter for someone else to receive GMOs/LMOs and products thereof in India for research and development purposes.
27.6.7	Form B-7	Transfer of GMOs/LMOs: After receiving approval from the IBC, applicants intending to transfer GMOs/ LMOs and products for R&D purposes must submit a Form B-7 to the RCGM for review and approval.
27.6.8	Form B-8	Authorisation letter of transfer of LMOs/GMOs: Letter of authorisation or permission to receive GMOs/LMOs and products thereof for the purpose of research and development, issued by the RCGM using Form B-8.

The FDA must primarily take into consideration any potential biosimilar in light of two statutory requirements: first, analytical validation of the structure, and second, the efficacy and safety must be proven by clinical research.

1. Characterisation of Biosimilar by Analytical Studies

The goals and guidelines that were set up to recognise the comparability with the reference biologic and the exhaustive exercise for any structural alterations that may have occurred during the manufacturing process or after translation was established.

The sequence of amino acids, the order in which structures are arranged, the degree of PEGylation and glycosylation, as well as the degree of variability between reference molecules and batches are all validated using analytical methods. When

TABLE 27.7
Important Format for Approval of Pre-clinical Studies, Research and Production of Biological Material

27.6.1	Form C1	Information of the Research: Through the IBC, the RCGM will be notified of the necessary information for the production of recombinant DNA products for use in health care and industry. These products are to be utilised in research involving GMOs and LMOs.
27.6.2	Form C2	Record of Information: After obtaining the Form C1, the RCGM issued the Form C2, which is considered to be the record endorsement against the application Form C1. This was done in order to accord the study involving GMOs/LMOs for the creation of rDNA products for use in healthcare and industry.
27.6.3	Form C3	Preclinical / safety studies Permission: The application for authorisation to use any recombinant DNA products that were generated with GMOs or LMOs and are intended for use in health care, industrial settings, or any other setting, must be submitted to the RCGM using Form C3.
27.6.4	Form C4	Grant of Permit for preclinical safety studies: After obtaining the Form C3, the RCGM issued the Form C4, which is considered the record endorsement against the application Form C3 to give the permission of pre-clinical research rDNA products for health care and industrial use.
27.6.5	Form C5	Submission of Pre-Clinical reports: After receiving Form C4, in which it was agreed that pre-clinical studies could be conducted on recombinant DNA products and that the results of those studies were to be reported to the RCGM using Form C5.
27.6.6	Form C6	Forwarding and Recommendation: Once the C5 Form has been received and the RCGM's requirements have been met, the application can be sent to DCG(I) for the appropriate phase of the clinical study.

compared with the reference product, the structure–activity–function links can be easily confirmed by *in vitro* or *in vivo* tests.

Advanced, high-tech analytical studies like spectroscopy methods also helped find impurities and structural characteristics. For example, nuclear magnetic resonance (NMR) or mass spectroscopy anticipated the tertiary and quaternary structures, whereas HPLC and gel electrophoresis anticipated aggregation, glycosylation trends, and purity. Both size-exclusion chromatography and enzyme-linked immunosorbent assays (ELISAs) are well-known methods for determining variations in molecular weight and size from the reference molecule. Size-exclusion chromatography was developed in the 1960s and ELISAs were developed in the 1970s. The term "drift" refers to any variation from the reference or approved molecules, and biosimilar properties are restricted to those of the reference molecules, leading to the conclusion that they are "highly similar." Any extra components of the structure added to the reference molecules, as well as their implications on the activity and safety, need to be discussed. Post-translational modification, which can result in modifications to the C and N terminals, as well as changes to the excipient, is also something that is taken into consideration. Therefore, in order to establish the pharmacodynamic (PD), clinical immunogenicity, human pharmacokinetic (PK), efficacy, and safety investigations, the FDA has clearly defined the "highly similar" or "formulation or minor structural differences" and "totality of evidence" approach. Clinical studies are carried out in order to provide evidence that a strategy is effective and safe; nevertheless, the FDA retains the discretionary power to waive off the requirement for clinical testing if it is either justified or deemed to be required.

2. Validation of Biosimilar Preclinical and Clinical Studies

In accordance with the provisions of Section 351(a) of the FDA regulation, the analytical investigations and a bare minimum of human pharmacokinetic and pharmacodynamics study are required in order to re-confirm the product's resemblance to the licensed reference product. Comparing the clinical immunogenicity evaluation of the biosimilar to that of the reference molecule is critical, and the clinical immunogenicity assessment should be undertaken by anticipating the risk associated with the biosimilar until the FDA waives this requirement.

Due to the fact that fusion proteins, heterogeneous biologicals, and monoclonal antibodies do not have a pharmacodynamic property that is continuous or comparable, clinical efficacy trials are required to prove their effectiveness. After receiving clearance for a restricted use, post-market surveillance and minor clinical trials are used to evaluate the immunogenicity of the product. The Food and Drug Administration (FDA) contains rules that allow for the extrapolation of the safety of biosimilar using reference biologicals, and such biosimilars are exempt from the clinical trial.

3. Interchangeability

Interchangeability is a concept that refers to switching between numerous products of reference molecules and is common in the EU. Despite this, the EU does not promote the use of interchangeable multiple reference medicines or moving from one biological drug to multiple or another biosimilar. In contrast to the USFDA guideline, the provisions of interchangeability are more concise and clearly written in accordance with the guideline that was developed in 2017. According to the US Food and Drug Administration, biosimilars can only be licensed for use for a period of two years at a time and there is no room for interchangeability; in India, there is no such rule in place.

4. Pre-submission Meeting between the Applicant and the FDA

This is an official quorum, and the arranged meeting is held between the developer and the FDA to analyse the biosimilar; sometimes, the FDA gives attention to a part-off application that is submitted after the deadline. The meeting is normally held two months before the application is due.

5. Application Submission of Biosimilar Drugs

On the basis of the conversation that took place during the pre-submission meeting and discussion, the application was turned in to the Centre for Drug Evaluation and Research (CDER).

6. Day 74 Letter

Within the 74 calendar days that followed the first filing and acknowledgement of any further review filing difficulties, the application was considered to be its final form.

7. Mid-cycle meeting and Any Other Communication

After the mid-cycle review, the Centre for Drug Evaluation and Research (CDER) within the FDA provides the applicant with the necessary information, whether it be in the form of an information letter (IR), in cases where additional information is needed, or a discipline review (DR), in cases where a shortcoming has been identified. CDER contacted the applicant or may have called the applicant during the first two weeks after the mid-cycle meeting to provide an update on the status of the meeting.

8. Late-cycle Meeting

The late cycle meeting is the last review, and the applicant is told about the conclusion in accordance with the process. The late-cycle meeting is called at least 12 calendar days before the meeting of the Committee and, during this meeting, a decision is made on the emergency Risk Evaluation and Mitigation Strategies (REMS) plan for the product.

9. Wrap-up Meeting

The FDA holds an internal meeting to decide what, if any, regulatory action is necessary to ensure the safety, quality, and efficacy of the proposed product in light of the information required by Section 505 of the Food, Drug, and Cosmetic Act.

27.27 THE EU'S APPROVAL PROCEDURE FOR BIOSIMILAR DRUGS

Biosimilar guidelines were first developed in the EU in 2005 by the European Medicines Agency (EMA), and they cover a wide variety of goods in the field, including monoclonal antibodies, gene therapy, therapeutic proteins, cell therapy, and more. The analytic profile must be properly adhered to, and the regulatory guideline must closely resemble the reference molecule. The recommendation also favoured less extensive testing of biosimilar drugs in humans. First, biosimilar drugs must be chemically, structurally, and functionally equivalent to the reference substance. Second, they should be of equivalent value, reliability, and performance. Although both the WHO and EMA have quality considerations in common, the EU rule requires that the medical product be approved in the EU, whereas the WHO has advised accepting any approved reference molecules.

The European Medicines Agency (EMA) has approved many biosimilar drugs that have been successfully used in the treatment of a number of diseases, such as somatropins, epoetins, and filgrastims, and there is always room for refinements from the initial products and the continuous evolution takes into account the evolution of quality profile during the product lifecycle.

The EMA has created a regulatory pathway for the approval of biosimilar products that is distinct from the generic pathway for the approval of many biosimilars, including erythropoietins, granulocyte-colony stimulating factors, insulins, growth hormones, low-molecular-weight heparins (LMWH), and alpha interferons.

BIBLIOGRAPHY

Basic Principles on Global Clinical Trials 27 September 2007, Notification No. 0927010. Available from: https://www.pmda.go.jp/files/000157900.pdf.

Clini Experts, New Delhi. Available from: https://cliniexperts.com. Accessed 4 October2023.

EMA-DNA and Host Cell Protein Impurities Routine Testing Versus Validation Studies, 1997.

EMA Guideline on Similar Biological Medicinal Products Containing Biotechnology Derived Proteins as Active Substance: Non-Clinical and Clinical Issues, London, 2006 (CHMP/BMWP/42732).

EMA Guideline on Immunogenicity Assessment of Biotechnology-Derived Therapeutic Proteins, London, 2007 (CHMP/BMWP/14327).

EMA Guideline on Similar Biological Medicinal Products, London, 2014 (CHMP/437/04 Rev 1).

EMA Guideline on Similar Biological Medicinal Products Containing Biotechnology-Derived Proteins as Active Substance: Non-Clinical and Clinical Issues, London, 2014 (EMEA/CHMP/BMWP/42732/2005 Rev1).

Guidelines and Handbook for Institutional Biosafety Committees (IBSCs) (2nd revised edition), Department of Biotechnology, Govt. of India, May 2011.

Guidelines for Preclinical Evaluation of Similar Biologics in India, Dept. of Biotechnology, Govt. of India. Available from: http://dbtbiosafety.nic.in/Files2/Guidelines_SimilarBiologics.pdf.

Guideline for Safety Study of Biological Products, KFDA, 2010.

Guidelines on Similar Biologics: Regulatory Requirements for Marketing Authorization in India. Available from: http://dbtbiosafety.nic.in/Files%5CCDSCO-DBTSimilarBiologicsfinal.pdf.

ICH Guideline on Preclinical Safety Evaluation of Biotechnology-Derived Pharmaceuticals (S6), 1997 and Addendum, 2011.

ICH Q1 A(R2)- Stability Testing of New Drug Substances and Products, 2003.

Kant L, Mourya DT. Managing Dual Use Technology: It takes Two to Tango. *Science and Engineering Ethics* 2010 March, 16(1):77–83. doi: 10.1007/s11948-008-9062-9. Epub 2008 Apr 26. PMID: 18438721.

Quan H, Mao X, Chen J, Shih WJ, Ouyang SP, Zhang J, Zhao PL, Binkowitz B. Multi-Regional Clinical Trial Design and Consistency Assessment of Treatment Effects. *Statistics in Medicine* 2014 June 15, 33(13): 2191–205. doi: 10.1002/sim.6108. Epub 2014 Feb 11. PMID: 24515845.

Recombinant DNA Safety Guidelines and Regulations, Dept. of Biotechnology, Govt. of India, January 1990. Available from: http://dbtbiosafety.nic.in/guideline/pdf/guidelines _90.pdf.

Schedule Y- Drugs and Cosmetics (2nd Amendment) Rules, 2005. Department of Health. Available from: http://dbtbiosafety.nic.in/act/schedule_y.pdf.

Sekhon BS. Biosimilars: An Overview, Dove Express, on 14 March 2011. Available from: http://www.dovepress.com/biosimilars-an-overview-peer-reviewed-article-BS.

Singh G., Budhwar V, Choudhury M, Singh S. Regulatory of Regulation on Genetically Modified Microorganism and Their Relation Bioterrorism in India Bull. *Journal of Pharmaceutical Sciences* 2022, 4: 565–584.

The Drugs and Cosmetics Act, 1940 & Rules, 1945, Department of Health, Govt. of India. Available from: http://indianmedicine.nic.in/writereaddata/mainlinkFile/File222.pdf.

Thulasi LK, Sreekant Reddy CP, Alagusndaram M., Jaychandra RP. Regulatory Approval of Biosimilar Marker Perspective. *International Journal of Advanced Pharmaceutics* 2014, 4: 245–258.

Wang J, Shein-Chung C. On the Regulatory Approval Pathway of Biosimilar Products. *Pharmaceuticals* 2012, 5: 353–368.

World Health Organization (WHO), Guidelines on Evaluation of Similar Biotherapeutic Products (SBP), 2009.

World Health Organization (WHO), Guidelines on the Quality, Safety and Efficacy of Bio-Therapeutic Protein Products Prepared by Recombinant DNA Technology, 2013.

28 Regulations of Biopharmaceuticals Using Living Microorganisms, Genetically Modified Foods, and Vaccine Development

28.1 INTRODUCTION

In the early 1980s, the idea of biotechnology and derived products was structured; later, this concept was propagated all over India. Both the notion of genetic engineering and the product that was developed from biotechnology helped to revolutionise the process of drug development, which resulted in an increase in the number of treatments that could save lives. The regulatory authorities are working to come up with rules and regulations to ensure that pharmaceuticals of this type are safe. Because their manufacture involves the use of living cells, many biopharmaceuticals, including some plant-derived medications, are referred to as biologic drugs, biologics, biopharmaceuticals, or recombinant therapies. These terms are used indiscriminately because the products are extensively used in the diagnosis, treatment, and prevention of diseases. As the few patents covering the first generation of biopharmaceutical drugs expire or are about to expire in the near future, it is anticipated that additional biopharmaceutical drugs will become available for purchase on the market. The challenges that come up concern the manufacture of the product, as well as concerns about its safety and other legal concerns. The use of genetically modified foods and pharmaceuticals is at the centre of many debates, and the regulatory authorities are under intense pressure to regulate critically, to assess the facts according to the principles that they should be scientifically acceptable. One of these criteria is that preclinical safety evaluation programmes must be in place.

Guidelines for dealing with these products have been developed by a variety of regulatory organisations, including the World Health Organization (WHO), the

DOI: 10.1201/9781003397854-12

European Medicines Agency (EMA), Health Canada, the Korean Food and Drug Administration (KFDA), and the Ministry of Health in Malaysia, among others.

The International Conference on Harmonization of Technical Requirements for Registration of Pharmaceuticals for Human Use (ICH) has also provided helpful information for biological treatments, but this guidance is not particularly relevant to biosimilars. In December 1989, the Ministry of Environment and Forests notified and categorically described "Rules for the manufacture, use, import, export, and storage of hazardous microorganisms or genetically engineered organisms or cells" under the Environment (Protection) Act (EPA) of 1986. This was done in order to contain any potential hazards to the environment that could be caused by the release of Genetically Modified Organisms (GMOs). The majority of the regulatory standards and criteria for pharmaceuticals generated from biotechnology were formed by following the rules established by the European Union, Japan, and the United States. The majority of countries have adopted a practical guideline by adhering to an adaptable, scientifically possible strategy. Other guidelines, such as those concerning preclinical safety and clinical development, in addition to marketing permission, have also been implemented. This process is ongoing, and the regulator is working to maintain equilibrium while taking into account the global scenario.

Toxicologists and regulators want to uncover the answers to two questions through the process of preclinical safety review: first, what dose should be utilised for therapeutic benefit, and second, how much may be given in total without producing toxicity?

Toxicologists aim to assess how a substance may affect different organs within the human body. This involves understanding the potential toxic effects on organs such as the liver, kidneys, heart, lungs, and others, depending on the nature of the substance. Toxicologists seek to determine whether any organ intoxication resulting from exposure to a substance is transitory (temporary) or permanent. This information is crucial for understanding the potential reversibility of adverse effects and the overall impact on long-term health.

Toxicologists assess the safety margin, which is the difference between the effective dose (the dose that produces the desired effect) and the toxic dose (the dose that causes adverse effects). A wider safety margin indicates a greater level of safety. If the toxic dose is close to the effective dose, it may raise concerns about the potential for adverse effects. The clinical monitoring therapeutic index is another term for the safety margin and refers to the range between the therapeutic (effective) dose and the toxic dose. This index helps guide clinical monitoring practices to ensure that the substance is administered within a safe and effective range. The expression "last, but not least" emphasizes the importance of the safety margin and its determination in toxicological assessments. It underscores the significance of considering safety factors in addition to therapeutic effectiveness.

These days, biopharmaceutical research and development follow the same guidelines as the diagnostic, therapeutic, and preventative uses of biomolecules. This chapter focuses on the key and most fundamental aspects of the regulation of vaccine or GMO food development.

28.2 REGULATORY AGENCY IN INDIA FOR GMO/LMO

The Drugs and Cosmetics Act of 1940 and the Environment (Protection) Act of 1986 are the two provisions of legislation in India that together constitute the country's implicit regulatory framework for recombinant drugs. The purpose of this task force was to harmonise the regulatory guidelines and work towards developing an acceptable regulatory guideline that takes into account Indian concerns while also making an effort to streamline the regulatory process. On the basis of the advice, the draft guidelines are all exclusive to products that are developed from living GMOs, or the final product may or may not contain the living modified organisms (LMOs). This is an excellent step that the government is taking towards the promotion of the growth of indigenous products, including the manufacture and marketing of those products. Importing products made with LMOs also requires strict adherence to this regulation. The Ministry of the Environment, Forest and Climate Change (MoEFCC) notified the 1989 Rules (also known as Rules 1989) governing the production, use, import, export, and storage of genetically modified organisms, dangerous microorganisms, and cells which fall under the jurisdiction of the Environment (Protection) Act of 1986. The enforcement of these rules took effect in April, 2006, signifying its official initiation

The regulations are effective for any production or study that involves releasing genetically modified organisms (GMOs) into the environment, as well as for large-scale production that use such organisms in their processes. The other competent authorities, such as the Institutional Biosafety Committee (IBC), the Review Committee on Genetic Manipulation (RCGM), and the Genetic Engineering Appraisal Committee (GEAC), are constituted in accordance with the rules and regulations. Each of these committees has particular authority limits. In addition, The Drugs and Cosmetics Act of 1940 and the Rules of 1945 were subject to periodic amendments by the Drug Controller General of India (DCGI) in order to facilitate the regulation of recombinant pharmaceutical products.

In order to simplify the process of regulating recombinant products and ensure their safety, purity, potency, and efficacy, the Department of Biotechnology (DBT) developed a set of recommendations. These guidelines can be found here. According to Rule 1989 of the DBT, the requirement of pre-clinical, clinical, and validation data for the recombinant DNA (rDNA) vaccine, diagnostics, and other biological products, as well as relevant data, must be submitted to the RCGM/GEAC and DCGI. The DBT guidelines stipulate that a certain number of committees must be formed, and each member of the committee must adhere to their own boundaries.

The following individuals make up the committees.

1. The Recombinant DNA Advisory Committee, often known as the RDAC.
2. IBC, which stands for the Institutional Biosafety Committee.
3. The Review Committee on Genetic Manipulation (also known as the RCGM)
4. The Committee for the Approval of Genetic Engineering Appraisal Committee (GEAC)
5. The State Biotechnology Coordination Committee, often known as the SBCC
6. A committee at the district level, known as the DLC.

It is usual for there to be ambiguity regarding biopharmaceuticals because there are various concerns to consider, such as patient compliance, environmental safety, patient safety, and regulation, among other things. Resolving the issues, the empowerment was delegated to various agencies like GEAC, which was involved in all issues related to environmental regulations, including the implementation of the Environment Protection Act, 1989, and the use of large-scale production of biologicals, whereas the DCGI looked at product safety and efficiency, clinical trials, market authorisation, and synchronised regulatory processes. GEAC was involved in all issues related to environmental regulations, including the use of large-scale biological production. Again, Dr R A Mashelkar served as the committee's chairman. In 2004, the Director General of the CSIR established a committee with the objective of providing more authority, greater responsibility, and greater clarity with regard to the roles of the GEAC and DCGI in addressing concerns over LMOs and indigenous products. Following the committee's recommendation of simplified and more rationalised regulatory procedures, which were then separated into five categories, the Government ultimately decided to adopt such procedures in 2006.

Protocol I: A pharmaceutical product that was developed, manufactured, and finally marketed indigenously is derived from a Living Modified Organisms (LMOs), but the end product is not an LMO.

Protocol II: A pharmaceutical product that was created, made, and finally marketed. Indigenously generated LMOs were used in the manufacturing process, and the end product was an LMO.

Protocol III: Pharmaceutical products that are being imported and marketed as LMOs, and the end product is also considered to be an LMO.

Protocol IV: This calls for the importing of bulk medicinal products, disguised as LMOs, with the end result also being LMOs.

Protocol V: Importing a bulk medicinal product classified as an LMO even though the end result will not be an LMO.

In order for the product to be made available on the market, the applicant is required to comply with the terms of "The Drugs and Cosmetics Act", 1940. This will involve the examination of the manufacturing facilities, the issuance of a temporary licence to produce trial batches, the shipment of products from five trial batches to either Central Research Institute (CRI) in Kasauli or CDL in Kolkata for testing, the receipt of the test report by DCG (I), or, finally, the clearance to manufacture and market the product.

During the process of marketing, both DCG (I) and GEAC have the authority to impose conditions of surveillance on the product. The initial marketing time allowed by the EPA can be anywhere from two to four years, and this period can be extended as long as an application is submitted. The applicants may be required to generate post-market surveillance data and submit it to DCG (I) and GEAC if this requirement is issued.

28.3 LEGISLATURE OF THE CATEGORY I PRODUCT, I.E., A PHARMACEUTICAL PRODUCT WHICH IS DEVELOPED, MANUFACTURED, AND FINALLY MARKETED AND INDIGENOUSLY DERIVED FROM LMOS BUT THE END PRODUCT IS NOT AN LMO

The new recommendations state that the GEAC does not play a role in the regulation of LMOs that are classified as belonging to risk groups 1 and II while GEAC does not play a role in the authorisation of Phase III clinical trials for risk groups III and above.

The amendment of Rule 1989 is not required as the MoEFCC has the authority to utilise the exemptions outlined in Rule 20. This rule stipulates that the MoEFCC may provide exemptions to occupiers who are involved in the handling of specific microorganisms or genetically altered organisms, thereby exempting them from compliance with Rules 7-11 as deemed essential.

1. As a consequence, LMOs that are classified as belonging to risk groups 1 or II might not require clearance from the GEAC.
2. In addition, the precise rule that stipulates previous approval of GEAC for human clinical trials on recombinant pharmaceutical products may be found in 1999 when DBT guidelines were issued for generating pre-clinical data for recombinant DNA (r-DNA)-based vaccines, diagnostics, and other biologicals. These guidelines were written exclusively for the purpose of generating pre-clinical data for r-DNA-based vaccines, diagnostics, and other biologicals. In the case of therapeutic proteins, there is no role for the GEAC to play in Phase III clinical trials; hence, the DBT guidelines need to be updated appropriately to reflect this fact.
3. The roles of RCGM and DCGI will remain the same under Protocol I; there will be no shift in either of these responsibilities (Figure 28.1).

As per the Drugs and Cosmetics Rules (8th Amendment), vide notification no. G.S.R.944 (E), it was noticed that pre-clinical toxicity studies for animal toxicology, teratogenicity, prenatality, reproduction, mutagenicity, and carcinogenicity are less strict for drugs that have already been approved. Also, the regulatory bodies are writing up the requirements for similar biologics, or "mimic biologicals."

Biopharmaceuticals' Rules and Regulations

1. The Environment Protection Act, 1986 and the EPA Rules, 1989.
2. The Industries (Development and Regulation) Act, 1951.
3. The New Industrial Policy and Procedures Act, 1991
4. Drugs and Cosmetics Act, 1940; Rules, 1945
5. Pharmaceutical Policy, 2002.
6. Recombinant DNA Safety Guidelines, 1990
7. Recombinant DNA Safety Guidelines and Regulations, 1994.

8. Guidelines for Safety in Biotechnology, Revised, 1994
9. Revised Guidelines for Research on Transgenic Plants, 1998 (j): Guidelines for gathering pre-clinical and clinical data for rDNA vaccines, diagnostics, and other biologicals, 1999.
10. It's a constant process to change the rules (Figure 28.2).

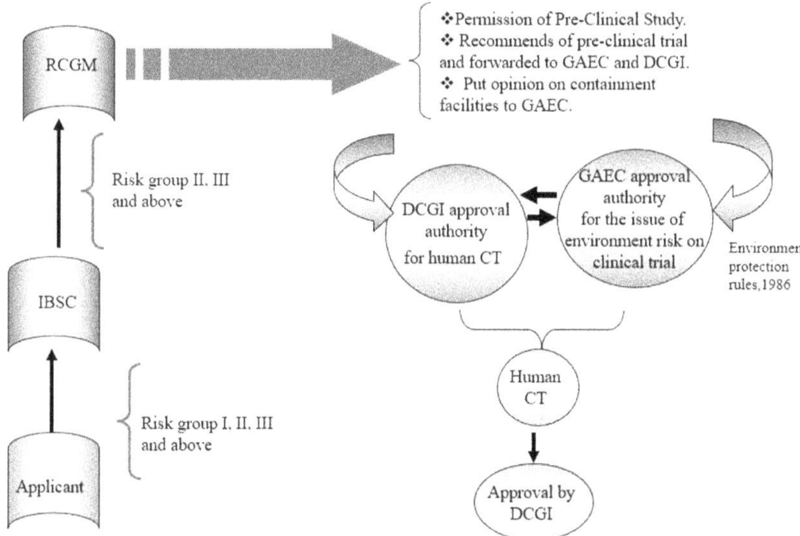

FIGURE 28.1 Process of the research and development of drugs from living modified organisms.

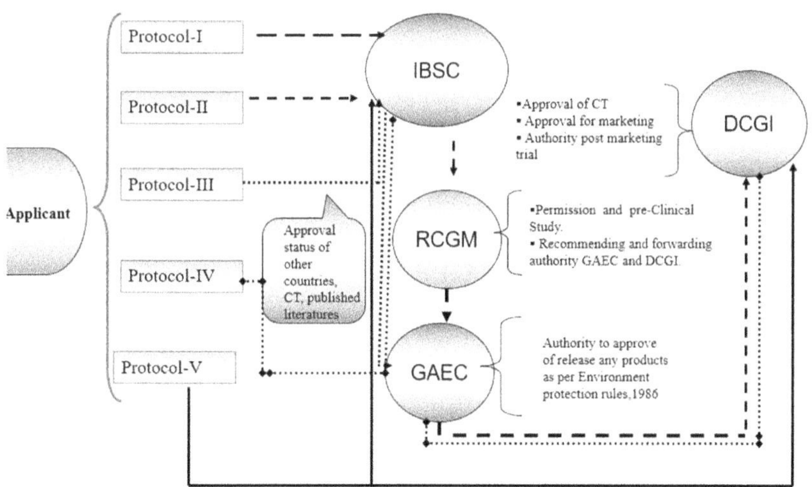

FIGURE 28.2 Approval procedure for according the characters of living modified organisms (Protocols II to IV).

28.4 DEVELOPMENT OF VACCINE

A set of guidelines with a higher standard of scrutiny has been adopted for the clearance of vaccines in India. The DCGI is the only regulatory authority in India, and they have established a well-defined process with published guidelines. Additionally, the ethical bodies are included in it for clinical trials.

The Drugs and Cosmetics Act of 1940 and the Drugs and Cosmetics Rule of 1945 both govern the vaccines that are available in India; there is no separate regulation for it. Vaccines fall under the purview of Schedule Y of the aforementioned regulations, just like new pharmaceuticals. In accordance with Schedule Y, clinical trials of the vaccine should be carried out. In India, conducting Phase I studies using new vaccines is not normally allowed, and researchers are obliged to submit data from Phase I studies that were carried out in other countries. The Phase I repeat research is going to be carried out in India, and then the Phase II and Phase III trials are going to have to be finished with the approval of DCGI and at a clinical trial site that has been approved by DCGI. After the completion of the Phase III trial, the vaccines are eligible to be approved for sale and distribution.

The COVID-19 pandemic has knocked on our door, and we need to develop an emergency vaccine as soon as possible to prevent one million deaths and a social and economic collapse. In conjunction with the efforts being made around the world, the Government of India has issued an urgent appeal for the generation and production of vaccines, and it is closely monitoring all of the parts of regulation pertaining to the development of vaccines. As a result, key decisions have been made to keep the emergency situation under control. When the Government of India declared on January 16, 2021, that free vaccination against COVID-19 would begin in India, the world witnessed the largest immunisation programme ever. This was accomplished with the assistance of billions of Indians and the sincere hope that it would save countless lives (Figure 28.3).

28.5 VACCINE TYPE

The following vaccines are available in India:

1. Live, attenuated: measles, mumps, and rubella (MMR), varicella, yellow fever, rotavirus, influenza.
2. Inactivated: hepatitis A, influenza, polio, rabies. COVID-19 vaccine
3. Crude or purified antigens derived from living or killed cells: diphtheria and tetanus toxoids, polysaccharides.
4. Conjugates: Hemophilus type b, pneumococcal, meningococcal.
5. Recombinant DNA-derived: hepatitis B, human papillomavirus.

Drugs and vaccines that target diseases like HIV, malaria, tuberculosis, and cancer pose a significant public health jeopardy and are therefore given special consideration on a case-by-case basis, with expedited clearance processes as outlined above and in accordance with regulatory authorities.

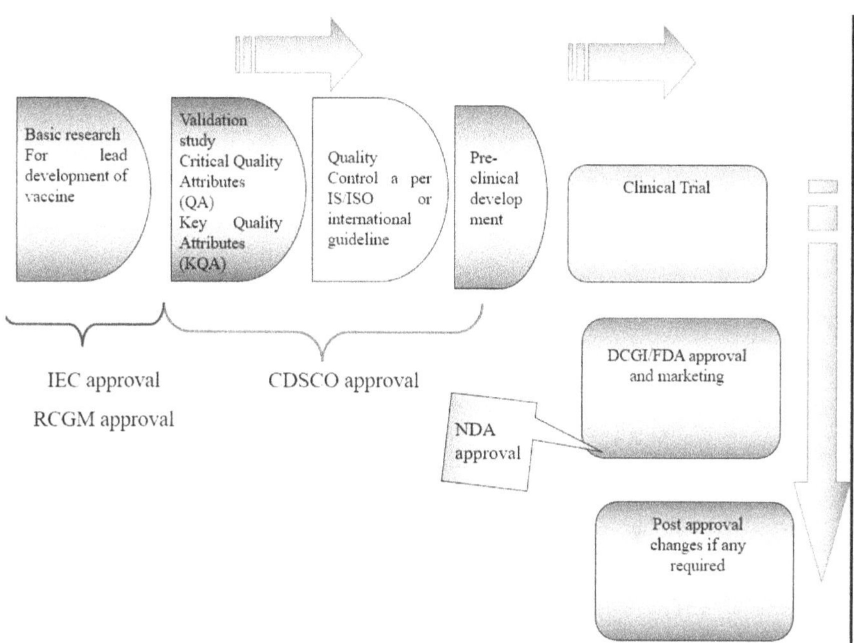

FIGURE 28.3 Phase development of vaccine.

28.6 REGULATORY PROCEDURE FOR APPROVAL OF VACCINE

In Step 1, the developed lead candidate is established and revalidated. This can include cloned, monoclonal, or polyclonal antibodies.

Step 2: Vaccine validation is essential since the final product stimulates the same antibody and the mechanism must be established.

Step 3: Quality control and standardisation are essential in order to guarantee that the product that was generated does not contain any contaminant.

Step 4: Preclinical development should include establishing toxicity, determining dose, and locating the site of action in both rodent and non-rodent models, transgenic animals, and homologous protein models, among other models. This should be done.

Step 5: The most important aspect of the vaccine development process is the clinical trial. The clinical study needs to include the multicentric trial as well as the trial in a foreign country (Figure 28.4).

The approval process for new vaccines follows the same four phases as the approval process for new drugs, namely Phases 1, 2, 3, and 4. However, the incubation period for vaccine clinical trials is kept longer than it is for new drugs in the event that any immunogenic reaction is noticed for an extended length of time. The approval of the RCGM under the Department of Biotechnology is necessary for any companies or institutes that want to import genetically modified or foreign materials for research and development purposes. On the other hand, the approval of GEAC is necessary for any companies or institutes that want to use genetically modified or foreign materials for commercial purposes. In accordance with the Foreign Trade (Development and Regulation) Act, 1992, if any of the aforementioned standards are violated, the company, the institutes, or the individual importer may be subject to disciplinary action (Figure 28.5).

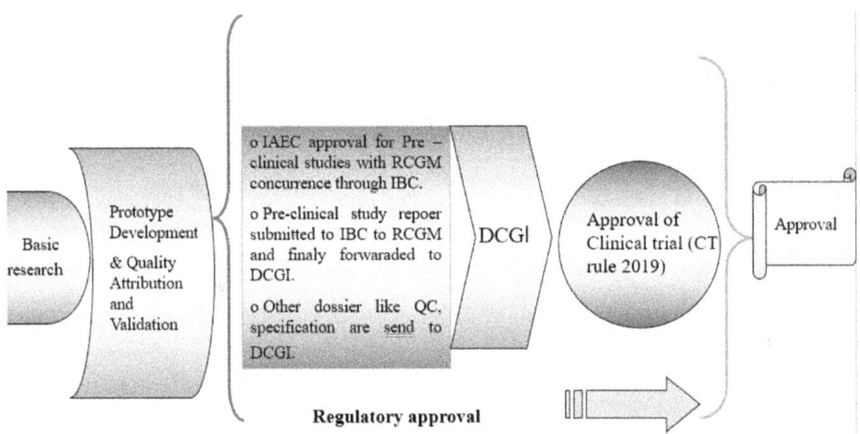

FIGURE 28.4 Regulatory procedure for permission for the clinical trial of vaccine.

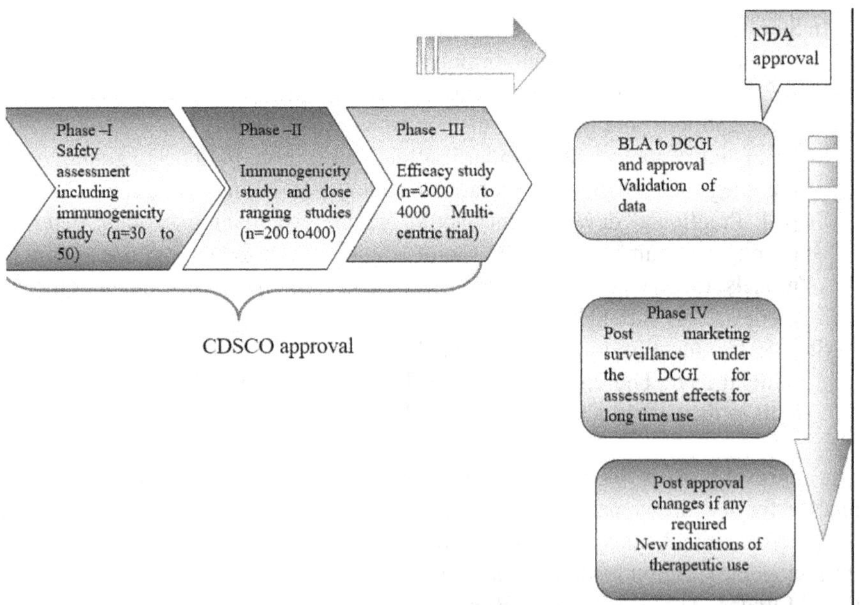

FIGURE 28.5 Procedure for clinical trial of vaccine.

During public health emergencies or the presence of serious or life-threatening illnesses, regulatory agencies, such as the U.S. Food and Drug Administration (FDA), may issue Emergency Use Authorizations (EUAs). An EUA allows the use of certain medical products, including IVDs, vaccines, and drugs, during emergencies based on an evaluation of the available scientific evidence. The FDA has programs for expedited review, such as the Fast Track, Breakthrough Therapy, and Priority Review designations. These designations aim to facilitate the development and expedite the review of drugs, vaccines, and other medical products intended to address serious or life-threatening conditions.

Biological license approval is generally the final step in the regulatory process for vaccines and certain biologics. Accelerated approval mechanisms may be used to speed up the licensure of products that demonstrate a significant therapeutic advantage over existing treatments.

Phase I clinical trials are the initial stage of testing in human subjects to assess safety, dosage, and potential side effects. In emergencies, such as a pandemic, regulatory agencies may prioritize and expedite the review of Phase I data to facilitate quicker access to promising medical interventions. Expedited review mechanisms are often applied to medical products addressing serious or life-threatening illnesses with unmet medical needs. These mechanisms are designed to bring potentially beneficial products to patients more quickly, while maintaining rigorous safety and efficacy standards.

The scenario of the approval procedure in India is somewhat different because India is not on the FDA list, so the export of any investigational new product can be done without IND. However, if India is marked after the joint trial with the listed countries recognised by the European agency or obtains export approval from the FDA, it is mandatory to submit the abbreviated dossier and letter to the FDA, providing the necessary documents get approvals from Indian regulatory authorities and clearance from Ethics Committees before the developed product can be exported. Safety and toxicity studies are described in Chapter 27 of this volume.

28.7 PENAL AND LEGAL REPERCUSSIONS FOR DISOBEYING THE REGULATION

28.7.1 The Law of Torts

The beauty of the Indian constitution is that every individual is endowed with a certain number of legal rights, and the law has appropriately bestowed upon everyone the responsibility and obligation to respect the legal rights held by others. A person is considered to have committed a tort if it is discovered that they interfered with the pleasure of another individual within the scope of their legal rights. Explained in a more clear and concise manner, the term "breach of duty" refers to tort. On the other hand, the tort law in India is not conditional and is still in the process of growing. In this case, the law of torts is inferred from the question of whether or not the maker of the therapeutic product may be trusted.

28.7.2 Consumer Protection Act, 1986

The Act was passed in order to make it easier for consumers to have their complaints addressed and resolved. It is guaranteed that the consumer's rights will be respected. In this case, the Consumer Protection Act, 1986, is inferred because of the issue of counterfeit, possibly toxic medicines, IVDs, or vaccines being marketed with the mark, as well as the violation of consumer rights associated with purchasing counterfeit commodities.

28.7.3 The Drugs and Cosmetics Act, 1940

If a counterfeit or contaminated drug is sold or exhibited, the maker, seller, stockist, or promoter of the medication could face legal action.

28.7.4 The Law of Contracts

In this situation, the law seems to imply that the contracting party may be accountable for selling items that are defective.

28.7.5 Criminal Law

It is believed that acts of gross negligence and acts of indulgence to spare the infection of a disease that is threatening life will result in legal responsibility.

28.8 GENETIC MODIFIED FOODS [GENETICALLY MODIFIED ORGANISMS (GMO)]

Foods that have been genetically engineered (also known as genetically modified organisms, or GMOs).

Article 51A(h) of the Indian Constitution states that cultivating a scientific temperament is one of the essential tasks of a citizen of the country. This provision is one of the many reasons why the Indian Constitution is so important for ensuring the independence and equality of all people. However, it is also true that fundamental responsibilities are purely voluntary and citizens cannot be compelled in the form of legal requirements or obligations committed to the state or society. Also, I'll put another legality that is stated in the directive principles, where the designated and for-the-right of the framers gives more value to economic freedom and social freedom as citizens of the country. Because of this, we can draw the conclusion that the application of GMO foods cannot be implemented in a coercive manner; rather, the issue is entirely dependent on the preferences of farmers. As a result of the government's awareness of the problems, various committees and organisations were established, and the responsibilities of each committee were outlined in their respective charters. The insertion of DNA from one organism into another organism or any other change of an organism's DNA to obtain a desired feature is what is meant by the term GMO.

28.9 REGULATORY BODIES APPROVAL FOR GMOS

28.9.1 Institutional Biosafety Committees (IBC)

Legality is bound to be responsive to any research that is involved in the issue of researching genetically modified organisms. The IBC is constituted with the approval of the DBT, and as a result, the IBC is regarded as a statutory entity that is operated by the institutes. It is responsible for the appropriate application of biosafety rules, regulations, and guidelines. The rules for the manufacture, use, import, export, and storage of hazardous microorganisms or genetically engineered organisms or cells, 1989, were notified by the MoEFCC, Government of India, in accordance with the "Environment (Protection) Act, 1986." These rules define who is responsible for ensuring compliance on the part of the principal investigator as well as the committee.

28.9.2 Review Committee on Genetic Manipulation (RCGM)

More functionally, the RCGM is the regulatory authority where the IBC reports and functions as the DBT nominee to monitor any research using GMOs and small-scale field trials. This is because the RCGM reviews genetically modified organisms (GMOs) and small-scale field experiments.

28.9.3 The Genetic Engineering Appraisal Committee (GEAC)

This committee is the DBT's highest decision-making body and is responsible for all environmental GMO releases. The comments and views are sent in to DCGI for the IVD kits, vaccines, or biopharmaceuticals that are being tested, but is the competent authority for major agricultural trials (Table 28.1).

In India, foods containing GMOs are subject to regulation by a number of different guidelines, each of which has its own designated area.

28.9.3.1 The Environmental Protection Act of 1986 (often known as the EPA).

28.9.3.2 Rules pertaining to the "Manufacture, Use, Import, Export, and Storage of Hazardous Microorganisms, Genetically Modified Organisms, and Cells" (1989 Rules).

28.9.3.3 The "Recombinant DNA Safety Guidelines," published in 1990 by the Department of Biotechnology's guidelines (also known as the "1990 DBT Guidelines"). 28.13.3.4 Revisions to the "Safety in Biotechnology" Guidelines (1994 DBT Guidelines).

28.9.3.5 Revised Guidelines for "Research in Transgenic Plants and Guidelines for Toxicity and Allergenicity Evaluation of Transgenic Seeds, Plants, and Plant Parts" (1998 DBT Guidelines).

28.9.3.6 Guidelines for Toxicity and Allergenicity Evaluation of Transgenic Seeds, Plants, and Plant Parts.

28.9.3.7 Seed Policy, 2002

TABLE 28.1
Role of Different Authorities to Control the GM Foods

Sl No.	Activities	Authority
28.1.1	Any research involving GMO (genetically modified organisms) should be conducted in a laboratory, glasshouse, or polytunnel to ensure that the environment is controlled.	RCGM (Review Committee on Genetic Manipulation)
28.1.2	Experiment in the field, experiment with the environment, or release to the environment	RCCGM and GEAC (Genetic Engineering Approval Committee) with concurrence of the other expert panel, if required
28.1.3	GMO crops that have been transformed into foods through processing or are otherwise treated as foods	FSSAI (Food Safety and Standards Authority of India)
28.1.4	Acceptance of processed foods for release into the commercial market	FSSAI
28.1.5	Environmental risk evaluation of genetically modified foods	GEAC

28.10 CARTAGENA BIOSAFETY PROTOCOL

The first worldwide regulatory framework that functioned for the safe use of LMOs, the Cartagena Protocol on Biosafety was developed under the jurisdiction of the Convention on Biological Diversity (CBD). India was one of the 143 countries that signed the agreement before it was officially adopted on January 28, 2000. In India, the "Biosafety Protocol" was implemented on January 17, 2003, and it went into effect on September 11, 2003 across the entire country.

28.10.1 A Concise Overview of the "Biosafety Protocol"

The DNA experiment is categorised in the protocol according to its inherent characteristics.

28.10.1.1 Category I is defined as routine recombinant DNA research carried out inside a laboratory with RCGM approval required and IBC validation of the procedure. These kinds of tests are under the purview of the IBC.

28.10.1.2 Category II is designated as experiments which are carried out in both laboratory and glasshouses studies with transgenes, evaluating for response to abiotic stressors through resistance/tolerance to herbicides and pesticides. Approval from the RCGM is also necessary for this category of experimentation.

28.10.1.3 Categories III and IV are designated from trials in the greenhouse to environmental release in field trials, with the anticipation of major adjustments in the ecosystem. The clearance of the GEAC is essential for this kind of trial. The MoEFCC and the Department of Biotechnology (DBT), both under the jurisdiction of the Government of India, are the primary organisations tasked with carrying out the requirements outlined in the laws. The responsiveness of DBT is relevant in situations where the guideline has been applied, and it covers practically all significant issues, including transgenic crops, the intentional release of genetically modified organisms (GMOs), plants, animals, and products into the environment, as well as the transportation and importation of GMOs. Additionally, the DBT was responsible for directing the prospective toxicities of the environment, and it mandated that toxicity and allergenicity data be collected from ruminants such as goats and cows after eating transgenic plants (Figure 28.6).

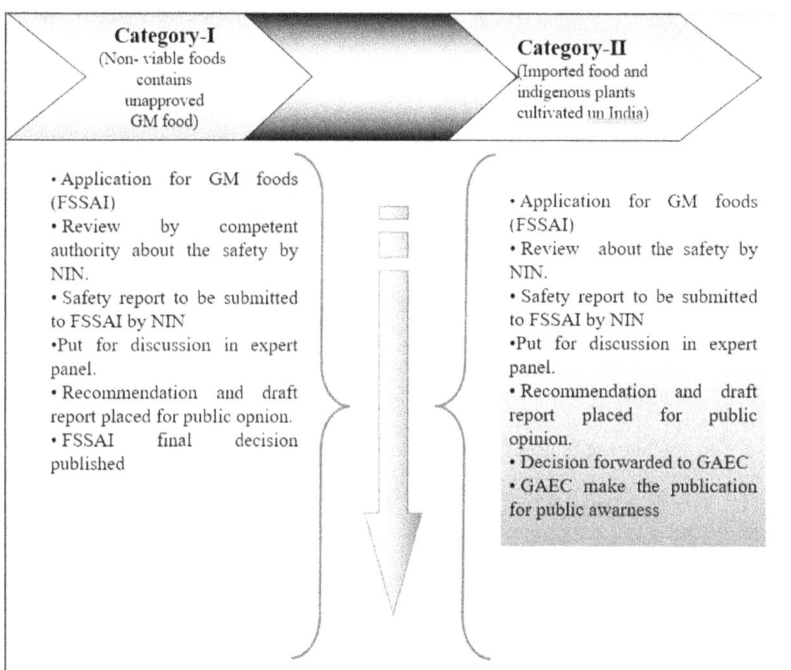

FIGURE 28.6 Application for GM foods for safety assessment.

28.11 DATA REQUIRED FOR APPROVAL OF GM CROPS/FOOD

28.11.1 Part 1

28.11.1.1 The nature of genetic alteration and the effects of the insect-resistance gene *cry 1AC* against the fruit and shoot borer, the *nptII* kanamycin-resistance marker gene, and the spectinomycin-resistance marker *aadA* gene.
28.11.1.2 Expression as well as Stability
28.11.1.3 The Environmental Safety Assessment
28.11.1.4 The possibility of genetic exchange with wild relatives
28.11.1.5 The degree of outbreeding and the circulation of pollen
28.11.1.6 The possibility of the GM food's genes being transferred to other plants.
28.11.1.7 The possibility of the GM food's genes being transferred to other organisms. 28.15.1.8 The possibility of increased weediness in the transgenic plants
28.11.1.9 The effect on organisms other than the ones intended, including the effect on the soil

28.11.2 Part II

28.11.2.1 Evaluation of GM food and its safety
28.11.2.2 Evaluation of toxicity and allergenicity (testing on skin and mucous membranes)
28.11.2.3 Fate related to digestion (*cry1AC*, *nptII*)
28.11.2.4 An examination of the composition of the GM food
28.11.2.5 Feed to rabbits, fish, chickens, goats, and cattle.

BIBLIOGRAPHY

Ahuja V. Regulation of Emerging Gene Technologies in India. *BMC Proceedings* 2018 July 19, 12(Suppl 8): 14. doi: 10.1186/s12919-018-0106-0. PMID: 30079105; PMCID: PMC6069684.

Baldrick P. Safety Evaluation of Biological Drugs: What Are Toxicology Studies in Primates Telling Us? *Regulatory Toxicology and Pharmacology* 2011, 59(2): 227–236.

Chimata MK, Bharti G. Regulation of Genome Edited Technologies in India. *Transgenic Research* 2019 August, 28(Suppl 2): 175–181. doi: 10.1007/s11248-019-00148-z. PMID: 31321702.

CLSI EP25-A, Evaluation of Stability of In Vitro Diagnostic Reagents; Approved Guideline, CLSI, Wayne, PA, 2009.

DBT Guidelines for Assuring the Quality of Pharmaceutical and Biological Products Prepared by Recombinant DNA Technology. In WHO Expert Committee on Biological Standardization. Forty-first report, Geneva, World Health Organization, 1991, Annex 3 (WHO Technical Report Series No. 814).

Drugs & Cosmetics Rules, 1988 (8th Amendment).

EMEA Guideline on Immunogenicity Assessment of Biotechnology-Derived Therapeutic Proteins, London, 2007 (CHMP/BMWP/14327).

EMEA Guideline on Similar Biological Medicinal Products Containing Biotechnology Derived Proteins as Active Substance: Non-Clinical and Clinical Issues. London, 2006 (CHMP/BMWP/42832).

EN 13640, Stability Testing of in Vitro Diagnostic Reagents.

Environment Protection Act, 1986 and Rules Framed Thereunder (Environment Protection Act, 1986 and Rules Framed. Available from: http://envfor.nic.in.

Guidelines for Generating Pre-clinical and Clinical Data for rDNA Vaccines, Diagnostics and Other Biologicals, 1999.

ICH Guideline on Preclinical Safety Evaluation of Biotechnology-Derived Pharmaceuticals (S6, 1997).

ISO 18113-1:2009 In Vitro Diagnostic Medical Devices — Information Supplied by the Manufacturer (labelling) — Part 1: Terms, Definitions and General Requirements.

Laws: ITC (HS), 2012 Sechdule-1 Import Policy, GSR, DGFT, Govt. of India.

Rules for the Manufacture, Use, Import, Export & Storage of Hazardous Microorganisms, Genetically Engineered Organisms or Cells, 1989.

29 Laws, Enforcement of Environmental Protection Act
Role of Institutional Biosafety Committee

29.1 INTRODUCTION

The rapid growth of biotechnology in India and around the world, as well as its applications in contemporary medicine and agriculture, grabbed the attention of researchers interested in safety and application issues. This technology, which is more commonly referred to as rDNA technology, allows for the transfer of genes from one species to another, which allows modern biotechnology to both improve and develop genetically modified species.

Genetically modified organisms (GMOs), including those developed using recombinant DNA (rDNA) technology, are subjects of ongoing research and discussion. The goal of using rDNA technology is often to enhance certain traits in crops, such as improving nutritional content or making them more resistant to pests. However, the safety and potential environmental impacts of GMOs are areas of concern and are typically rigorously assessed before their approval for commercial use. If there have been new developments or studies since my last update that suggest a negative influence of rDNA technology on people and the environment, it would be essential to review the latest scientific literature and regulatory reports to gain a comprehensive understanding of the issue.

As for the specific claim about the outbreak of nut allergy in soybeans in Brazil due to the combination of beans with a nut gene, it's crucial to verify the source of this information and check if it has been corroborated by reputable scientific studies or regulatory agencies. Misinformation and misconceptions can sometimes circulate, and it's important to rely on scientifically validated information when assessing the safety of biotechnological processes like rDNA technology.

The mailman's toxicity was reported as a result of genetically engineered plants with tolerance to glyphosate. Glyphosate is a herbicide commonly used in agriculture, and genetically engineered plants are often modified to be tolerant to it, allowing for effective weed control. The mention of eco-friendly pesticide technology could refer

DOI: 10.1201/9781003397854-13

to efforts to develop and use pesticides in a more environmentally sustainable manner. The International Agency for Research on Cancer (IARC) highlighted potential cancer hazards associated with glyphosate. This assessment has raised concerns and triggered debates about the safety of glyphosate in various regions.

In contrast to the IARC assessment, the European Union (EU) report did not reach a conclusion regarding whether glyphosate is carcinogenic to humans. The EU's regulatory stance on glyphosate has been a subject of discussion and scrutiny. The World Health Organization (WHO) is mentioned as indicating that the study did not ensure the level of risk. It suggests that WHO may have reservations or additional considerations about the study's findings or methodology. The European Food Safety Authority (EFSA) is cautious of cancer and deemed the level of risk irrelevant to the risk level. This implies that EFSA may have a more conservative stance on glyphosate's potential carcinogenicity. The statement suggests that the identified level of risk has not been implemented in the EU. This could mean that, despite differing assessments, specific regulatory actions may not have been taken based on the identified risk level.

The natural phytoestrogens genistein and daidzein found in soybeans are primarily responsible for the soybean's ability to imitate oestrogen. Research conducted in the laboratory demonstrated that even a trace amount of genistein and daidzein was sufficient to promote the growth of breast tumours. Glyphosate-tolerant soy, an example of GM soy, led to an increase in the levels of the phytoestrogens genistein and daidzein, which, in turn, caused breast cancer.

Concerns have been raised about genetically modified (GM) corporations, as well as foods generated from biotechnology, medicine, the ability of government authorities to oversee cross-border shipment, research, and the sensible application of modern biotechnology. The IBC is responsible for keeping an eye on laboratories that use deoxyribonucleic acid (DNA) technology to ensure that research is carried out in a responsible and risk-free manner.

29.2 IMPLEMENTATION OF THE CARTAGENA PROTOCOL'S IBC REQUIREMENTS

It was the first international pact that was legally implemented to provide safeguards related to the conservation of biodiversity and the application of genetically modified organisms (GMOs) in agricultural settings. In addition to this, the convention is responsible for enforcing the international policy and the legally binding transboundary movement of GMOs from one country to another. The international agreement was first adopted on January 29, 2000, and it was put into effect on September 11, 2003.

The protocol is an international agreement for the conservation of biological variety and access to the possible risks of living microorganisms and the appropriate application of biotechnology. The agreement was developed in order to ensure that the correct procedures are followed in research. Adopting the precautionary developed procedures and the advance information on the importing of Living Modified

Organisms (LMOs) were both agreed upon in the protocol. This was done so as to ensure that countries are, in fact, importing.

The protocol also agreed to the exchange of information with the LMO and to provide assistance with its implementation. Regulatory agencies and a central repository for biosafety that are harmonised have been established.

29.3 CONVENTION ON BIOLOGICAL DIVERSITY (CBD)

Both the release of LMOs and their use in practice are subject to strict regulations, with the primary goal being the preservation of biological variety in a sustainable form. The CBD was introduced in order to maintain a healthy and safe environment by preventing the cloning of animals and the emergence of new species. The CBD became legally binding on December 29, 1993, through India.

29.4 UNITED NATION TREATY AND RESPONSIBILITY: STOCKHOLM SUMMIT 1972

Under the aegis of the United Nations, for the first time ever, a conference was organised in 1972 to debate a topic such as the regulation of pollution in the natural environment. This meeting was known as the United Nations Summit on the Human Environment. A total of 473 nations get together in an international conference to talk about issues related to environmental pollution. The Water Pollution Act of 1974 was the first act of legislation that expressly addressed the problem of environmental pollution. This was followed by the Air Pollution Act of 1981, which was established to address air pollution. In 1986, the Environment Protection Act, (EPA 1986), went into effect.

The aforementioned expression pertains to any substance, whether in solid, liquid, or gaseous form, that exists in a concentration that has the potential to cause harm to both the environment and human beings. This condition is indicative of an ecological imbalance. Moreover, it is imperative to provide a comprehensive definition of materials or substances that, upon their integration with air, water, or land, result in a modification of their inherent characteristics to an extent that renders the utilisation of these resources by humans and other living organisms detrimental and potentially fatal to health. Consequently, it is crucial to prioritise the avoidance of such materials or substances under all circumstances.

29.5 ENFORCEMENT OF BIODIVERSITY IN INDIA

Under the authority granted to it by Article 253 of the Indian Constitution, the Government of India passed the EPA 1986 in the aftermath of the Bhopal disaster. The Act's goal is to serve as an "umbrella" piece of legislation, meaning that its intent is to offer a framework for the Central government to coordinate the actions of numerous central and state authorities that were established under earlier laws, such as the Water Act and the Air Act. This Act's purpose is to fulfil the aforementioned goal.

TABLE 29.1
Important Articles of the Convention

1	Article I. (Objectives)	The protection of biological diversity and the fair distribution of the advantages derived from genetic resources, as well as the development of appropriate technologies
2	Article 2. (Definition of terms)	Outlines some of the more prevalent terms "Biological diversity," "Biological resources," "Biotechnology," "Country of origin of genetic resources," "Country providing genetic resources," "Domesticated or cultivated species," "Ecosystem," "*Ex-situ* conservation," "Genetic material," "Genetic resources," "Habitat," "*In-situ* conditions," etc.
3	Article 3. (Principle)	According to the Charter of the United Nations and the principles of international law that govern environmental policies implemented by sovereign nations.
4	Article 4 (Jurisdictional scope)	Acts of national jurisdiction pertaining to the biological variety of connected subjects.
5	Article 5. (Cooperation)	Collaborate with one another and be encouraged by the national authority in order to solve problems with a shared interest in doing what is in the best interest of the preservation of biological variety and its ability to be sustained.
6	Article 6. (General Measures for Conservation and Sustainable Use)	The actual carrying out of the national conservation strategies, plans, or programmes for the protection of biological variety.
7	Article 8 (*In-situ* Conservation)	Strictly regulate, manage, or restrict the release of living modified organisms emerging from biotechnology that have a negative effect. On environmental protection and the sustainable use of biological diversity, while also considering the hazards to human health. It is imperative that invasive alien species that pose a threat to ecosystems, habitats, or species not be allowed to enter the country, that they be controlled, and that they be eradicated.
8	Article 9. (*Ex-situ* Conservation)	Acknowledgement from countries that conduct the importing and adoption of appropriate steps to conserve biological diversity *ex-situ* along with regulation of preventative measures to protect ecosystems and conserve *in-situ* populations of species as biological resources from natural settings. In most cases, the notification is published within the first ninety days following receipt of the foreign material.
9	Article 10. (Sustainable Use of Components of Biological Diversity)	The decision to preserve the best interests of the community while still allowing for traditional uses of biological resources and minimising negative consequences on biological diversity is part of the decision to use biological resources in a sustainable manner. This decision also encourages customary uses that are in line with cultural traditions.
10	Article 11. (Incentive Measures)	In order to protect biological diversity and make sure it is used in a way that is ecologically sound, it is necessary to take measures that are applicable, economical, and socially acceptable.

(*Continued*)

TABLE 29.1 (CONTINUED)
Important Articles of the Convention

11	Article 14. (Impact assessment and minimising Adverse impacts)	Evaluating the planned projects, to see whether there is a possibility of any negative consequences on biological diversity, as well as how such effects may be resolved or mitigated, is a necessary step. Also, assessing the possibilities of exchanging knowledge within the framework of bilateral, regional, or multinational agreements that fall under their purview in order to regulate the biological variety. Also, how to launch emergency responses when there is an immediate threat to biological diversity.
12	Article 15. (Access to genetic resources)	Natural resources are the property of the states, and access to genetic resources is governed by the laws of individual nations. The conclusion reached by this convention is that the genetic resources being offered by an importing country have been acquired in compliance with this Convention. In order to access the genetic resources, both parties are required to first provide prior information and then reach an agreement on how the requirements would be implemented. Both the exporter and importer of genetic resources must be scientific endeavours in their respective countries. A financial disclosure of mutual research and direction for legislative, administrative, or policy measures is necessary, and this part plays an important role in that.
13	Article 16. (Access transfer of technology)	In order to achieve the goal that the private sector promotes access to, joint development of, and the transfer of technology, each contracting party is obligated to implement legislative, administrative, or regulatory measures, as necessary.
14		The Parties to the contract are obligated to make it easier for information to be shared, using any and all sources that are open to the public, which is pertinent to the protection and responsible utilisation of biological variety. This should be done while keeping in mind the unique requirements of developing nations. The act of sharing technological, scientific, and socioeconomic outcomes of studies, along with data pertaining to training and surveying programmes, specialised expertise, and indigenous and traditional knowledge, both independently and in conjunction with the technologies mentioned in Article 16, can be classified as an exchange of information. In addition to that, wherever it is possible, it will incorporate the return of information.
		The parties to the contract must, through suitable international and national agencies, encourage international technical and scientific collaboration in the field of preservation and sustainable use of biological variety.
16		Each party involved in the contract should, to the best of their ability, enact legal, administrative, or regulatory steps to ensure the significant involvement of those parties involved in the contract, with a particular emphasis on developing nations that supply the genetic resources for such research.

(Continued)

TABLE 29.1 (CONTINUED)
Important Articles of the Convention

	In the domain of ensuring the secure transfer, manipulation, and utilisation of any living modified organism derived from biotechnology, which has the potential to adversely impact the preservation and sustainable utilisation of biological diversity, it is incumbent upon the involved entities to assess the need and mechanisms for a protocol that delineates suitable protocols. These protocols should encompass various procedures, with a specific emphasis on obtaining prior informed consent. This examination is to take place in the context of the parties' consideration of the need for the protocol.
17	The provisions of this agreement shall not impair the rights and responsibilities of any Contracting Party derived from any existing international agreement, with the exception of situations in which the exercise of those rights and obligations would cause substantial damage or pose a serious threat to biological diversity.
18	In order to guarantee that the conference of the parties and its subsidiary bodies get prompt guidance on the execution of this convention, the establishment of an additional body for the provision of scientific, technical, and technological support is hereby enacted. This council will be comprised of experts from a wide range of fields and will encourage involvement from all parties. It is required to be made up of government representatives who are knowledgeable in the applicable field of competence. At regular intervals, it must update the conference of the parties on its progress in all areas of responsibility.
19	If a disagreement arises between Contracting Parties about the meaning or application of this Convention, the parties involved shall attempt to resolve the matter via negotiation. If the parties involved can't settle their differences through arbitration, they can all decide to go to litigation.
20	The parties to this convention shall work together to develop and ratify any necessary protocols. The conference of the parties is the body responsible for ratifying any proposed protocols.
21	The Convention or the Protocols could be changed. Every participating party must enact legislation, establish administrative measures, or develop policies, as needed, to ensure the active involvement of contracting parties, especially developing nations, that supply genetic resources for biotechnological research. This should be done within the respective contracting parties, provided it is feasible. The Parties are obligated to consider the need for and the requirements of a protocol that outlines appropriate procedures, such as, in particular, advance informed agreement, in the field of the secure movement, handling, and utilisation of any living modified organism that is the result of biotechnology and that may have a negative effect on the conservation and sustainable use of biological diversity. The Parties will also consider whether or not such a protocol is necessary.

The term "environment" is defined to include water, air, and land, as well as the interrelationships that exist between water, air, and land, as well as between water, air, and land, and human beings and other living animals, plants, microorganisms, and property. This gives the Act a potentially wide scope of application.

This Act's overarching goal is to safeguard and enhance environmental conditions, including those of water, air, land, humans, other animals, plants, microorganisms, and property. This Act also has a number of other goals that are related to the environment. In addition, the protection of the natural environment is guaranteed by constitutional law. Article 48A stipulates that the state must make efforts to maintain and develop the environment, as well as to preserve the forests and wildlife of the country. Additionally, Article 51A mandates that each individual citizen must protect the environment. The EPA 1986 governs all of India, including Jammu and Kashmir, and is applicable throughout the entire country.

The authority to prevent and limit the use of hazardous materials and place of industries is granted by Sections 3–6 of the Act, as is the power to notify standards and acceptable levels of air, water, and soil pollutants for different places and purposes. These provisions can be found in the Act.

The authority to prevent and restrict the handling of hazardous materials and the location of industries, as well as to establish rules for controlling environmental pollution, and to disclose standards and the upper limits for contaminants of air, water, and soil for various places and purposes, are all granted by the Act (Sections 3–6).

According to Sections 10 and 11, of the Act the appointed person or agency is authorised to conduct inspections, can enter the premises, and can take samples for analysis.

In accordance with the provisions of Section 5, the central government has the ability to issue written directives to any person, officials, or authority, requiring them to comply of the act. It is possible that there might be a shutdown, a prohibition on the provision of electricity, an operation, or a process; a suspension in the supply of electricity, water, or any other service; or regulation of the supply of power, water, or any other service of non-compliance. It is the government's responsibility to establish act under Section 6 to carry out the Act's purpose.

A person is considered to be operating an industry, operation, or other activity if they do not permit the emission or discharge of environmental pollutants in quantities that are more than the acceptable criteria (Section 7). Organization or establishment are required to provide the relevant information to the relevant authorities, and those who handle hazardous substances are required to comply with the procedural precautions outlined in Section 8.

29.6 CASE STUDY: TAJ MAHAL CASE

M.C. Mehta v. Union of India 1996 (4) SCALE (SP) 29 is a case that was brought before the Honorable Supreme Court of India in order to protect India's cultural heritage, the Taj Mahal, from industrial pollution. The case resulted in the government taking appropriate action within the confines of the law.

29.7 INSTITUTIONAL BIOSAFETY COMMITTEE (IBC) AND EMPOWERMENT

The committee was established in accordance with the directives issued by the Department of Biotechnology in order to eliminate the power recommendation and simplify the movement of biological material, trans-boundary transit, handling, and use of living modified organisms (LMOs), all of which have the potential to have negative impacts. The IBC is in charge of ensuring that biological diversity is preserved while also making responsible use of it, taking into account its potential impact on human health. The development of IBC concurrency and the outcome of an international treaty such as the Convention on Biological Diversity (CBD) 1992, the Cartagena Protocol on Biosafety (CPB) 2003, the Nagoya Protocol on Access and Benefit Sharing (ABS) 1992, and the Nagoya Kuala Lumpur Protocol on Access and Benefit Sharing (ABS) 1992 are examples of such international agreements.

In the beginning of 1983, the Department of Biotechnology, Government of India, came up with the safety rules for the purpose of reducing the risk of adverse effects on one's health. In the year 1990, the r-DNA Advisory Committee came out with the Indian recombinant DNA (r-DNA) biosafety guidelines to perform research on GMOs. These guidelines were amended in the years 1994 and 1998 after they were initially established. Guidelines and instructions pertaining to large-scale operations and the environmental and health concerns linked with biotechnology research were established in the year 1990. The revised guidelines from 1998 further expanded the scope of the development of r-DNA technology to include GMOs, vaccines, diagnostics, and transportation for laboratory research and large-scale usage. Additionally, the guidelines directed both the process and the goal of quality control for biologically produced products that were made using r-DNA technology. Additionally, the new guideline included a description of the toxicity and allergenic tests that must be performed on any transgenic seeds, plants, or plant parts. The incremental guideline for restricted field trials and regulations on the restricted trials of genetically engineered plants were both released in 2008. These guidelines covered topics such as the transport, harvest or termination, post-harvest technology, and management. Additionally, the guideline outlined criteria for safety, labelling, documenting, and records, as well as corrective actions in the event that accidental releases occurred.

The EPA 1986 prohibits the manipulation or use of any harmful microorganisms as well as genetically altered creatures or cells. This law went into effect as a preview. The rules apply in a broad manner to the following aspects:

1. The transaction of microorganisms in any form, including but not limited to their sale, storage for the purpose of commercial exploration, and any other form of handling.
2. Cells or organisms that have been modified genetically, together with related compounds, for the purpose of exporting and importing.
3. The production, processing, warehousing, and packaging of items that have been genetically modified.

4. The production and manufacture of pharmaceuticals, foodstuffs, and other medicinal products with the use of genetically modified microorganisms.

   The understanding of the work and mandate of IBC, the following regulation is very important and legibly enforced accordingly.
5. EPA 1986.
6. Eighth Amendment to Drugs and Cosmetics Act, 1988 and Notification of Rules for Implementation, 1989.
7. Guidelines for Research, Trials and Commercial Applications on Biotechnological Products, 1990.
8. Guidelines for Research in Transgenic Plants, 1998.
9. Guidelines for Research for Clinical Products, 1999.
10. Protection of Plants and Farm.
11. New Drugs Policy, 2002.
12. Seeds Policy, 2002.
13. Guidelines and Standard Operating Procedures (SOPs) for Confined Field Trials of Regulated, Genetically Engineered (GE) Plants, 2008.
14. Guidelines for the Safety Assessment of Foods Derived from Genetically Engineered Plants, 2008.
15. Protocols for Food and Feed Safety Assessment of GE crops -2008.

The IBC only has the capacity to make recommendations, and it does not possess the absolute power to approve any and all recommendations in accordance with the surrounding legislation as stated. In addition, the inter-ministerial laws are consistent with any decisions that have been made, such as the Ministry of Environment, Forest and Climate Change, serving as the regulating and focal agency for the control of the production, use, import, export, and storage of genetically modified or dangerous microorganisms through enforcing regulations, such as the Biological Diversity Act of 2002 and the Environmental Protection Act of 1986. In a similar vein, the Ministry of Agriculture and Farmer Welfare is the focal agency for execution of the Plant Quarantine Order, 2004 issued by the NBPGR and the Seed Policy, 2002. The GM Policy in Foreign Trade Policy (2006–09) Act designates the Directorate General of Foreign Trade (DGFT) as the agency under the Ministry of Commerce and Industry that is responsible for regulating the export and import of genetically modified (GM) food products. For the use of genetically modified organisms (GMOs) in food items and pharmaceuticals, the Food Standard Safety Act of 2006 and the Drugs and Cosmetics Act of 1972 are under the authority of the Ministry of Health and Family Welfare (Table 29.2).

29.8 INSTITUTIONAL BIOSAFETY COMMITTEE (IBC)

IBCs oversee all biosafety-related r-DNA technology research. The Institutional Biosafety Committee is recognised by the Department of Biotechnology (DBT) and is in compliance with regulations and legislation. The DBT brought in biotechnology department personnel and a medical officer to assess risks. At least once every six months, the DBT must submit a report to the RCGM.

TABLE 29.2
Government Stakeholder and Responsibilities

1	Ministry of Environment, Forest and Climate Change	The conservation and protection of the environment, as well as the authority to release any LMOs for the purpose of protecting human health or the environment, are of utmost importance.
2	Department of Biotechnology (DBT)	Support for the advancement of biotechnology and the provision of services relevant to biotechnology research
3	Ministry of Agriculture	Post-release support for agriculture development, GM technology, and agronomic advantage.
4	Ministry of Health and Family Welfare	Human health protection policies.
5	Ministry of Commerce and Department of Custom	Enforcement of trade-related matters, particularly import/export policies

The decision-making processes of the IBC pertaining to the regulation of genetically modified organisms (GMOs) and the facilitation of access to imported GMOs. Moreover, the decision could be made by taking into consideration factors such as the approval of medicinal recombinant DNA (r-DNA) products. Prior to executing the IBC job, it is imperative to have a comprehensive understanding of the delegation requirements and the legal framework of the country in which the decision, forwarding, and suggestion are adopted.

29.9 THE MANDATE OF THE INSTITUTIONAL BIOSAFETY COMMITTEE

Using r-DNA technology or possibly hazardous biotechnological research as examples, the IBC is the first legislative Committee to operate from the premises committee where the institutional obligation is established. All biotechnological research falling under r-DNA technology is to be reported to RCGM by the IBC on a semi-annual basis.

All biosafety protocols have been examined, assessed, and monitored by the IBC committee. According to the r-DNA criteria, the Review body will analyse, assess, and monitor the projects, and if necessary, will advance the application to the next higher body, the RCGM. Since the IBC committee is not a permanent statutory body, its membership is rotated every three to five years.

29.10 RESPONSIBILITIES OF THE CHAIRPERSON OF THE IBC

The law stipulates that the person who is in charge of the organisation automatically holds the position of chairman. However, the enforcement obligations of biosafety are vested in the head of the Institute or the authority that has been given by the head of the Institute. The delegation of the post may be acceptable. The primary responsibilities consist of the following:

29.17.1 Conduct frequent meetings of the IBC at a minimum interval of every six months and to review or monitor any recombinant research initiatives that are going to Institution.

29.17.2 After the members of the DBT and any other external organisations have discussed and put the policy into effect.

29.11 REVIEW OF THE PROJECT UNDER THE SPECIFIED CATEGORY AND CLEARANCE

The guidelines are applied to the projects, and each one is evaluated and classified according to the level of risk it poses. The timely transmission of the recommendations and observations to RCGM is ensured. The embodied panel is also responsible for providing advice, ensuring that all other permission requirements are met, and assessing the socioeconomic benefits of the project that is being carried out.

29.11.1 Understanding the Risk Assessment of the Associate Project

The IBC is responsible for conducting an assessment of the project's potential risks in order to investigate both the intended and unintended implications of the genetic manipulations that were carried out. Handling and keeping the microorganism that is going to be examined requires a certain level of personal knowledge in addition to a certain level of containment facilities.

29.11.2 Training on Biosafety

The IBC is also entrusted with the role of providing training to members of the organisation so that they are capable of accepting responsibility and accountability for the management of experiments in high-risk categories. The committee is also responsible for ensuring compliance with the applicable regulations and submitting a report to RCGM regarding the education and awareness of all workers who are participating in the high-risk experiment.

29.11.3 Establishing a System for Health Monitoring

Another obligation that is placed in the research worker is the responsibility of recognising the related hazards that come with addressing the risk of microorganisms. It is needed to provide regular interval clinical reports of the investigator, as well as current health status, to the RCGM.

29.11.4 Adopting Various Forms of Contingency Planning

In addition to this, the committee looks through the strategy that was turned in by the primary investigator for the accidental release measure of r-DNA products and the procedure of mitigating any potential emergencies. The copies should be provided for notification to all regulatory bodies within the system, such as the State Biotechnology Coordination Committee (SBCC) or the District Level Committee (DLC), as well as the RCGM and the GEAC.

29.11.5 Role of DBT Nominee

The DBT nominee is an ex-officio member of the committee and was appointed by the DBT to function as a representation for the purpose of ensuring that all required guidelines are adhered to, and that the committee conducts the experiments in accordance with the rules. In addition, the DBT nominee is responsible for ensuring that all reports are sent to RCGM/DBT on a semi-annual basis and that all experiments relating to the risk microorganisms are conducted in accordance with the rule are adequately communicated to the DBT nominee or the DBT/RCGM.

29.11.6 Principal Investigator

About the nature of the experiments that are being carried out, the principal investigator (PI) is associated with the recombinant DNA is to be informed and appraised of the experiment by the IBC. IBC is obligated to ensure that the proposal is admissible before beginning any research effort or filing a request to the RCGM for concurrence.

The PI is responsible for adhering to the guidelines outlined in the biosafety standards. Regarding genetically modified organisms, it is the responsibility of the PI to determine the appropriate level of containment for the research and, in accordance with the DBT Guidelines, to develop the necessary experimental protocols. Physical and biological confinement, research technique, and the origin of any DNA or vector/host systems are all evaluated in light of the IBC's requirements before any studies are carried out. The principal investigator is also responsible for obtaining authorisation for the studies and ensuring that any potential biohazards are mitigated, that the experiment is carried out safely in the laboratory, that appropriate preventative medical procedures are followed, and that the recombinant microbe is finally released.

29.12 IBC ACCOUNTABILITY OR DNA RESEARCH WORK

Evaluate the potential risks associated with the selected gene, including its known functions, interactions, and any potential unintended effects. Ensure a clear scientific rationale for the choice of the gene, considering the purpose of the research and the desired outcomes. Assess the safety of the vector used for gene transfer, considering its stability, potential for unintended consequences, and any known risks associated with the vector. Evaluate the method of gene transfer, considering the efficiency, specificity, and potential off-target effects. Assess the suitability of the host organism for receiving the transferred gene, considering factors such as compatibility, stability, and the potential for ecological impact. Investigate potential post-translational effects of the transferred gene within the host organism, including alterations in metabolic pathways and unintended consequences. Consider the implications of scaling up experiments, including potential changes in risk factors and the ability to control and contain the modified organisms. Conduct an environmental impact assessment to anticipate any potential ecological consequences of large-scale experiments. Implement appropriate containment measures to prevent accidental environmental discharge. Develop and communicate emergency response plans in the event of an accidental release, addressing both short-term and long-term consequences. Ensure that transportation protocols adhere to safety standards and regulations to prevent accidental spills or contamination during shipping. Provide comprehensive documentation regarding the transported materials, including emergency response information. Thoroughly characterize the gene products post-translationally to identify any potential risks or unintended effects. Consider the long-term effects of the modified organisms on the environment and ecosystems. Ensure that the research hypothesis is clearly defined and that experiments are designed to test specific hypotheses. Consider the reproducibility of the experiments and the reliability of the results. Encourage peer review of research plans and results to enhance scientific rigor and validity.

29.12.1 Attributes Shared by All Donor Organisms

Understanding the risk evaluation begins with having a thorough understanding of the donor organism. In most cases, DNA with a clear identifty and an established phenotype or a promoter is chosen. After the insert or recombination, if the donor gene creates any biologically active protein or post-translational alterations that are the poisons or any virulence characteristic, and in such instances, it is highly crucial to keep all of the further consequences.

29.12.2 Characteristics of the Host/Recipient Organisms

Characteristics of the host and recipient organisms are essential to have a good understanding of the host or recipient organism in order to properly evaluate the risks that are connected with the situation. The correct taxonomy of the host needs to be determined, and doing so is a prerequisite for establishing the safety (Table 29.3).

29.13 THE IBC POWER AND ENFORCEMENT OF "REVISED GUIDELINES FOR RESEARCH IN TRANSGENIC PLANT, 1998

1. Category I experiments consist of routine, uncomplicated recombinant DNA experiments that just need to be reported to the IBC in the proper format. Category II experiments encompass laboratory and greenhouse/nethouse investigations conducted inside a controlled environment. These operations involve the use of well-defined components of DNA which cause no harm to humans or animals, with the purpose of genetically modifying plants. The authorisation to conduct Category II

experiments is granted by the IBC. However, it is necessary to inform the RCGM of the IBC's decision prior to carrying out the experiment. The RCGM will then documented this information. Category III is categorically identified as the high-risk experiments and the risk associated with the impact on the biosphere by releasing transgenic traits into the open environment. Category III experiments are usually carried out in close conditions like a greenhouse and over a limited area. The approval of RCGM is mandatory for starting the experiment, whereas the release to the environment requires GAEC approval.

The pathogenicity, treatment, and communicability of the disease-causing pattern of the organism are important for the understanding of the IBC and, accordingly, the experiments are designed, following approved of the facilities available in the Institute. IBC has also accountable for any accident hazards (Table 29.4).

TABLE 29.3
Categorisation of Experiments According to the r-DNA Technologies.

1	Category I	This category is limited to cloning are involved self-strains or interspecies within the same exchanger group etc.
2	Category II	Category I experiments are not limited to laboratory level and large-scale use requires prior intimation to IBC. The containment levels II, III, and IV are required.
3	Category III	Any experiments involving gene cloning for vaccine production or toxin production by using infectious animals or plants or involving any viruses or self-fusion. Also, any field testing and environment release requires approval of IBC before any commencement of the experiment.

TABLE 29.4
Hazardous Classification of Microorganisms Based According on Their Pathogenicity

1	Group 1	In this category, neither prior notification nor approval is necessary. This category is restricted to cloning that involves only self-strains, interspecies, or strains of other species that belong to the same exchanger group, etc.
2	Group 2	In the event that the category I experiment is not restricted to the level of a laboratory, and in the event that it is intended for use on a broad scale, prior notification to the IBC is required. It is necessary to maintain containment at levels II, III, and IV.
3	Group 3	Using infected animals or plants, viral or self-fusion techniques, or cloning genes to manufacture vaccines or toxins is strictly forbidden.
4	Group 4	In addition, the approval of GAEC was necessary prior to the beginning of any experiment that involved field testing or environmental release.

29.14 AN OVERVIEW OF THE PLANT QUARANTINE (REGULATION OF IMPORT IN TO INDIA) ORDER, 2003, INDIA

Regulations governing the import and export of plants or agriculture products may have preventive enforcement the infectious pathogens and the vectors that carry them, known as quarantine regulations. Whereas the GEAC is the institution in responsible, overseeing imports of seeds between states as well as the necessary permissions. Let's analyse the National Seed Policy's governing regulations from 2002 to gain a better understanding of accountability. Before being released onto the market, each and every genetically modified variety is required to undergo biosafety testing in accordance with the regulations that were established by the EPA in 1989. In accordance with the law, IBC is authorised to carry out inspections at the time of planting, as well as during the growing and harvesting seasons. With the approval of the Genetic Engineering Approval Committee (GEAC), the National Bureau of Plant Genetic Resources (NBPGR) is the organisation that has a mandate to transfer genetically engineered materials.

Certificates to import transgenic plants are issued by the exporting country's competent authority; prior to importation, the agronomic value must be evaluated through ICAR's All-India Coordinated Project Trials for at least two growing seasons; biosafety clearance and seed act registration must also be obtained. It is interesting to note that, in accordance with the Plant varieties protection Act and post-market monitoring (performance in the field), transgenic varieties can eventually achieve the same status as non-transgenic varieties after commercial cultivation. In addition, the Ministry of Agriculture and state departments of agriculture are responsible for conducting all of the necessary research for a trial period of at least three to five years.

In addition to this, the IBC is expected to have knowledge of the Destructive Insects and Pests Act, 1914, specifically Section 3 of Article 9 of Article 4, which states that the IBC is the first responder to identify and take the appropriate steps to quarantine contaminated weed species or pests that are regarded as being detrimental to agricultural seeds or materials. The task has also been allocated to enforce the threatening effects that will have on interstate boundary transport as well as the consequences that will have on geoclimatic and ecological variation.

Any transport that was considered to be infested, any transport that was infected with a pest, or any transport that was polluted by dangerous weeds was prohibited by Section 3 of the Destructive Insects and Pests Act of 1914. Any business that imports agricultural products is required to provide a phytosanitary certificate issued by the country from which they originate. The certificate and the order to import plants and plant goods were both granted by the specialised committee of the Ministry of Agriculture, which is responsible for the export and import of seeds and planting materials.

A risk assessment of pests is also required in accordance with the rules that have been set. This assessment must include the probable classification of pests, evaluation, mitigating methods, and environmental risk. Additionally, the legislation is implemented for the confirmation by the phytosanitary specialists who are deputed to the export country for the purpose of evaluation, inspections of pre-shipmen, post-harvest treatment technologies, and the quarantine procedure. Permits are being handed out, including this one, on the basis of the suggestion made by the expert committee. These permits are valid for a period of six months, and their validity can be extended. However, the certificate cannot be changed and cannot be transferred; the only thing that can be changed is the entrance point of import.

The permits are not transferable and cannot be altered in any way, with the exception of the change of access points that is permitted. Only through the announced points of entry are shipments permitted to be brought into the country. Imports are subject to inspection by the plant protection adviser or other authorised personnel. In order to enable the inspection-related responsibilities, such as providing information, samples, and consignments, the importer is expected to pay the relevant charges. In addition, the importer is responsible for facilitating these duties. The packaging must pay particular attention to the containment of any leakage that may occur while the product is in transit. Insects are included in the scope of the act's special provisions, together with the ground, the soil, and the sand; microbial cultures; biocontrol agents; and microbial cultures. Seed may be imported when it has been grown and inspected by the plant protection adviser or a representative who has been designated. The post–quarantine procedure needs to be followed, and the advisor to the plant protection officer has complete authority to order the destruction of the consignment if any exotic diseases or pests are discovered. It is necessary that the article for genetically modified seeds and planting supplies mention the various agronomic and transgenic benefits of the product.

The authorities that imports materials for the purposes of research are the IBC and RCGM, whereas the import of LMOs for industrial and commercial exploration is controlled by GEAC. Figure 29.1

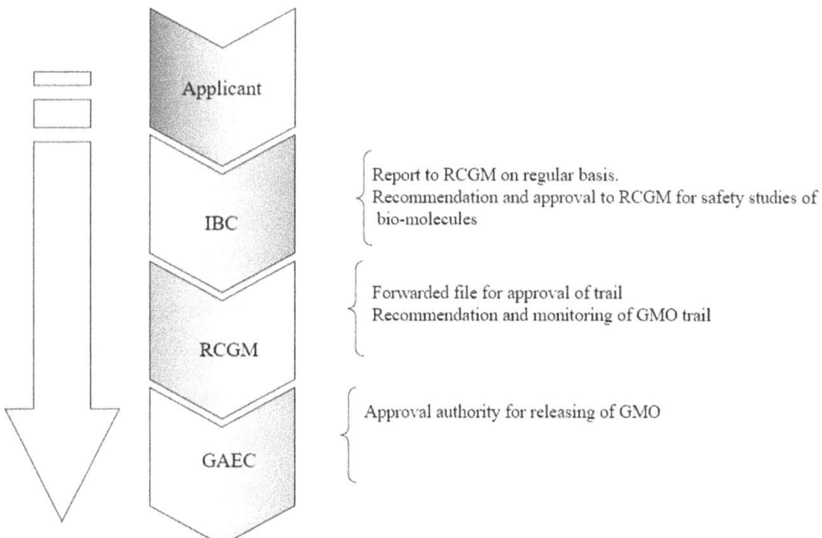

FIGURE 29.1 Regulation of the GMO corporations.

29.15 IBC INTERSTATE ROLE—SHIPPING OF PLANT MATERIAL AND SEEDS

There are a number of public regulations that have been effectively implemented, all with the goal of promoting the conservation of the ecosystem. Although many Public Interest Lawsuits (PIL) are brought in accordance with the letter of the law, many such cases are nonetheless brought about like Animal and Environment Legal Defence Fund - Vs. - Union of India & Ors. (1997) 3 SCC 71; M.C. Mehta –Vs. - Union of India & Ors 1986(2) SCC 176; Rural Litigation and Entitlement Kendra & Ors –Vs.- State of U.P. & Ors AIR 1987 SC 359; 1987 (1) SCR 641; and many other cases like this. The judicial system has acted in the appropriate manner to save the environment by implementing the laws that had been passed. In Chapter II of the Biodiversity Act of 2002, it was stated unequivocally that any biological resource for commercial use, biosurvey or bio-utilisation for commercial use shall not be obtained by any Indian citizen or by any corporate, association, or organisation registered in India, unless prior notification to the relevant State Biodiversity Board has been given.

This was a directive that was intended to be taken very seriously. When the topic of biodiversity activity was brought up, the phrase "extended" to include microorganisms, plants, and animals, was found to be equally applicable to the habitats that they occupy.

IBC has a fiduciary responsibility to avert the destruction of natural habitats caused, in part, by unnecessary farming practices and, in the same way, those brought on by excessive human exploitation of cultivated plant genetic resources. The introduction of non-native species into an ecosystem can lead to an increase in disease risk, a phenomenon known as bioinvasion. Explanation and cultivation of alien or exotic species that have been moved outside of their natural environment, whether on purpose or by accident, are subject to critical evaluation, despite the fact that not all alien species are associated with the production of dangerous effects. The World Conservation Union has previously issued a list of foreign species, and many foreign species have had a negative impact on agriculture and the ecosystem by growing more quickly than native species, altering the habitat in a way that is incompatible with the ecosystem, or causing the spread of diseases.

IBC is highlighted as having a fiduciary responsibility to prevent the destruction of natural habitats. This responsibility implies a duty to act in the best interests of environmental conservation and sustainable land use. Unnecessary farming practices are identified as a contributing factor to the destruction of natural habitats. Such practices may include unsustainable land use, deforestation, or other activities that negatively impact ecosystems. The human exploitation of cultivated plant genetic resources is mentioned as another factor leading to habitat destruction. This may refer to activities such as overharvesting or unsustainable use of plant varieties, affecting biodiversity. The introduction of non-native species is discussed in the context of bioinvasion, leading to increased disease risk. The phenomenon of bioinvasion occurs when non-native species are introduced into an ecosystem, potentially causing ecological imbalances.

The World Conservation Union has identified certain alien species that have had a negative impact on agriculture and ecosystems. These species may grow rapidly, alter habitats in incompatible ways, or contribute to the spread of diseases. The economic significance of invasive species like lantana and carrot grass is discussed, revealing major trends. Invasive species can have economic repercussions, affecting agricultural productivity and ecosystem health. *Mikania* and *Chromolaena* species are cited as examples that have taken over parts of India, particularly in the Northeastern Himalayan and Western Ghats regions. The invasion of these species contributes to the destruction of native vegetation. Several species, including *Eupatorium glandulosum, Parthenium, Mimosa, Ulex europaeus, Euphorbia royleana, Prosopis juliflora,* are mentioned as among the most invasive. These species can pose significant threats to local ecosystems and agriculture.

India is very precise and strictly enforces the quarantine restrictions, which are a legally serious offence. These regulations are enforced by the Plant Protection, Quarantine, and Storage Department, although there is a lack of information, and no exclusive regulation has been put in place to combat invading alien species. According to the Plant Quarantine Order 2003, approximately 61 species of plant (including 12 species of fungus), 14 species of insect, and 36 species with regional distribution were determined to be invasive. In addition to this, the order made it abundantly plain that 28 species endemic to India have been identified as causing ecological disruption in other biogeographical zones. The IBC is responsible for approving and evaluating applications for the cultivation of such species, and it has the authority.

In Chapter IV of the Constitution of India, it is stated that the protection of the environment is included as part of the fundamental duties. In contrast, Section 57 of the Biodiversity Act vested duty to individual persons of the companies for any offences committed. Indian research institute(s) could be indirectly prosecuted under the biopiracy act, but there are no specific grounds on which to impose liability on the individual offender who transfers biological resources to foreign institutes or enterprises.

29.16 EXAMPLE OF BIOPIRACY CASES

29.16.1 Bt Brinjal Biopiracy Case

Accusations and subsequent legal action were taken because of the production of GM Bt brinjal utilising indigenous types of brinjal. The accusation is that this activity harms the biodiversity of the country.

29.16.2 Haldi as Wound Healing Agent

According to a United States patent (number 5,401,504), turmeric is effective in wound healing. The United States Patent and Trademark Office (USPTO) cancelled the patent as a consequence of a challenge brought by the Council of Scientific and Industrial Research (CSIR) of India in New Delhi. This challenge was based on the existence of prior art and supported by documentation demonstrating that India has been using haldi for wound healing for a significant amount of time.

29.16.3 The Bt Cotton Incidence

The only genetically modified organism to be granted approval in India in 2002 was created by the Maharashtra Hybrid Seeds Company (MAHYCO), a joint venture between Bayer and Monsanto. Permission was given on the grounds of increased income for farmers, decreased consumption of insecticides, and other similar beneficial factors. The results of many field surveys were inconclusive regarding the question of whether or not Bt cotton is superior to regular cotton. Agriculture ministers from Andhra Pradesh and Karnataka made statements in 2002–2003 regarding the failure of Bt cotton. In addition, an independent survey conducted by the Research Foundation for Science, Technology and Ecology (Delhi), Gene Campaign (Delhi), and Greenpeace India surveys also revealed that Bt cotton is not superior to normal cotton.

Biodiversity Heritage Sites (BHS) are protected under the definition of Biodiversity Acts in Section 2, and they are responsible for ensuring both ecological and human health. The formulation of the concept of *sui generis*, which means “of its own kind” or “unique,” was mandated in order to safeguard indigenous ways of knowing, innovating, and working with biological resources.

29.17 THE LEGAL IMPLICATION OF THE INTERSTATE SHIPPING OF PLANT MATERIAL AND SEEDS IN INDIA

Before going into detail, just remember that Article 48A of the Constitution of India (42nd Amendment Act, 1976) stated explicitly that the “State shall endeavour to preserve and enhance the environment and to safeguard the forests and wildlife of the country," while Article 47 of the Constitution enforces the state duty for the protection of health. In addition, Clause (g) of Article 51A stipulated that it is “a fundamental duty on every citizen of India to protect the environment,” where “environment” refers to natural features, including lakes, rivers, forests, and wildlife.

The demand for an increase in food production has scientists using a wide variety of strategies, including the use of current science, the development of new crop categories, and the use of novel seeds. Scientists may manage environmental protection in an effective manner, including human and animal health, biosafety, and the enhancement of crop output. It is essential to balance protecting agricultural biodiversity with the needs of local farmers and their communities. A regulatory mechanism is essential to enforce the seed industry’s other obligations so that farmers are not exploited. The breeder’s, foundation, registered, and certified seed requirements are mandated by Indian law. The Protection of Plant Varieties and Farmers' Rights Act, 2001 (PPVFR Act) mandated the conservation, gathering, exploration, characterisation, and evaluation of plant genetic resources for the purpose of ensuring the nation's food and nutritional security.

The Seed Act of 1966 is a foundational law that governs the production, distribution, and sale of seeds in India. It aims to ensure the availability of quality seeds to farmers and regulate the seed industry. The Seed Rules of 1968 provide detailed regulations and procedures under the Seed Act of 1966. They specify the standards and requirements for seed certification, labeling, and packaging. The Seed (Control) Order of 1983 is likely an amendment or additional order related to the Seed Act. It might provide further control measures and guidelines for the seed industry.

1. Plants, Fruits & Seeds (Regulation of Import into India), 1989: This regulation focuses on the importation of plants, fruits, and seeds into India. It likely includes measures to ensure that imported materials meet certain quality and safety standards.
2. PPV & FR Act (2001): The Protection of Plant Varieties and Farmers' Rights Act of 2001 (PPV & FR Act) is designed to protect the rights of plant breeders and farmers. It includes provisions related to the registration and protection of new plant varieties.
3. Essential Commodities Act, containing Seeds (1955): The Essential Commodities Act of 1955 empowers the government to control the production, supply, and distribution of essential commodities. This may include seeds, ensuring their availability and preventing hoarding.
4. National Seed Policy (2002): The National Seed Policy of 2002 outlines the government's approach and objectives regarding the seed sector. It likely includes strategies for promoting seed quality, availability, and research and development.
5. Seed Bill (2004): The Seed Bill of 2004 is a legislative proposal that may aim to amend or update existing seed laws. Bills are often introduced to address emerging issues or to modernize regulatory frameworks.
6. New Policy on Seed Development (1988): This policy likely represents an update or new direction in seed development strategies introduced in 1988, emphasizing the government's approach to seed-related issues.

Under the Seed Act of 1966, a regulated standard has been established for the germination and purity of seed. Although the Seeds (Control) Order, 1983, was responsible for enforcing the quality restriction of seeds, the Essential Commodity Act, 1955, provided additional help to farmers on the condition that seeds be considered an essential commodity. A licence is required in order to engage in the business of selling, exporting, and importing seeds, as stated in the Rule. This legislation applies to any individual, organisation, or firm.

NBPGR is the authorised agency to certify the cargo and permit it to be subject to the authorisation under conditions as stated by RCGM. IBCs have the capability of interstate shipping with the knowledge of RCGM in accordance with the Plant Quarantine (Regulation of Import into India) Order, 2003 with the subject to labelling, packaging, and shipment requirements. IBC is responsible for carrying out the instruction given by the Government of India and does so accordingly. The importation of GMOs and LMOs for R&D purposes was mandated by Notification No.

2(re-2006) I 2004-2009, which introduced the Biosafety Protocol in Chapter 2 of the 2003 order. The scientist or research organisation makes a clear reference or declaration in the consignments that the product is genetically modified or derived from living modified organisms (GMOs or LMOs).

The Foreign Trade (Development and Regulation) Act, 1992, is a significant piece of legislation in India that aims to provide the development and regulation of foreign trade. It may cover various aspects related to imports and exports, trade policies, and regulatory frameworks. The punitive provisions within the Act likely specify the penalties or consequences for individuals or entities that contravene the provisions of the Foreign Trade Act. It's mentioned that the punitive provisions have been in effect since July 6, 2006. This date indicates when the specific legal measures and penalties related to contraventions became applicable. There's a reference to scientists and researchers, suggesting that they have specific responsibilities under the Foreign Trade Act.

The information provided does not specify the exact nature of these responsibilities, but it mentions the expectation that scientists and researchers should have a clear understanding of the necessary approvals from Biosafety. Biosafety typically refers to the measures and precautions taken to prevent the unintentional release of genetically modified organisms (GMOs) and to protect human health and the environment. Scientists and researchers involved in activities related to biotechnology or genetically modified organisms might be required to obtain approvals from Biosafety authorities to ensure compliance with safety and environmental regulations.

29.17.1 Category I: Involving Routine R-DNA Research

The research involves the use of DNA from non-pathogenic or non-infectious viral, bacterial, or fungal organisms with the intention of manipulating or inserting it, cloning it, or giving it expression in higher organisms like *Escherichia coli*. Confirmation that the final product, or the experimental end product, is safe for humans and the environment must be obtained before moving forward. As a consequence of this, there is no rule that is enforced on any fundamental necessity, such as the BSL category.

29.17.2 Category II: Involving Routine R-DNA Research Obtained from Pathogenic Organisms

This is comparable to Category I, with the exception that the DNA was extracted from potentially infectious or pathogenic species, but the final outcome of the manipulation was not harmful. A level II or BSL II containment facility was necessary for such an experiment, and the final product was determined not to be contagious or pathogenic.

29.17.3 Category III: Involving Pathogenic R-DNA Research

This class of microorganisms is hazardous, and some of them may even be pathogenic, which means they could be hazardous to human health or the environment. Experiments involve working with DNA, which at the time of its alteration in the lab could represent a health risk to human participants in the form of a disease or an infectious agent. There is a comparable probability that the disease will spread through the air as there is that it will spread through a vector. Experiments that fall into this category include things like cloning antibiotic resistance genes into pathogenic organisms, studying mutant organisms, conducting infectious research, and transfecting oncogenes, among others. In order to carry out studies of this nature, several mandates have been set, such as the required containment levels III and IV, safety, etc.

29.18 UNDERSTANDING THE SACREDNESS OF INDIAN CONSTITUENTS FROM A LEGAL STANDPOINT

The Central Government provided security against hazardous chemicals, accidents, and environmental damage and enforced the remedial measures by Article 25 of the EPA Act, although the same legislation imposes the remedial measures of the hazardous substance handling. Gene technology is defined as the use of cell hybridisation, cloning, or gene manipulation of the heritable material, according to clause rule 3 (3) of Rule 3, and this technique is regulated by rule 2 (3) of Rule 2.

This action demonstrates the manipulation of inheritable material because it is the LMO that is used to format agricultural products, foodstuff items, and linked items that contain GMOs. The restrictions do not only apply to those working in the food industry, but they also apply to pharmaceutical products and services that make use of LMOs. GEAC and RCGM formulated a set of safety guidelines for research involving GMs, vaccines, and diagnostics where the r-DNA technology is used in 1998. This guideline was not only limited to research but also extended to the transportation, release, and safety aspect of GMO plants, including import and export. It was enforced by the DBT, Government of India, and the necessary preparations are made.

BIBLIOGRAPHY

Bøhn T, Cuhra M, Traavik T, Sanden M, Fagan J. Compositional Differences in Soybeans on the Market: Glyphosate Accumulates in Roundup Ready GM Soybeans. Food Chemistry 2014, 153: 207–215.

GM Soybeans Are No More Allergenic Than Conventional Soybeans. Available from: http://academicsreview.org/reviewed-content/genetic-roulette/section-3/3-1-gm-soybeans-and-allergens/. Accessed March 2020.

Guidelines and Handbook for Institutional Biosafety Committees (IBCs) Department of Biotechnology, Ministry of Science & Technology Biotech Consortium India Limited, New Delhi Second Revised Edition 2011. Available from: https://biosafety.icar.gov.in/wp-content/uploads/2015/05/IBCs_Guidelines_Handbook.pdf.

Huda, J. An Examination of Policy Narratives in Agricultural Biotechnology Policy in India. *World Affairs* 2018, 181(1): 42–68. doi: 10.1177/0043820018783046.

Indian Council of Agricultural Research Biosafety Portal. Available from: https://biosafety.icar.gov.in/. Accessed March 2020.

Mario DL. Effects of Soy Phytoestrogens Genistein and Daidzein on Breast Cancer Growth. *The Annals of Pharmacotherapy* 2001: Sep; 35(9): 1118–21.

Microbial Diversity and the 1992 Biodiversity Convention. *Biodiversity and Conservation* 1996, 5: 473–491. doi: 10.1007/BF00056392.

National Guidelines for Stem Cell Research. 2017. Indian Council of Medical Research & Department of Biotechnology Published by the Division of Publication and Information on Behalf of the Secretary DHR & DG, ICMR, New Delhi.

Nordlee JA, Taylor SL, Townsend JA, Thomas LA, Bush RK. Identification of a Brazil-Nut Allergen in Transgenic Soybeans. *The New England Journal of Medicine* 1996, 334: 688–692.

Palitha TBK. Clare S. The Convention on Biological Diversity: Bridging the Gap Between Conservation and Development. *RECIL* 1992, 1: 278–288.

Singh G, Budhwar V, Choudhury M, Singh S. Regulatory of Regulation on Genetically Modified Microorganism and Their Relation Bioterrorism in India Bull. *Journal of Pharmaceutical Sciences* 2022, 4: 565–584.

The Greenpeace Study Was Conducted in Dharwad, Haveri, and Raichur districts of Karnataka. Source: 'Bt Cotton: Future Imperfect. 13 April 2003. Available from: http://www.financialexpress.com/fe. Accessed March 2020.

Tiwari A., Tikoo SK., Angadi SP, Kadaru SB, Ajanahalli SR, Rao MJV. *Market-Driven Plant Breeding for Practicing Breeders*. Singapore: Spinger Nature, 2022.

30 Orphan Drugs and Regulatory Approval

30.1 INTRODUCTION

Terms like "rare" diseases, where there is limited or no therapy or specialised therapy, gave rise to the birth of orphan drugs. There are approximately 7,000 rare diseases and their total incidence is less than 6–8%, and virtually no company will produce medicine for treatment of such diseases because they would be non-profitable, as they would benefit such small numbers in the population. Orphan pharmaceuticals are medical substances used for the purpose of diagnosing, preventing, or treating rare conditions that provide a substantial risk to life or result in severe impairment.

After implementation of the Kefauver-Harris amendment (1962) in the USA, the drug discovery process became costlier to prove their therapeutic efficacy as well as their safety. Thus, drug companies shifted research and development towards the treatment of common diseases which affect larger populations, making such drugs profitable. This shifting research direction means that the rare or orphan diseases like Cohn's disease and Hansen's disease have little or no drug treatments.

In the late 1970s and early 1980s, understanding the burden of co-morbidity and mortality and the greater recognition of the number of people suffering from such rare diseases, the USA formed the National Organization for Rare Disorders (NORD) in 1982. The efforts of NORD and the pressure from many non-governmental organisations (NGOs) and families of sufferers from rare diseases, the Act passed into law as the Orphan Drug Act (ODA) in 1983.

30.2 ORPHAN DRUG POLICY IN INDIA

Many developing countries, including India, have no standard definition of rare diseases and their prevalence. Because of limited epidemiological data on rare diseases, the burden of morbidity and mortality associated with rare disease could not be determined. However, in India, about 5–8% of the population, corresponding to 80–100 million people, are suffering from rare diseases, mostly genetic in nature, including Wilson disease, Norrie disease, leishmaniasis, cystic fibrosis, and arthrogryposis. The rare diseases that affect the highest numbers of Indians include Alpha-1 antitrypsin deficiency, Graves' disease, and Parkinson's disease, where only limited treatment is available.

The National Policy for Treatment of Rare Diseases (NPTRD) of India, formed in 2017 under the directive of the High Court of Delhi in the case of Mohd. Kalim v. Employees State Insurance Corporation & OR's (W.P.(C) 8445/2014) ("Mohd. Kalim

DOI: 10.1201/9781003397854-14

Case"). Furthermore, in the petition of Mohd. Ahmed (Minor) v. Union of India & OR's W.P.(C) No. 7279 of 2013 ("Mohd. Ahmed Case"), the Delhi High Court directed the Delhi Government to provide the Mohd. Ahmed's cost of therapy treatment for Gaucher disease, which is expensive, while the petitioner's father is a rickshaw puller. It is noteworthy to add that, during the proceedings of a case pertaining to a rare disease in the Delhi High Court on November 30th, the constitutional duty of the state to guarantee availability of life-saving medications was emphasised. Consequently, the court issued an order for the formation of the National. Legal challenges prompted the suspension of actions by the NPTRD, leading to a re-evaluation of drug R&D policies for rare diseases. The lack of consultation during the formation of NPTRD and the subsequent involvement of the Health Ministry and National Health Mission indicate a shift in the governance and implementation of policies related to the treatment of rare diseases.

The petitioner also pointed out that the regulation of the New Drugs and Clinical Trial Rules, 2019 ("New Drugs & CT Rules") constrained the CDSCO from allowing the entry of any medicine from foreign countries without conducting local clinical trials. The terms "orphan drugs" or "orphan diseases" are applicable when the drug's use is for the treatment of fewer than two lakh people (200,000–400,000 people) in India and included 300 diseases in NPTRD which seeks to assist patients who are undergoing treatment for rare diseases. WHO defines a rare disease as a disease or condition with a disorder affecting ≤1/1,000 of the population whereas the European Union limited the number to <1/2,000 and the FDA limited it to <200,000 individuals at a single time point.

30.3 LIMITATION AND UNAVAILABILITY OF ORPHAN DRUGS

30.3.1 Unavailability of Treatment

Despite progress on drug discovery, the orphan drug sector is badly neglected as successful or safe treatments are not available for most of the orphan diseases. Advances in radiology, molecular biology, or pathology even after the diagnosis of the disease still mean that treatments are unavailable. Non-specific treatment or nonapproved therapeutics for specific treatments and a few therapies for ≤ 300 orphan diseases are available, although more than 6,000 rare diseases exist. Moreover, any developed orphan drugs are not free-access-to-all because of strict regulation and their high cost.

30.3.2 Costly Treatments

Orphan drugs are not economic because the drug market is small; to recoup the costs of research and development and achieve a profit, most pharmaceutical companies charge high prices. Many orphan medicines are costly like Kalydeco (ivacaftor) for treatment of cystic fibrosis and the monoclonal antibody eculizumab for treatment of typical haemolytic uraemic syndrome (aHUS), which are priced at £189,000 and £340,000 per patient per year, respectively. The high cost of the medicine means that it could not be distributed by the Government.

30.4 GOVERNMENT CALL FOR CONTROLLING THE PRICES OF ORPHAN DRUGS

The Government of India has taken significant action through legislation for controlling the price of orphan drugs to reduce treatment costs. Legislation like the Orphan Drug Act (ODA) extended the incentives to encourage the development of orphan drugs to treat rare diseases. The incentives included protection of exclusive rights for six to seven years and protection from the import of orphan drugs. This is a reason that the orphan drug sector is free from fear of competition and increased prices. Furthermore, despite initial reluctance, there has been a significant positive shift in the landscape for orphan drugs. The increased market share, availability of drugs, and a substantial rise in orphan drug designations suggest a more supportive and encouraging environment for addressing rare diseases within the pharmaceutical and healthcare industries.

Some orphan drugs may not offer a complete cure for rare diseases, but their financial success in the market is notable. The high market turnover and cost of these drugs reflect the economic viability of developing treatments for rare diseases, despite the challenges associated with limited patient populations. The substantial increase in the market share of the orphan drug sector in 2020 further underscores its growing importance in the pharmaceutical industry.

Another important issue that many old or off-label drugs use a tag of "orphan drugs" status even if they have not demonstrated any scientific validation. An inexpensive off-patent drug, approved for the treatment of some other diseases, but used for "off-label" treatment for an orphan disease, increased its marketability considerably. After being endorsed with the tag of orphan drug, it can enjoy exclusive marketability for seven to ten years in the USA like the off-label molecule imatinib used to treat chronic myeloid leukaemia and priced at USD 100,000 a year per patient in developed countries. On the other hand, India controls the exorbitant prices by allowing generic manufacturers to manufacture generic drugs, thus supplying this drug at lower prices. Furthermore, by encouraging generic drugs and implementing the price control order, the exorbitant prices of any drug are controlled. The Indian Government encourages local drug manufacture, public sector undertakings (PSU for the manufacture of generic drugs affordable to common people for the treatment of rare diseases.

30.5 INCREASED OPPORTUNITIES FOR FURTHER DRUG DEVELOPMENT FROM ORPHAN DRUGS

Many orphan drugs give a clue for future drug development. Chenofalk (chenodeoxycholic acid), an off-label drug used for low-cost treatment of hypo-bile acid syndrome; in 2008, the drug manufacturer Leadiant obtained the rights to the molecule, formulated its own iteration, and renamed it CDCA Leadiant. In a strategic move in 2014, the company successfully persuaded the European Union to designate its particular iteration as an "orphan drug," granting Leadiant exclusive marketing privileges for a period of ten years, and immediately the price per patient for a course of treatment increased from €500 per annum to €150,000 for a year's treatment. A drug like Daraprim was used for treatment of toxoplasmosis infection in people with HIV infection, and the mother company Turing Pharmaceuticals, owned by the infamous Martin Shkreli, increased the unit price from US$14 to US$750.

30.6 CHALLENGES OF THE DEVELOPMENT FOR AN ORPHAN DRUG IN INDIA

30.6.1 Lack of Epidemiological Data

The concentration of rare disease treatment in tertiary care hospitals in metropolitan cities doesn't always translate to comprehensive awareness among medical staff. Limited awareness contributes to poor epidemiological data, hindering efforts to understand and address rare diseases effectively. There is a need for improved data collection, increased awareness, and specialized training for healthcare professionals to better manage rare diseases despite their low frequency.

30.6.2 Diagnosis of Rare Diseases

Of the rare disease, ≥ 80% are caused by genetic abnormalities, and there is a poor diagnosis system, making it a considerable challenge to identify the demographic pattern of the disease. It is difficult to diagnose and takes several years because of the limitations of established testing procedures or the unavailability of diagnostic facilities. Genetic screening related to orphan diseases is time consuming and expensive.

Most physicians have limited awareness of the testing procedure and genetic testing, which is an expensive and time-consuming process. In the US, diagnosis of orphan diseases takes an average of 7.6 years, compared with 5.6 years in the UK. Rare diseases are poorly understood by both the general population and the medical community and sometimes misdiagnoses increase the suffering of the patients and delay orphan drug development.

30.6.3 Challenges in Research and Development

The development of orphan drugs has many challenges. First, the limited and fundamental knowledge of the disease pattern delays the orphan drug development. Second, the limited number of patients, which restricts the scope of clinical trials which are usually done in large populations. Third, the safety and quality of the drugs or diagnostic tools for an orphan disease is another issue which needs to be approved before the drug is in use.

30.7 REGULATION OF ORPHAN DRUGS IN THE USA

30.7.1 Evolution of the Orphan Drug Act (ODA)

Orphan drugs have a limited market and hence limited profit. The FD & C Act, 1962 and amendment of orphan drugs legislation had not made a significant impact on the orphan drug sector and only four drugs were approved in 1965. In 1992, legislation noted that most pharmaceutical company associated with drug development are focused on maximising profits to recoup their R and D costs.

Eventually, advocacy for the patients by many NGOs and the National Organization for Rare Disorders (NORD) criticised the public policy in the early 1980s. The Bayh-Dole Act (PL No. 96-517, 1984) was implemented in 1980 and provisioned special assistance from the government to the pharmaceutical companies for development of orphan drugs and established the Orphan Drug Act in 1983.

30.7.2 The Orphan Drug Act (ODA) of 1983 in the USA

The Act was enacted with the goal of increasing orphan drug development; before the Act, only a few orphan drug molecules had been approved. In response to the Act, many drugs were re-approved as orphan drugs to attract market share. In 1997, Congress enforced a 50% tax waiver to Research and Development costs for orphan drug developer and seven years exclusivity for sale, which were definitely beneficial to the pharmaceutical companies to reduce costs and increase the returns from orphan drugs. The exclusivity of the licence led to monopoly of the selling of the drug without the fear of market competition, which led to disproportionately high prices of the drugs. Most people could not afford such prices for the orphan drugs. Before 1985, orphan drugs could not be patented when the seven years' exclusivity clause expired but deletion of certain clauses in 1985 led to patentability of orphan drugs. Since certain biotech medications have difficulty getting patents, the orphan drug exclusivity designation was only granted to medications that were not patented. Market exclusivity became a difficult situation for the general population and expired before conclusions were reached about the drug's efficacy. Thus, in 2013, the ODA was enacted with limited exclusivity for the orphan drug.

30.8 REGULATION OF ORPHAN DRUGS IN INDIA

An "orphan drug" is defined as a drug that can be used to treat a patient populations of not more than 5 lakh persons in India. More than 30 million Indians suffer from orphan diseases and India is one of the most lucrative global markets for orphan drugs. Many drugs have been approved as orphan drugs. The USFDA approved about 400 US orphan drugs, while the EMA approved more than 90 drugs which are not available in India. Access to Indian orphan drugs is poor because of the lack of innovation, high drug costs, stringent drug regulations, and fewer drug approvals. Many orphan diseases have been reported in India, like leishmaniasis, cystic fibrosis, Wilson disease, arthrogryposis, and Norrie disease, etc. The Organisation for Rare Diseases India (ORDI) was established in February 2014, and many other related NGOs have been established like the Foundation for Research on Rare Diseases and Disorders, Down Syndrome Federation of India, Alzheimer's and Related Disorders Society of India, and the Haemophilia Federation of India advocate for increased research, availability, and cost-effectiveness of orphan drugs. Currently, no regulations are available exclusively for orphan drug and the scarcity of regulation of orphan drugs definitely affects the Indian drug market.

30.9 REGULATORY AND APPROVAL PROCESS FOR ORPHAN DRUGS IN INDIA

Orphan drugs receive special considerations, including a fast-track approval process, fee waivers for clinical trial filings, and an expeditious review process that aims to grant approval within three years. These measures are in place to facilitate the development and availability of treatments for rare diseases, acknowledging the importance of addressing the unmet medical needs of patients with these conditions. The special provisions for the approval of orphan drugs are as follows: -

1. The Directive 12-01/14-DC pt. 47, dated July 3, 2014, provisioned the waiver of clinical trials for orphan drugs where no alternative therapy is available, and the drug established is considered safe or is used by another country.

   Example: Afatinib is the drug treatment of choice for treatment of advanced or metastatic non-small cell lung cancer with epidermal growth factor receptor mutation, and is regarded as an orphan drug. The drug was approved on the basis of safety data on a very small population (47 patients).

   Obinutuzumab in combination with chorambucil is a treatment for untreated chronic lymphocytic leukaemia (an orphan disease) and is approved in many countries, like the US, Australia, and Sweden. The drug was approved by CLA without the need for a local clinical trial.
2. Accelerated approval process of orphan drugs and the fee waiver for filing a clinical trial.
3. Sponsor company can apply for an expeditious review process after establishing the safety of the drug and even when not all clinical trial phases had been completed.
4. Waiver of local clinical study and Phase IV on satisfaction of the CLA.
5. Accelerated approval post-marketing trials is required for validating anticipated clinical benefits. Example: Aflibercep is used for treatment of second-line metastatic colon cancer and such therapy is not available in India. The drug was approved to be imported without the requirement of local clinical trials, on condition that Phase IV trial, i.e., post marketing surveillance data are required for two years.
6. The approval procedure is similar to new drug development, except as stated

30.10 REGULATORY AND APPROVAL PROCESS OF ORPHAN DRUGS IN THE EUROPEAN UNION (EU)

Orphan drug regulatory guidelines in the EU were enforced in December 1999 by the Regulation (EC) No. 141/2000. According to the regulation, a dedicated committee was formed with regard to Orphan Medicinal Products. Competent persons were appointed by the European member states and patient associations and assigned to examine the application and approval of orphan drugs. The committee included patient representatives to ensure, according to Directive 141/2000 EU Regelation, that the suffering patients are equally eligible to receive the same treatment as normal patients. Enforcement of the regulation of Directive 141/2000 motivated the manufacturer to develop orphan drugs by the use of government incentives. The Committee on Orphan Medicinal Products (COMP) operates under the umbrella of the European Medicines Evaluation Agency (EMEA) with 28 members from each state of union, plus three members being nominated by the European Commission along with three representatives of patient associations. Like the USA and India, the EU also encourages the development and price discounting of orphan drugs.

1. The EU provides procedural assistance to pharmaceutical companies manufacturing orphan drugs.
2. The EU authorises centralised marketing.
3. Exclusivity of market rights for ten years
4. National incentives to the company from the European Commission.
5. Application fee exemptions/discounts like, for example, pre-authorisation inspections and discounted fee for marketing authorisation for new medicinal products fee.
6. Post authorisation and protocol assistance activities, including full reduction for the annual fee.

A total of 208 orphan medicines have been approved up to 2020, among which some drugs have been withdrawn on the grounds of safety or the EU did not consider them to be orphan drugs, rather than nutritional supplements, dietary products, or medical devices.

BIBLIOGRAPHY

Davis H, Smith J. Orphan Drug Law Matures into Medical Mainstay. *International Journal of Rare Disorder Research* 1999, 33: 11–16.

File No: 12-01/14-DC pt. 47. July 3, 2014. Waiver of Clinical Trial in Indian Population for Approval of New Drugs Regarding, Central Drugs Standard Control Organization Directorate General of Health Services, Ministry of Health and Family Welfare, Government of India. Available from: http://www.cdsco.nic.in/writereaddata/oo7.pdf. Accessed 22 September 2017.

Fiona M, Morton S. The Problems of Price Control. Cato Review of Business and Government. Available from: https://www.cato.org/publications/commentary/problems-price-controls. Accessed 20 March 2021.

Gajra BB, Limbachiya S. Absence of Regulations for Orphan Drugs in India: Ignorance of the Government. 2015. Available from: https://aapsblog.aaps.org/2015/05/13/absence-ofregulations-for-orphan-drugs-in-india-ignorance-ofthe-government. Accessed 24 March 2021.

Global Pharma Looks to India: Prospects for Growth. Available from: https://www.pwc.com/gx/en/pharma-life-sciences/pdf/global-pharma-looks-to-india-final.pdf. Accessed 20 March 2021.

Kesselheim AS. Innovation and the Orphan Drug Act 1983–2009. *Regulatory and Clinical Characteristics of Approved Orphan Drugs* 2015: 1–12.

Minutes of the Meeting. Meeting of Pharma Stakeholders with DCG (I) to Explore the Possibilities of Providing Cheaper Medicines, Therapies for Treatment of Rare Disease. 2016. Available from: http://www.cdsco.nic.in/writereaddata/Minutes%20Of%20Meeting%20Stakeholders%2004_05_2016.pdf. Accessed 24 March 2021.

National Policy on Treatment of Rare Diseases. Available from: https://mohfw.gov.in/sites/default/files/Rare%20Diseases%20Policy%20FINAL.pdf. Accessed 20 March 2021.

Nishith Desai Associates. Patented New Drugs and Orphan Drugs Out of Price Control in India. Mumbai, 2019. Available from: http://www.nishithdesai.com/information/news-storage/news-details/article/patented-new-drugs-and-orphan-drugs-out-of-price-control-in-india.html. Accessed 20 March 2021.

Nishith Desai Associates. Orphan Drugs & Rare Diseases: India, Mumbai, 2020. Available from: Nishith Desai & Associates / Indiahttps://pharmaboardroom.com/legal-articles/orphan-drugs-rare-diseases-india/. Accessed 24 March 2021.

Pharmaceuticals Export Promotion Council of India. Available from: http://www.pharmexcil.com/content/search/orphan. Accessed 24 March 2021.

Pradhan Mantri Jan Arogya Yojana. Available from: https://www.pmjay.gov.in/about-pmjay. Accessed 20 March 2021.

Rare Diseases: Common Issues in Drug Development. Guidance for Industry Rare Diseases. August 2015. Available from: http://www.fda.gov/downloads/Drugs/GuidanceComplianceRegulatoryInformation/Guidances/UCM4584 85.pdf. Accessed 24 March 2021.

Reddy DS, Pramodkumar TM, Reddy Y, Sirisha K. Orphan Regulations for Orphan Drug Development in India. *Asian Journal of Pharmaceutics* 2014, 8: 130–132.

Sharma A, Jacob A, Tandon M, Kumar D. Orphan Drug: Development Trends and Strategies. *Journal of Pharmacy and Bioallied Sciences* 2010, 2: 290–299.

31 Regulatory Approval Process of *In-vitro* Diagnostics

31.1 INTRODUCTION

In India, *in vitro* diagnostic kits and reagents are subject to the regulations laid out in the Drugs and Cosmetics Act of 1940 and the Drugs and Cosmetics Rules of 1945. In India, the Ministry of Health and Family Welfare, which is overseen by the Drug Controller General of India, is in charge of ensuring that IVDs adhere to standards on their efficacy, quality control, and safety.

The Drugs and Cosmetic Act of 1940 defines an *in vitro* diagnostic device (IVD) as a medical device, either single or in combination, which the manufacturer intends to be used for the *in vitro* examination of specimens derived from human bodies with the primary goal of providing data for compatibility, monitoring, or diagnostic purposes. This definition applies whether the IVD is used by itself or in combination with other medical devices.

Legitimately all *in vitro* diagnostic devices have been intended to be used outside of human or animal bodies for the purpose of diagnosing any disease or condition in human beings or animals that is included in clause (b) subclause (i) of Section 3 of the Drugs and Cosmetics Act, 1940. This clause specifies the diseases and disorders that can be diagnosed using IVDs. IVDs are periodically registered as a device in accordance with subclause (iv) of clause (b) of Section 3 of the Drugs and Cosmetics Act, 1940. People should not confuse the two types of diagnostic kits categorised by CDSCO as "Notified Diagnostic Assay" and "Non-notified Diagnostic Assay" and which required a licence in order to be imported into India or sold there. Malaria, tuberculosis, dengue, typhoid, chikungunya, syphilis, cancer markers, blood glucose test strips, glucose reagents, and other items are examples of non-notified *in-vitro* diagnostic kits. Notified diagnosis assays include detection kits for HIV, HBsAg, HCV, and blood groups.

31.2 REGULATION OF IMPORTATION OF DIAGNOSTIC KITS TO INDIA

The Drugs and Cosmetics Act and Rules cover import of *in vitro* diagnostic kits as well as covering other aspects of the industry. According to the Drugs and Cosmetics Act and Rules, an import licence is necessary for any drug that is either not specified in Schedule X. (Figure 31.1):

DOI: 10.1201/9781003397854-15

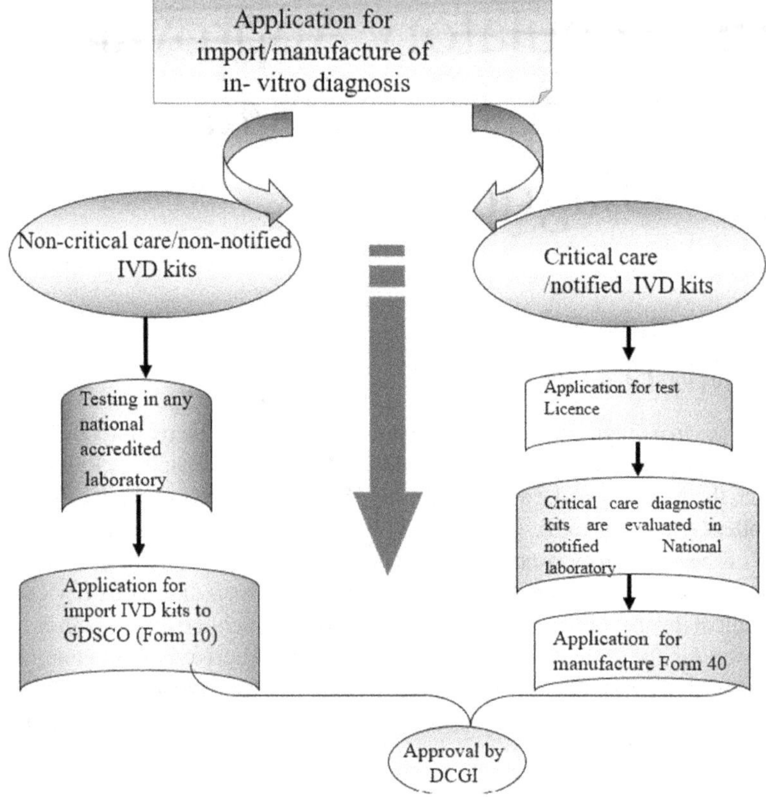

FIGURE 31.1 Importing of *in-vitro* diagnostics in India.

31.3 INDIGENOUS MANUFACTURING OF DIAGNOSTIC KITS

The domestic production of IVD kits is one of the most difficult challenges that must be overcome. Unfavourable conditions, an absence of understanding regarding regulatory requirements, and the scientists involved all contribute to the failure of the ideas. India's *in vitro* diagnostic technologies are limited and underdeveloped. Because of a lack of understanding of self-reliance, increasing competence gaps, a delay in technology indigenisation, and dependence on imports, the indigenous *in vitro* kit industry has not flourished.

Over 75% of the diagnostic tools used in medicine come from abroad, and the majority of these tests are quite expensive. It is often the common people who bear the financial burden of tests that are not widely used. Limited funding is allocated to research and development, despite India's need for diagnostic kits that are straightforward, of high quality, and reasonably priced, resulting from innovation and research.

The CDSCO has jurisdiction over IVD kits made in the country since they are under the purview of the Drugs and Cosmetics Act. In order to gain registration for an IVD kit with the CDSCO, the manufacturer must submit documentation detailing the production process, research and development, stability data, testing protocols

TABLE 31.1
Specific Regulations

21(d)	Free Sales Certificate from the country of origin is required in order to register for business in India.
24(i)	The applicant must possess a valid wholesale, retail, stock, or distribution license in India.
24(ii)	A signed agreement from the manufacturer and an undertaking in Form 9.
24(iii)	As of the amendment that took effect in 2005, it is not necessary to get an import licence in order to bring in non-notified diagnostic kits.
24 (A)	Power of attorney (POA) in the favour of under loan to startup manufacturing by Indian agents which has been legally attested by the Indian Embassy of the concerned nation.
25	The same legitimate manufacturer also makes these other products, although they make them in a different factory.
26(iii)	Sampling at random and testing of imported *in vitro* diagnostics for compliance with import in preparation for testing in CDL
26(vi)	Retail invoices
27A/28A	Verification of the registration and import licence's validity.
31	In order to meet the country's shelf life requirements, 60% of all products must be imported to India.
38	Statement regarding drugs and *in vitro* diagnostics that are imported
65	Conditions are required to fulfil to get registration for storage, distribution, and sale of the IVD kits.
109(A)	Labelling

for raw materials and completed products, in-house specifications, labelling details, and evaluation reports.

31.4 THE REQUIREMENT OF IVD KITS AND QUALITATIVE PARAMETERS

Qualitative parameters of ID kits are well defined and according to the ISO or IS protocol usually followed for the testing of the IVD kits which are described below.

31.4 REGULATORY PROCEDURE FOR APPROVAL OF THE IVD KITS

31.4.1 Step 1: First, the developed product needs to undergo validation, which involves demonstrating that it is effective in accordance with either the ISO standards or the regulatory guidelines that are recognized in India.

31.4.2 Step 2: Requires applicants to provide the required documentation to the DCGI/CDSCO including a detailed description of their facilities and dossiers for their products.

31.4.3 Step 3: Once the requirements of the DCGI have been met, the indenter is needed to deliver the three test batches to the DCGI/CDSCO, and the DCGI/CDSCO will then send a sample to the NIB, Noida, and NICD in New Delhi in order to validate the claim.

31.4.4 Step 4: Included data on accelerated stability as well as real-time stability, which necessitated the submission of the DCGI/CDSCO. The consideration takes into account IVD kits that have been stable for at least a year.

TABLE 31.2
IVD Kits Protocol as per ISO

Protocol	Category
ISO 23640:2011	Evaluation of the stability of *in-vitro* diagnostic medical equipment, such as reagents, calibrators, control materials, diluents, and buffers, as well as reagent kits
ISO 23640:2011	Evaluation of the stability of *in-vitro* diagnostic medical devices, also referred to as IVD reagents, comprising reagents, calibrators, control materials, diluents, buffers, and reagent kits. *In-vitro* diagnostic medical equipment, as well as instruments for measuring quantities present in samples of biological origin.
ISO 15193:2009	This study focuses on using *in-vitro* diagnostic medical equipment for the purpose of measuring various parameters within biological samples.
ISO15198:2004	Validation and quality control of *in-vitro* diagnostic medical equipment
ISO 16256:2012	Reference technique and *in-vitro* diagnostic testing system for antimicrobial compounds against infectious diseases caused by yeast and fungi.
ISO/TS 17822-1: 2014	The protocol for a qualitative *in-vitro* evaluation based on nucleic acids, including the detection and identification of the pathogens. Part I: Provide the General Requirements, Terminologies, and Definitions.
ISO 18113-1:2009	Manufacturer-provided information pertaining to the labelling of the product. Part 1: Terminology, Diagnosis, and General Requirements.
ISO 18153:2003	*In-vitro* diagnostic medical equipment, including the reagents to determine the values of the catalytic concentration of enzymes, as well as allocated calibrators and control material.
ISO 19001:2013	Medical instruments for *in-vitro* diagnosis, including information about the reagents used in *in-vitro* staining, can be found in the field of biology.
ISO/CD:20186-1	Molecular *in-vitro* diagnostic tests, including specifics for the preliminary investigation of cellular RNA and blood samples. Part I: The Total Amount of RNA Extracted from Individual Cells.
ISO/CD: 20186-2	Molecular *in-vitro* diagnostic tests, including specifications for preliminary screenings of blood and genomic DNA. First Section: DNA from Isolated Genomes
ISO/CD:20186-3	Molecular in-vitro diagnostic tests, comprising particular protocols for the preliminary evaluation of blood and RNA from cells Part III: Isolated Circulating Cell-Free DNA from Plasma
ISO/DTS:20658	The protocol that must be followed during a medical laboratory examination, comprising the mandated steps of sample collection, transportation, receipt, and management.
ISO:20776-1:2006	Evaluating the effectiveness of antimicrobial susceptibility test devices and assessing the susceptibility of infectious agents Diagnostic test systems for *in-vitro* diagnosis and clinical laboratory testing and *in-vitro* diagnostic test methods and clinical laboratory testing Part 1: Reference technique for assessing the *in-vitro* effectiveness of antimicrobial medicines against aerobic bacteria capable of fast growth that are associated with infectious illnesses

(*Continued*)

TABLE 31.2 (CONTINUED)
IVD Kits Protocol as per ISO

Protocol	Category
ISO/NP:20776-1:2006	Testing how resistant infectious agents are to antibiotics and reviewing how well antimicrobial sensitivity test devices work and *in-vitro* diagnostic test methods and clinical laboratory tests testing to see how susceptible contagious agents Part II: Antimicrobial Susceptibility Test Device Performance Evaluation
ISO:20776-2:2007	Testing carried out in clinical laboratories and in vitro diagnostic testing systems includes the testing of infectious pathogens for their sensitivity to antimicrobials and the evaluation of the efficacy of antimicrobial susceptibility test equipment. Part II: Antimicrobial Susceptibility Test Device Performance Evaluation
ISO/NP: 20916	Good practice for studying IVD for clinical effectiveness.
ISO/NP:21474	Multiplex Molecular Testing: IVD Kit Requirements and Terminology
ISO: 18113-2	*In-vitro* diagnostic (IVD) reagents, calibrators, and control materials are required to come with accompanying labels and instructions for use.
ISO: 18113-3	Labels and operating instructions must be included with every IVD device as a required part of the packaging.
ISO: 18113-4	*In-vitro* diagnostic (IVD) reagents, calibrators, and control materials for self-testing are required to come with accompanying labels and instructions for use.
ISO: 18113-5	Prerequisites for the labels and operating instructions that must be included with IVD devices that are used for self-testing

31.4.5 Step 5: The indenter is needed to submit an application for a manufacturing licence, which will then be inspected by a joint inspection team comprised of representatives from the respective state and DCGI/CDSCO authorities.

31.4.6 Step 6: The licence will be issued once all requirements have been met (Figure 31.2)

31.5 IMPORTING OF IVD KITS/REAGENTS TO INDIA

In order to obtain an import licence and a registration Form 10, one must comply with the Drugs and Cosmetics Act, 1940, and the Rules of 1945. In addition, the application must meet the necessary criteria before repackaging or manufacturing IVD kits. Certificate of Registration with Schedules D I and D II issued by Section 41. There must be full conformance between the Plant Master File (PMF) and the Device Master File (DMF). In addition to the test licence, the product number, lot number, batch number, testing principle, testing technique, repeatability, sensitivity, positive predictive value, negative predictive value, and the results of the tests should all be included in the reports detailing the results of the tests and evaluations. Importation of IVD kits in modest quantities is permitted with a test licence (Form 11), and applications are submitted using Form 12. The commercial use of the test

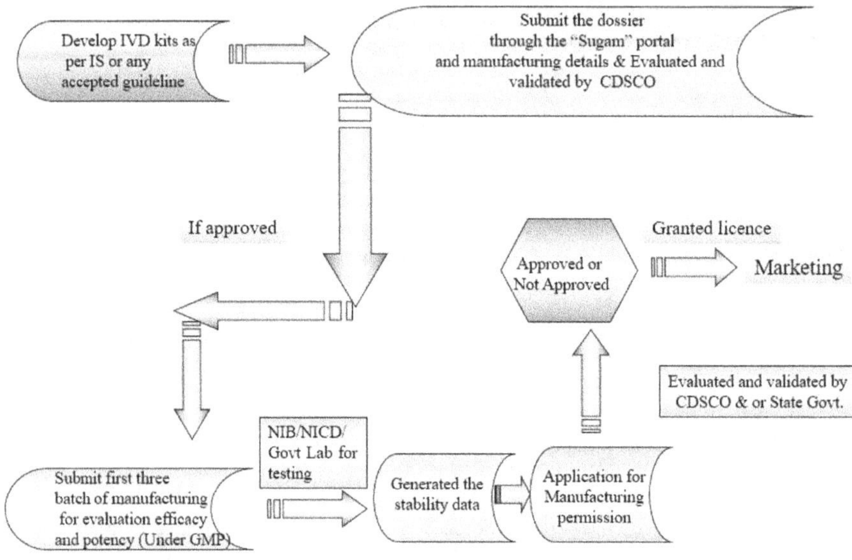

FIGURE 31.2 Regulatory procedures of IVD kits and the approval of manufacturing in India.

licence issued for testing and clinical trials in addition, the Form 12 is used to apply for a testing licence, together with the necessary costs, a notarised agreement if a third-party IVD is used, ethical committee permission, etc. In order to use IVD kits for animal diagnostics, a NOC from the Government of India's Department of Animal Husbandry, Dairy, and Fisheries is required. When importing IVD kits for influenza, the DG-ICMR's expert judgement is necessary. Performance Evaluation reports for three batches of Indian non-notified kits, such as those for malaria, TB, typhoid, dengue, chikungunya, syphilis, and cancer, must be presented alongside import licence applications. The minimum sensitivity for a notified IVD kit is better than 99% for tests like anti-HIV Rapid/ELISA, HBsAg, and HCV, while the specificity is less than 98%. The import, manufacturing, sale, distribution, and use of tuberculosis serodiagnostic products are all prohibited according to the Gazette Notification(s) GSR431(E) and GSR433(E) dated June 7, 2012, under Section 10A and Section 26A of the Drugs and Cosmetics Act, 1940.

The Drugs and Cosmetics Act of 1940 does not apply to the detection of microorganisms in food, animal feeds, environmental samples like water or soil, alcoholic beverages (wine, beer), etc. Instead, there are separate regulatory bodies in charge of this. Original labels on all IVD kits must contain the information required by Rule 96, including the date of manufacture, the date of expiration, the recommended storage conditions, a warning statement, and a statutory declaration. The Drugs and Cosmetics Act of 1940 makes it illegal to import IVD kits without a valid import licence. Form 8 (the application to import an IVD) is filled out by the applicant, while Form 9 (the Indian vendor's or company's undertaking) is included with the application. Form 12 was used to send the final approval registration certificate to the correct address when as per Rule 25 A of the Drugs and Cosmetics Act of 1940 had been met. The corporation must also be registered, which can be done by filing a Form 41 after submitting a Form 40 application.

Applications for registration certificates for IVD manufacturing in India are submitted using Form 40, and applications from international manufacturers are submitted through authorised agents in India. The Registration Certificate in Form 41 and the Indian company's power of attorney are attested by the appropriate Indian consulate.

31.6 DESIGN AND MANUFACTURING AND MANUFACTURING SITES' INFORMATION (CONTROL FILE OR MASTER FILE)

The device design, particularly of indigenous origin, is critical, and the principle of the instrument operating with the design for application of an *in vitro* diagnostic medical device is recorded in the master file or control file. The master book is expected to contain all of the required information, such as antibodies, enzymes, antigens, and nucleic acid primers. In the device master file, the specifics of the manufacturing process, including quality control processes for the in-process and finished products, packing, and validation, must be described. The document is necessary in order to do the quality audit as well as the other evaluations. In the master file, you are required to provide a discussion of the other manufacturing sites, and "manufacturing sites" refers to the locations where the essential technology is produced. The summary sheet must contain all of the test procedure, results, and conclusion in order to be considered an essential part of the master file, which is an important document. The rationale behind accepting the results, as well as the conformity statement and certificate, should be included in the master file and comparison are to be made with Compare these to any applicable standards. In the absence of a standard, the acceptance of the results must be rational and correct according to logical reasoning. Additionally, any industry guideline, professional update, or in-house standard may be referred to in the event that the recognised standard is not available. Acceptability and conclusive data must adhere to logical standards, and there must be a data summary sheet present to be mentioned. When there is non-standard availability of *in-vitro* diagnosis, a device of a mimic or similar type of devise are used *in-vitro* diagnostics can be used, instead of the standard.

31.7 ADDITIONAL INFORMATION REGARDING IVD KITS

Other types of information and details are required as well. These types of information include the study procedure, analytical technique, reports of investigation, and conclusions. In addition, the technique for data analysis, the certificate of conformity, the standards, a summary of the findings of the tests and the acceptance criteria need to be mentioned.

31.8 VALIDATION AND VERIFICATION OF IVD KITS

It is necessary to establish the validation and conformity of the final *in-vitro* diagnostic medical device. In order to enrol, one must first complete all of the quality control tests and adoption procedures. Each and every quality control test and procedure for implementation must be listed. Conformance with standards or equivalents, conformance with reference techniques, conformity with the in-house validated test method, and ultimately compression with established *in-vitro* diagnostics are the primary requirements for product validation and verification.

31.8.1 Medicinal Substances

Any medicinal compounds that are incorporated in the medical device must be mentioned, as well as the source of the molecules, instructions, safety, and applications.

31.8.2 Validation of Analytical Procedures

In-vitro medical tests are largely classified as quantitative, semi-quantitative, or qualitative, and analytical validation is done appropriately. It is interesting to note that the procedures for validating a chemical assay and a biological device are distinct from one another.

31.8.3 The Precision of the Measurements

31.8.3.1 Accuracy

Accuracy can be defined as the genuineness and exactness of the measurement device. Accuracy can be defined as the definite words and is used to describe how close something is to being true. The measurement is typically impacted by issues such as systematic inaccuracy, bias, random error, and analysis techniques.

31.8.3.2 Reproducibility

Variability is one of the most important concerns that arise during the process of analysis, and one might detect variability in the results whenever the analysis is carried out using a different day, lot, site, operator, or instrument. This category of variable data is referred to as "Intermediate Precision," and it serves as an assurance of the reproducibility of the data that are presented as ranges. In the dossier, the declaration of conformity data, the certificate of conformance data, the standard that was used, a description of the data, and conclusions should all be included.

31.8.4 Analytical Sensitivity

It is required to specify information relating to analytical techniques, such as the method, validation, matrix preparation, and minimum and maximum cutoff values. The type of procedure, analyte facilities, and instruments all play a role in determining the analytical procedure's level of sensitivity. The limit of blank, often known as LOB, refers to the value at which a blank sample (one that does not contain any analyte) is run and the standard deviation value is determined from the mean value. In order to achieve analytical validation, diagnostic medical devices of Classes C and D are required almost exclusively. The minimal concentration that an instrument is able to determine is referred to as the limit of detection (LOD). Limit of quantisation, also known as LOQ, refers to the values at which the values of the LOD are considered to be within the precision and/or correct range and have fulfilled the requirements of the objective of analysis. .

31.8.5 Analytical Specificity

Specificity refers to the analytical results that are acceptable despite the absence of any effects or interference and is referred to as "specificity." When determining the analytical specificity, it is important to take into account the effects of cross-reactivity, as well as the impacts of any additional reagents and chemicals originating from exogenous or endogenous sources. The reagent/chemical involved, either from exogenous or endogenous sources. Some of these reagent /chemical are present in other drugs, examples therapeutic agents or anticoagulants; items that are ingested, such as food or alcohol; internal sources, such as stabilisers or preservatives; the physiological status of the patients, such as haemoglobin, biliburin, and proteins; precursors or end metabolites that mimic the structure of hepatitis virus A or B; and other substances, which potentially modulates the analytical specificity

31.8.6 Measuring Limit and Metrological Traceability of Standard

When discussing the assay's measurement range, it is important to refer to the process that has been defined. It is necessary to include a description of the investigations in the dossier, and this summary must include discussion of linearity, nonlinearity, limit of detection, and all other derived techniques.

It was necessary for the summary of the test to include information regarding the quantity of samples, specimens, replications, and replicates that were carried out during the process of setting up the test. In addition to this, the chemical dilution factor of the concentrated samples, as well as the metrological impacts, the method variables, and the validation procedure, need to be mention.

31.8.7 Software Verification and Validation

The software design, development process, and validation of the software are required to be included in the dossier. Additionally, a comparison with other standard devices or devices that are comparable to the one being validated is necessary. Every software is to be registered to CDSCO as per Medical Device Rules, 2017. In addition, it is essential to have accurate data regarding the simulation conditions in order to comprehend about the software works. Additionally, it is necessary that the operating system, hardware specification, configuration, and data protection are mentioned in the dossier.

31.9 *IN-VITRO* DIAGNOSIS LICENSING IN INDIA

In the dossier, either the source antigen or the source antibody should be indicated, and a characterisation report should also be submitted alongside the dossier. The process control variable and the methods of impregnation or coating of antigen or antibody to the basement material strips, cards, or ELISA wells, such as nitrocellulose paper, etc., should also be described in the dossier. Additionally, it is necessary to stipulate the submission of the manufacturing process and a detailed flow diagram of the individual components in the dossier. It is necessary to discuss the method of testing, the specifications, and the analytical validation, including sensitivity, specificity, and the limit of detection. When a diagnostic was imported into the country, it was necessary to disclose both the National Control Authority test report and the country of origin. A minimum of three consecutive batches are required, and the specifications of each testing parameter must be mentioned for each batch. In addition to this, the kit is needed to provide a test report for each component, as well as information regarding the volume of the pack, its test number, and its labelling. The test certificate, together with the data from the laboratory in India and the report, should contain the specifics of the sensitivity and specificity tests. It is necessary to have instructions regarding the methods for handling, accident measurements, potentially hazardous situations, storage, and quarantining.

31.10 PREREQUISITES FOR THE ISSUANCE OF A LICENCE TO PERMIT THE MANUFACTURE OR IMPORT OF *IN-VITRO* DIAGNOSTIC PRODUCTS IN INDIA

Along with their filled-out forms, manufacturers of medical devices that fall under the category of "in-vitro diagnosis" are required to submit the necessary documents. The form MD 24 is used for the granting of approval for clinical investigation of any medical device that is likely to undergo it in order to prove the predicted claim that is filed by an authorised agency or a manufacturer. If the medical device contains any drug, it must first pass a battery of pre-clinical toxicological tests in order to be considered safe for human use. These tests include animal toxicology, teratogenicity studies, reproduction studies, perinatal studies, and mutagenicity and carcinogenicity tests. If a drug has been approved for use, is currently on the market in India, and is backed by sufficient and acceptable data that demonstrates its safety, then the drug may be excused from the need to undergo pre-clinical toxicity testing. The form MD25 is a grant of authority for import or manufacturing of medical devices This grant is only valid for designated or approved medical devices; it is not permissible to predicate medical devices or medical devices that are currently the subject of a clinical trial.

CLA accept submissions once every six months for the first two years, after which they will only accept yearly submissions. The person who has been granted permission to use Form MD25 is required to report any potentially unexpected major adverse events to the CLA within 15 calendar days of becoming aware of the events. The application to import or manufacture a novel *in-vitro* diagnostic medical device, which can be done by appointing an authorised agent or a manufacturer, by appointment by using to CDSCO Form MD26. Form MD27 is known as the "Permission Grant to an Authorised Agent or a Manufacturer" document. This document is necessary in order to import or manufacture novel *in-vitro* diagnostics.

The following documents are required for an import licence in Form 10 for notified *in-vitro* diagnostics.

TABLE 31.3
Documents Required for an Import Licence in Form-10 for Notified *in-vitro* Diagnostics

1	Covering Letter: Make sure to explain the reasoning in a clear way, together with the indexing and page number.
2	Authorisation letter: A letter of authorisation for the director, company secretary, or partner of the Indian Agent firm responsible for issuing the authorised signatory excise power.
3	Form 8: A fully filled-out form that has been duly signed and stamped by the authorised agents and the applicant
4	Form 9: A fully filled-out form that has been duly signed and stamped by the applicant, by the authorised agents, or that has been duly apostilled or notarised, signed, and stamped by the manufacturer.
5	Wholesale licence or manufacturing licence: A copy of the Indian Agent's signature that has been notarised is required.
6	Fees, together with the original T/R Challan, are required.
7	Copy of Registration: Form 41
9	Registration Certificate
10	Labels as per Rule 109 of the Drugs and Cosmetics Rules, 1945
11	Specifics on the applicant's postal address, as well as the mailing address of the applicant's authorised signatory

31.11 AN OVERVIEW OF THE RISKS AND PRECAUTIONS OF IVD KITS

The possibilities of the risk are mentioned in the device master file, and the controls of the risk that are related to the device are also required to be mentioned. The summary also includes a mention of the percentage of false positive or false negative results, which might be caused by the instability of the chemical, contaminated reagents, incorrect storage, or mishandling on the part of the user. At the conclusion of the risk assessment, the developers will need to provide evidence that the benefits of the project outweigh any related risks.

31.12 LABELLING OF IVD KITS

The labelling that is linked with the IVD medical device should normally be included in its own complete set within the device master file, as was covered in Chapter VI.

31.13 POST-MARKETING MONITORING INFORMATION (ALSO KNOWN AS VIGILANCE REPORTING) OF IVD KITS

It is also necessary to note in the dossier any adverse reactions or complaints that were received after clinical testing or when the product was being marketed. In addition, it is necessary to demand that the manufacturer take the necessary corrective action in order to resolve the adverse reaction.

31.14 PREREQUISITE FOR THE USE OF NOTIFIED IN-VITRO DIAGNOSTIC KITS AND REAGENTS IN THE COMPLETION OF FORM 41

TABLE 31.4
Items Must to be Included in Order to Submit a Full Form 41 and Participate in the Proposal Process

1	Covering Letter: Please specify the index and page number in cover letter's mention of the rationale of use of *in-vitro* diagnostics
.2	Authorisation letter: Authorised signatory excise power issued by the director/company secretary/partner of the Indian Agent firm
3	Form 40 must be fully filled out and submitted alongside all necessary supporting documentation.
4	Fee: Required payments to be made with the TR6 Challan
.5	A power of attorney for a foreign manufacturer must be provided to an Indian agent by the foreign manufacturer and confirmed by the Indian embassy in the country where the product being manufactured was originally produced.
6	Submit a notarised copy of the Indian Agent's wholesale or manufacturing licence.
7	Undertaking: It is required that both the Schedule D I and the Schedule D II be properly filled out, signed, and stamped with the name and designation of the manufacturer or Indian agent.
8	Regulatory certificates
9	Free sale certificate/marketing authorisation: The certificate must come from the country of origin and be properly notarised and apostilled.
10	Notarised Copy: Notarised copy apostilled and notarised copies of the quality control certificate must be provided for the legal and actual manufacturing location. In addition, certifications such as CE design certification, quality management certification, quality assurance certification, and declaration of conformity certifications are necessary.
11	Labels and pack insert: Notarised copy of the labels, IFU, and pack insert to be included in accordance with the requirements of Rule 109 of the Drugs and Cosmetics Rules, 1945
12	Products requiring a quality conformity certificate from NIB, Noida, including HIV, HCV, HBV, and blood grouping sera, are to be ordered in three consecutive batches. Any testing from a government-accredited laboratory is acceptable in place of the non-availability testing performed by the NIB.
13	To register or re-register a business, the manufacturer must submit a notarised undertaking to provide a complete plant master file.
14	To register or re-register an IVD, the manufacturer must submit a notarised undertaking of the Plant Master File and the IVD Master File.
15	Evaluation report: The National Control Authority of the country of origin shall submit evaluation reports detailing the evaluation.
16	Schedule DII: The annexure of source of the diagnosis of HIV, HCV, and HBV, as well as blood grouping sera, must be placed into Schedule DII.
17	Compliance of Complaint: In the event of re-registration, it is necessary to provide a statement of compliance and a notarised undertaking addressing complaints received.
18	Post marketing study (PMS) Study Report: Re-registration documentation, including PMS study reports notarised within the last three years.
19	Adverse events, serious adverse events, recalls, and complaints about the products Details of any adverse events, serious adverse events, recalls, and complaints about the proposed products that have been reported globally have to be stated, together with the process for investigation and the underlying cause.
20	Specifics on the applicant's authorised signatory's mailing address

31.15 REQUIREMENT FOR THE GRANT OF IMPORT LICENCE

TABLE 31.5
Necessary Informations Required in Order to Receive an Import Licence for Non-notified *in-vitro* Diagnostic Kits

1	The permission to sign on behalf of the excise authority is granted by the director/company secretary/ partner of the Indian Agent firm, along with the submission of legal documents like Form 8, Form 9, and others.
2	Form 8: A fully filled out form that has been officially signed and stamped by the applicant and by the authorised agents.
3	Form 9: A completed form that has been duly signed and stamped by the applicant by the authorised agents or that has been duly apostilled/notarised signed and stamped by the manufacturer
4	Wholesale Licence or Manufacturing Licence: The notarised copy of the Indian Agent's wholesale or manufacturing licence is required per section
5	Fees are required along with the original T/R challan.
6	Free Sale certificate/marketing authorisation: The certificate must be apostilled and notarised, and it must come from the nation of origin.
7	Notarised Copy: Apostilled and notarised copies of the quality control certificate for the legal and real manufacturing location. In addition, the certifications, such as the CE design certification, quality management certification, quality assurance certification, and declaration of conformity, are necessary.
.8	Quality Conformity: This is crucial for establishing the quality conformity of products and ensuring that the manufacturing process meets specified standards. Additionally, emphasizing the country of origin ensures compliance with relevant legal and regulatory requirements. .
9	Performance Evaluation Reports (PER): The PER reports from a NABL-approved laboratory are required to be submitted for three successive batches of IVD kits. These kits include markers for diseases such as malaria, tuberculosis, dengue, chikungunya, syphilis, and typhoid.
10	Quality conformity certificate: It is necessary to get quality conformity certificate products from NIB, Noida, such as a blood glucose test certificate, for three consecutive batches. In the event that testing from the NIB is unavailable, testing from any government-accredited laboratory is acceptable.
11	Veterinary IVD Kits: The Mandatory Requirement of a NOC from the Department of Animal Husbandry, Ministry of Agriculture.
12	Radioimmuno Assay Kit: This is an essential prerequisite in order to receive NOC from the Bhabha Atomic Research Centre (BARC).
13	Influenza Kit: The compulsory necessity of NOC from the DG, ICMR
14	Labels and Pack insert: A notarised copy of the labels, IFU, and pack insert in accordance with Rule 109 A of the Drugs and Cosmetics Rules, 1945, along with a Certificate of Analysis (COA), for the items that are being proposed.
15	Import Licence in Form 10: Certificate required for renewal or endorsement of an import licence.
16	Specific intended uses: The contents of the product list, in addition to the specified intended uses, are required.
17	Free Sales Certificate: Form 8, Form 9, and the FSC Free Sales Certificate are required, in addition to the correlation chart.
18	Specifications about the applicant's mailing address and the address of an authorised signatory for the application

31.16 REQUIREMENT FOR GRANT OF TEST LICENCE FOR *IN-VITRO* DIAGNOSTIC KITS/REAGENTS

TABLE 31.6
Test Licences for *In-vitro* Diagnostic Kits can be Obtained by Submitting a Completed Form 11 Together with the Necessary Information

1	Covering Letter: Purpose must be specified explicitly, along with the page number and the index.
2	A duly certified copy of the authorisation letter, issued by the director/company secretary/partner of the Indian Agent firm, is required.
3	The Form 12 must be properly signed and stamped by the authorised signatory of the applicant. It must also include the name and address of the testing places, as well as the name and address of the manufacturer. Identifying information regarding the product, including the package size is also required.
4	Fee paid in full amount (Rs. 100 for one product and Rs. 50 for each subsequent product) on TR-6 Challan
5	A detailed consumption breakdown, including an explanation for the recommended amount of each product
6	A copy of the proposed product's packaging insert or label is required.
7	Procedures for testing the proposed product, if any of these exist.
8	A legally enforceable contract stating that the proposed kits are not intended for sale or distribution in any form
9	Undertaking stating that the proposed kits are Not for Commercial Purpose
10	An authentic copy of the testing laboratory's NABL accreditation certificate, where appropriate.

BIBLIOGRAPHY

Checklist for Grant of Permission to Manufacture/Import of Bulk Drug Already Approved in the Country. Available from: https://cdsco.gov.in/opencms/resources/UploadCDSCOWeb/2018/UploadIndustryChecklist/checklistSND.pdf. Accessed 10 March 2021.

EMA Press Release: First Guidance on New Rules for Certain Medical Devices 2019 Feb 28. Available from: https://www.ema.europa.eu/en/news/first-guidance-new-rules-certain-medical-devices. Accessed 10 March 2021.

G.S.R. 78(E), Medical Devices Rules, 2017 Gazette of India Notification Dated 31 January 2017 by the Ministry of Health and Family Welfare, Government of India. Available from: https://www.emergobyul.com/sites/default/files/india-medical-devices-rules-2017.pdf. Accessed 10th March 2021.

In - Vitro Diagnostic (IVD) Devices Doc No.: CDSCO/IVD/FAQ/02/17 Central Drugs Standard Control Organization Directorate General of Health Services, Ministry of Health and Family Welfare, Government of India. Available from: https://cdsco.gov.in/opencms/export/sites/CDSCO_WEB/Pdf-documents/IVD/FAQs/FAQ_IVD_MDR-2017_2.pdf. Accessed 10 March 2021.

In - Vitro Diagnostic (IVD) Devices Doc No.: CDSCO/MD/FAQ/IVD/01/00, Central Drugs Standard Control Organization, Directorate General of Health Services, Ministry of Health Services, Ministry of Health Family Welfare. Govt. of India.

In-Vitro Diagnostic (IVD) Medical Devices Frequently Asked Questions Doc No.: CDSCO/IVD/FAQ/03/2022 Central Drugs Standard Control Organization Directorate General of Health Services, Ministry of Health Services, Ministry of Health Family Welfare. Govt. of India. Available from: https://cdsco.gov.in/opencms/export/sites/CDSCO_WEB/Pdf-documents/IVD/FAQs/CDSCO-IVD-FAQ-03-2022-.pdf. Accessed 10 March 2021.

ISO 18113-1:2009. In-Vitro Diagnostic Medical Devices — Information Supplied by the Manufacturer (labelling) — Part 1: Terms, Definitions and General Requirements. International Organization for Standardization, Switzerland.

ISO 15193:2002, In-Vitro Diagnostic Medical Devices — Measurement of Quantities in Samples of Biological Origin — Requirements for Content and Presentation of Reference Measurement Procedures. International Organization for Standardization, Switzerland.

ISO 15198:2004, Clinical Laboratory Medicine — In- Vitro Diagnostic Medical Devices — Validation of User Quality Control Procedures by the Manufacture. International Organization for Standardization, Switzerland.

ISO 15194:2009, In-Vitro Diagnostic Medical Devices — Measurement of Quantities in Samples of Biological Origin — Requirements for Certified Reference Materials and the Content of Supporting Documentation. International Organization for Standardization, Switzerland.

ISO/TC212: Clinical Laboratory Testing in Vitro Diagnosis Test System. International Organization for Standardization, Switzerland.

Jarow JP, Baxley JH. Medical Devices: US Medical Device Regulation. *Urologic Oncology* 2015, 33: 128–131.

Khare CP, Katiyar CK, Ed. *The Modern Ayurveda.* New York: Routledge. eBook. doi: 10.1201/b11722.

Liotta LA, Petricoin 3rd EF. Regulatory Approval Pathways for Molecular Diagnostic Technology. *Methods in Molecular Biology* 2012, 823: 409–420.

Lyon HO, Horobin RW. News from the Biological Stain Commission No. 11. *Biotechnic & Histochemistry* 2012 January, 87(1): 72–77. doi: 10.3109/10520295.2011.634376. PMID: 22176519.

Medical Device Diagnostic Division of CDSCO. Available from: http://cdsco.nic.in/forms/list.aspx?lid=1580. Accessed 10 March 2021.

Rathee P, Sehrawat R, Rathee P, Khatkar A, Akkol EK, Khatkar S, Redhu N, Türkcanoğlu G, Sobarzo-Sánchez E. Polyphenols: Natural Preservatives with Promising Applications in Food, Cosmetics and Pharma Industries; Problems and Toxicity Associated with Synthetic Preservatives; Impact of Misleading Advertisements; Recent Trends in Preservation and Legislation. *Materials (Basel)* 2023 July 3, 16(13):4793. doi: 10.3390/ma16134793. PMID: 37445107; PMCID: PMC10343617.

Saminathan J, Patel R. Current Regulatory Challenges and Approaches in Registering In-Vitro Diagnostics (IVD) in India. *Journal of Basic and Clinical Pharmacy* 2017, 8: S125–131.

US FDA. Guidance for Industry and Food and Drug Administration Staff. In Vitro Companion Diagnostic Devices. Available from: http://www.fda.gov/downloads/MedicalDevices/DeviceRegulationandGuidance/Guidance. Accessed 10 March 2021.

User Manual For e-Governance Solution for CDSCO Centre for Development of Advanced Computing. Central Drug Standard Control Organization (CDSCO), Delhi. Available from: https://cdsco.gov.in/opencms/export/sites/CDSCO_WEB/Pdf-documents/SUGAM_user_manual.pdf. Accessed 10 March 2021.

Index